The Nurse Practitioner in

Michelle Lajiness • Susanne Quallich
Editors

The Nurse Practitioner in Urology

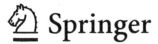 Springer

Editors
Michelle Lajiness
Department of Urology and
Department of Infectious Disease
Beaumont Health System
Royal Oak, MI
USA

Susanne Quallich
Department of Urology
University of Michigan
Rochester, MI
USA

ISBN 978-3-319-28741-6   ISBN 978-3-319-28743-0   (eBook)
DOI 10.1007/978-3-319-28743-0

Library of Congress Control Number: 2016936387

Printed on acid-free paper

This Springer imprint is published by Springer Nature
The registered company is Springer International Publishing AG Switzerland

Foreword

I accepted the invitation to write this prolusion with honor and alacrity because I want to be part of a book whose goal is to improve health care in America and the world over. I believe this book will do just that by arming the nurse practitioners and other health-care providers with an easy to read current knowledge and solutions for their day-to-day delivery of health care. After reviewing the content of this book, "The Nurse Practitioner in Urology," I was amazed by the numerous contributions and major advances made by the nurse practitioners in urology over the years, both in the field of general and subspecialty urology. It became obvious that the knowledge must be disseminated through a book that is both concise and practical. This book delivers on that premise, edited by two highly qualified and experienced senior leaders in urologic nursing: Ms. Lajiness and Quallich, who assembled the collected knowledge into this book. Further, these tandem assembled a cadre of contributors that are considered leaders in their own field. I envision this book very appropriate for students, newcomers, and established practitioners and general practitioners wishing to branch into a subspecialty.

This book is very timely as the field of urologic nurse practitioner is growing and maturing, yet there are not enough handy resources they can go to if they wish to improve their knowledge or to review a urologic topic of interest. This book will serve as a handy resource for budding nurse practitioners; as a reference for current practitioners, students, and practitioners who wish to improve their competencies and skills; and a guideline for those interested or already practicing a subspecialty. The book is loaded with basic information as well as tips and pearls for practitioners.

The urologic nurse practitioner has been established as a part of the urologic health-care professional team, well ahead of many other medical specialties. The demand for their service is more evident now than ever before because of increasing demand for health-care services. The demand is exacerbated by many reasons including population growth, increased longevity and aging population, the demand for improved quality and safety outcomes mandated by the government, and third-party carriers and shortage of physicians, to mention a few. The urologic nurse practitioners that have always been part of the team are now assuming more responsibilities in urologic practice. This partnership has been shown to improve patient accessibility, practice efficiency, and patient satisfaction. However such increased role calls for the urologic nurse practitioner to keep an up-to-date knowledge to ensure excellence in the practice of urology. This book will certainly serve that need.

Ananias C. Diokno, MD
Oakland University William Beaumont School of Medicine,
Rochester, MI, USA

Beaumont Health System (now Beaumont Health)
Royal Oak, MI, USA

Preface

Nurse practitioners have their background in primary care, which offers the opportunity for imaginative solutions for the day-to-day management needs of patients. Nurse practitioners in urology are able to offer these imaginative solutions within the context of a surgical specialty that blends medical management needs with surgical management needs. It offers the opportunity for NPs to blend the patient-centered problem-solving skills we develop as nurses with the specific needs of a variety of GU patients. In short, urology offers countless opportunities for the nurse practitioner to blend nursing, medical, and surgical care to meet the needs of their patient population. NPs are a dynamic, adaptive, and vital addition to the care management team of GU patients and can serve to improve access, manage chronic GU conditions, and increase patient satisfaction. This is becoming more important as the well-documented shortage of urologists continues, coupled with the continued aging of the US population who will need increased urologic care services.

There is a lack of literature that describes the role of the NP in specialty environments, and urology is no different in this regard. There have been few publications that address a role for a nurse practitioner specifically within urology. However, for those of us currently working with urology patients, it is clear that NPs are not only moving into the care of GU patients but excelling in the management of these patients, particularly those diagnoses that need chronic management and are less amenable to surgical solutions.

We have a combined 30 years of experience as nurse practitioners working in urology, and we hope that this book will give the reader insight into the rapidly expanding potential for the NP role within outpatient and ambulatory care urology. Nurse practitioners working in urology are not confined to general urology roles, although there are many NPs who manage general urology patients. Many NPs go on to specialize in urologic oncology, sexual dysfunction, incontinence, or stone disease. This book is meant to present the perspective of the nurse practitioner on managing urology patients. It is not a compendium of specific, detailed treatments for patients with a specific urologic issue – these details can be found in a variety of medical textbooks.

This book is meant to be a signpost of sorts, to give the reader direction about these individual GU topics and provide other resources that will help further refine both knowledge and skills from an advanced practice perspective. It is a collection of tips and tricks for patient management from this unique NP perspective and to offer additional resources for each topic that has that is addressed. This book high-lights the pathophysiology, assessment, and diagnostics specific to these GU conditions and promotes advanced critical thinking. It avoids recommending specific medications, but may address classes of medications as appropriate. Nurse practitioners, above all, avoid reinventing the wheel, and so we have recommended resources that we and our colleagues have found especially relevant and helpful in the Appendix.

Lastly, Chap. 21 is a reprint of a *Urologic Nursing* article that presents competencies for the NP working with adult urology patients. It is included here as a resource for the NP who is seeking to move into a urology environment, or for the nurse practitioner who wishes to progress in his/her current role toward the management of more complex urologic patients.

It is our hope that this book will serve as an introduction to the potential that nurse practitioners have to provide high-quality, cost-effective care for adult urology patients.

Royal Oak, MI, USA   Shelly Lajiness, MSN, FNP-BC
Rochester, MI, USA   Susanne A. Quallich, MSN, ANP-BC,
                                                                              NP-C, CUNP, FAANP

Contents

Contributors

Jeffrey Albaugh, PhD, APRN, CUCNS Sexual Health, John & Carol Walter Center for Urological Health, North Shore University Health System, Chicago, IL, USA

Gail M. Briolat, ANCP-BC Michigan Institute of Urology, St Clair Shores, MI, USA

Sherry M. Bumpus, PhD, RN, FNP-BC School of Nursing, Eastern Michigan University, Ypsilanti, MI, USA

Lindsey Cox, MD Medical University of South Carolina, Charleston, SC, USA

Julie A. Derossett, RN-BAS Division of Cancer Center Urology, Department of Urology, University of Michigan Health System, Ann Arbor, MI, USA

Luke Edwards, MD Department of Urology, Beaumont Health system, Royal Oak, MI, USA

Kaye K. Gaines, FNP-BC, CUNP Department of Medicine, C.W. Bill Young V.A. Medical Center, Bay Pines, FL, USA

Natalie Gaines, MD Female Pelvic Medicine and Reconstructive Surgery, Department of Urology, Beaumont Health System, Royal Oak, MI, USA

Jason P. Gilleran, MD Department of Urology, Oakland University William Beaumont School of Medicine, Royal Oak, MI, USA

Jason Hafron, MD Department of Urology, Beaumont Health System, Royal Oak, MI, USA

Laura J. Hintz, FNP-BC, CUNP Midwest Prostate and Urological Institute, Saginaw Center for Female Urology, Saginaw, MI, USA

Penny Kaye Jensen, DNP, APRN, FNP-C, FAAN, FAANP Salt Lake City Department of Veterans Affairs, Healthcare System, Salt Lake City, UT, USA

Pamela M. Jones, FNP-C Advanced Prostate Cancer Clinic, Michigan Institute of Urology, St Clair Shores, MI, USA

Christine D. Koops, RN, BSN Dynamic Measurements LLC Mobile Urodynamics, Grand Rapids, MI, USA

Michelle (Shelly) J. Lajiness, MSN, FNP-BC Department of Urology and Department of Infectious Disease, Beaumont Health, Royal Oak, MI, USA

John E. Lavin, MD Department of Urology, Beaumont Health System, Royal Oak, MI, USA

Katherine Marchese, ANP-BC, NP-C, CUNP, CWOCN Department of Urology, RUSH University Medical Center, Chicago, IL, USA

Silvia S. Maxwell, ACNP-BC Detroit Medical Center, Department of Urology, Detroit, MI, USA

MiChelle McGarry, MSN, RN, CPNP, CUNP Pediatric Effective Elimination, Program Clinic & Consulting, PC, Highlands Ranch, CO, USA

Staci L. Mitchell, FNP Department of Urology, University of Michigan Health System, Ann Arbor, MI, USA

Suzanne T. Parsell, ANP-BC, CUNP Division of Endourology, Department of Urology, University of Michigan Health System, Ann Arbor, MI, USA

Susanne A. Quallich, ANP-BC, NP-C, CUNP, FAANP Division of Andrology and Urologic Health, Department of Urology, University of Michigan Health System, Ann Arbor, MI, USA

Richard A. Santucci, MD, FACS, HON FC Urol(SA) Urology, Detroit Medical Center, Detroit Receiving Hospital, The Center for Urologic Reconstruction™, Michigan State College of Medicine, Detroit, MI, USA

Heather Schultz, FNP-C Department of Urology, University of North Carolina at Chapel Hill, Chapel Hill, NC, USA

Sarah R. Stanley, MS, MHS, PA-C Department of Urology, University of North Carolina, Chapel Hill, NC, USA

Leslie Saltzstein Wooldridge, GNP-BC, CUNP, BCIA-PMD Mercy Health Bladder Clinic, Muskegon, MI, USA

Transitioning Pediatric Urology Patients (and Their Families) to Adult Urology Care

MiChelle McGarry

Contents

Introduction

For many years, children with urological issues were cared throughout their life spans by pediatric urologists as their life spans averaged in the mid-20s at the latest; the "official" definition for the age of pediatric patient care is 0–21 years. Modern medicine has extended the life span of this population of children with complex urologic conditions, and now children who were pediatric urology patients are living well into adulthood. Dr. Rosalia Misseri (2013) of Riley Hospital for Children estimates that excluding hypospadias, there are 100,000 adult individuals in the USA living with genitourinary tract diseases that began before the age of 21 years.

M. McGarry, MSN, RN, CPNP, CUNP
Pediatric Effective Elimination, Program Clinic & Consulting, PC, Littleton, CO, USA
e-mail: michelle@peepclinic.com

© Springer International Publishing Switzerland 2016
M. Lajiness, S. Quallich (eds.), *The Nurse Practitioner in Urology*,
DOI 10.1007/978-3-319-28743-0_1

This has necessitated the transition of their care to adult urology providers. The universal goals of pediatric urologists are to preserve kidney function, preserve upper tract and lower tract function, provide for safe urine storage and drainage, and attain and maintain continence, fertility, sexual function, and genital cosmesis. The last three are usually not necessarily on the minds of the parents and patients until adolescence, but need to be a factor in all pediatric surgical and medical decisions made throughout the life span of the child. The actual transition of care is complex and unique to each child, family, diagnosis, pediatric care given, and pediatric urology provider team.

Ideally this transition from pediatric to adult care should be a process that aligns with the adolescent developmental process, specifically identity versus role conflict. But there can be many practical obstacles to this actually happening. Developmental delay of the patient, difficulties with the patient taking responsibility, difficulty with the parents relinquishing responsibility, a lack of adult providers knowledgeable and/or desiring to care for these kids as adults, and the reluctance of pediatric urology providers to relinquish their patient's care to adult urology providers can all be factors. Another obstacle is the coordination of other needed medical specialties such as nephrology, PT/OT, orthopedics, neurology, neurosurgery, or endocrinology. In the pediatric hospital model, all these specialties are housed in one system, and electronic medical records facilitate seamless care transitions between specialties. Many institutions promote multidisciplinary clinics where the providers come to the patients, providing not only convenience for the patient and families, but more opportunities for provider to provider communication and continuity of care. This includes access to ancillary team members such as social work, therapeutic play specialists, and pediatric psychologists.

Currently, this issue of transition of complex pediatric patients to adult care is being addressed at many levels. Kelleher et al. (2015) describe the issues with transitions of complex pediatric patients to adult care, citing the challenges of spina bifida patients in particular, who require management from urology, neurosurgery, orthopedics, and general medical services well into adulthood. There is guidance for this transition: "Federal Policy Supporting Improvement in Transitioning from Pediatric to Adult Surgical Services" (Kelleher et al. 2015; Box 1.1). Furthermore, the American Academy of Pediatrics (2011) states that "optimal health care is achieved when each person, at every age, receives medically and developmentally appropriate care." The process includes multiple entities, including the patient, family and/or other caregivers, the pediatric and adult providers and support staff, as well as adult and pediatric hospitals and insurance companies and the health-care system as a whole. With the passage of The Patient Protection and Affordable Care Act of 2010 (PPACA), children are able to remain on their parents' insurance until age 26, providing time to identify resources for coverage due to their disability.

Due to reconstruction of the GU tract, facilities need to have pediatric-sized instruments (such as cystoscopes) available at the adult hospital, introducing the need for planning and potential financial impact. Finally, radiologists who are familiar and comfortable with the appearance of genitourinary systems that have been reconstructed are essential.

Box 1.1 The Patient Protection and Affordable Care Act of 2010 Provisions That Benefit Adolescents with Chronic GU Conditions Transitioning to Adult Care

1. Adolescents and young adults are able to remain on their parents' coverage until age 26. This means that youths with chronic medical and surgical conditions will remain insured on commercial plans.
2. Health insurance plans are prohibited from discrimination based on preexisting conditions or health status. Youths that age out of their parents' insurance or purchasing individual insurance will not have any chronic health conditions held against them through denials, higher premium rates, or complete refusal to insure.
3. Annual/lifetime limits on dollars or benefits are excluded in the PPACA.
4. The PPACA sets the minimum Medicaid eligibility for young adults at 133 % of the federal poverty level (for those states expanding Medicaid).
5. The PPACA establishes rules and requirements for the availability of insurance exchanges for the purchase of insurance by individuals in each state. These exchanges provide for new coverage of preventive benefits and provide subsidies prorated based on income.

The most pediatric urology issues and diagnoses present very early in life or even prenatally, but they can also arise throughout adolescence. The conditions can be mild to life-threatening and also have a very variable effect on the child's psychosocial well-being depending on the specific disease process and how the family has coped with the disease and its effects. Their success in management depends on the support system in place to help them and the skill of knowledgeable providers.

Transitioning

Transition to adult care obviously happens frequently in pediatrics, but one component making the urology transition different is that the conditions are uniquely pediatric and until recently have been cared for solely by pediatric providers. Both cardiology and pulmonology disciplines have led the way in pediatric to adult care transitioning with specialized fellowships. The European model as described at the European Association of Urology (EAU) 25th Annual Congress: Abstract 811 (Presented April 19, 2010) has specialized providers in pediatric to adult care, including in urology. The newness of these transitions in urology can create stress, ambivalence, and resistance among members of the team, with the patient/family feeling fear about a new system that does not know them personally. They may feel they are being abandoned by the people "who saved their child's life," while the pediatric urology team may fear that all they have "fixed" will be undone.

Depending on the child's cognitive level, issues also begin to arise regarding confidentiality, informed consent, and patient/physician decision making versus patient/ physician/family decision making. These issues are vital in the process of ongoing care and benefit from being addressed at the same time as any physical issues are being addressed. The majority of parents/caregivers who have children with chronic disabilities that involve multiple systems have been fierce advocates for their children. While this is good, for them the process of letting go and having their children become as responsible as possible needs to start early and be directed by the care team. It can become very difficult for these families, and they can feel that they are losing control of their child's health care, which has consumed a large part of their own adult lives.

Subspecialty certification in Pediatric Urology began in 2008 for those urologists whose practice is a minimum of 75 % pediatric urology. Applicants approved by the Board to enter the process of subspecialty certification must be engaged in the active practice of pediatric urology and must hold a current unrestricted general certificate in urology issued by the American Board of Urology (http://www.abu.org/subspecialtyCert_PSCOverview.aspx). With the pediatric certificate of added qualification, pediatric urologists must not have non-pediatric patients comprising more than 25 % of their work in order for them to keep their specialty qualification. It is essential to note that if adult patients stay in a pediatric practice, there is reduced time to see pediatric patients, meaning that patients must be "aged out" of the pediatric urology practice.

Nurse practitioners (NPs) are uniquely qualified and positioned to help families with this preparation and transition process owing to their unique knowledge of child development, family systems, and disease processes. This process happens with families primarily through education within the context of the clinic visits, the strength of nurse practitioners. After training as either pediatric or family NPs, the transition to caring for patients within a specialty practice offers the opportunity for NPs to focus their training on the specific needs of pediatric GU patients.

Looking at the generalized process, it is important to start and keep a concise summary of all diagnoses, interventions, and surgical procedures. The actual surgical notes are important as there are different techniques, and which one was used originally and what any revisions were is important to future adult surgical decisions. There should be a notebook for each patient with all of this information for each child that the family/caregiver keeps and is added to with every visit and procedure so that it is complete with all surgical, procedural, and interventional information at transition. This avoids a time-consuming task to review years of care as a family presents for their last visit. A second vital issue is encouraging pediatric GU patients to enroll with a primary care provider; it is more likely for children to have a pediatrician than for adults to be able to identify a primary care provider. This is important, as pediatric providers are not trained or equipped to manage "adult" issues such as smoking prevention and cessation, obesity, type II diabetes, sexuality, birth control, or hypertension as they pertain to the adult patient.

There is a distinct need to develop transition plans for pediatric urology patients to move to adult urology providers. Some facilities have created formal plans that can be adapted to other environments. Riley Hospital for Children has a well-established program for urology transitioning, and Children's Hospital of Wisconsin website has a comprehensive section on general transitioning of pediatric to adult care including an e-book titled *Transition Health Care Checklist: Preparing for Life as an Adult* (http://www.chw.org/medical-care/transition-to-adult-care/). Toronto's Hospital for Sick Kids *Good 2 Go* is another successful program that is available on their website and has materials for transition of care for clinicians, patients, and families. This program is based on a shared management model between family, providers, and the young adult.

Several diagnoses necessitate the transition from pediatric to adult urology care: neurogenic bladder (caused by a variety of diagnoses, one being spina bifida), bladder exstrophy, hypospadias, epispadias, disorders of sex development, posterior urethral valves, cloaca, vesicoureteral reflux, ureteropelvic obstruction, nephrolithiasis, pediatric genitourinary tract cancers, undescended testes, varicoceles, and upper tract anomalies. The remainder of the chapter is a disease-by-disease review of the items for adult care providers to remember, assess, and measure for the most common pediatric genitourinary diseases that will require lifelong care.

Discussion of Specific Pediatric Genitourinary Conditions

Neurologic Conditions

Neurologic conditions include myelomeningocele, tethered spinal cord, cerebral palsy, sacral agenesis and spinal dysraphisms, and Hinman's syndrome (non-neurogenic, neurogenic bladder). Spina bifida is the most common birth defect in the USA (www.spinabifidaassociation.org), but all of these conditions have the potential to be part of a syndrome as well. Males and females with spina bifida are the largest population of persons with urogenital anomalies in the USA. There are many treatment options for them as adults, with clean intermittent catheterization (CIC) being responsible for the marked increase in life expectancy over the last 20 years. Other treatment interventions can include augmentation cystoplasties, botulinum toxin, catheterizable channel creation (Mitrofanoff), anticholinergics and other meds to increase bladder capacity, antegrade continence enema creations (ACE or MACE), and other older types of urinary diversions. The main issue for these patients is the inability to store and release urine safely and in a controlled manner.

The primary goal for the medical team is always protection of the upper tracts, but for patients and families, their goal is likely to be socially acceptable continence. These two goals can be directly opposed to each other at any time during the patient's life span. Due to the reconstructions that they undergo, both to protect upper tracts and to achieve the continence, these patients are at a lifelong risk for true infection that can cause urosepsis (not from colonization due to CIC), nephrolithiasis, stricture of their cathing channel (urethra or surgically created channel; stenosis of a surgically created channel is an expected occurrence), upper tract damage, and bladder cancer. To effectively monitor for the upper tract damage, the most important sequelae to avoid, they need serial urodynamics (with baseline communicated to the adult urology team), renal and bladder ultrasounds, and reassessment of continence, and any change in status also necessitates a spinal cord evaluation for new tethering. Awareness of the presence of a VP shunt and avoidance of infecting this are also essential.

For any child who underwent an augmentation cystoplasty, he/she needs lab work to assess for metabolic acidosis (specifically hyperchloremic acidosis), renal function, and vitamin B12 deficiency (if terminal ileum was used). The other things that the patient (and possibly caregivers) needs to be taught are signs and symptoms of bladder rupture, as well as that not catheterizing increases this risk, bowel obstruction due to adhesions, and bladder stones due to mucous from the bowel mucous settling in the bladder (46 % of patients have recurrent bladder stones (Wood 2015). Bladder malignancy is also increased in the population which has had an augmentation. The risk of bladder cancer in patients with bladder augmentations is higher than the general population, but it is unclear if this is related to the augment itself or the underlying disease process (Higuchi et al. 2010). The vast majority of these patients will be on anticholinergics or antimuscarinics, and monitoring for side effects of these medications is essential.

The final considerations for patients with neurologic issues are sexuality and fertility, and these may be best and most appropriately addressed in a transitional setting. It is also important to review birth control, STD prevention (remember, the risk for latex allergies is increased in pediatric urological patients due to frequent instrumentation; this has been decreasing recently due to early elimination of latex exposure), and sexual abuse prevention, especially considering the cognitive level of the patient.

Many young adult and teen spina bifida patients are sexually active, and healthcare professionals at all levels of care may be faced with issues regarding relationships and sexuality among young adults with spina bifida. Ideally these should be addressed with patients by adult specialists in these areas before sexual activity is initiated. Nevertheless, it is important to establish the information patients already have, even in the pediatric environment; some patients report they have never discussed sexuality issues with a provider and some report they would have discussed these issues if the provider had initiated the topic (Sawyer and Roberts 1999). Males with neurologic GU conditions will have possible issues with erections and retrograde ejaculation, while females will be able to conceive, but body habitus may be an issue and factor into potential delivery concerns as they become pregnant. Female spina bifida patients are less likely to use hormonal contraception and to be using no method of birth control (Cardenas et al. 2010). There is a higher incidence of precocious puberty and premature activation of hypothalamic-pituitary-gonadal axis in spina bifida girls than is seen with their healthy counterparts, and the timing of puberty may be earlier, at 10.9–11.4 years (Trollmann et al. 1998), making this a consideration in their ongoing care.

Obstructive Uropathy

Obstructive uropathy includes some degree of neurogenic bladder; these children are all born with renal disease. Posterior urethral valves are the most common diagnosis in this group and occur exclusively in males. These patients demonstrate some degree of chronic kidney disease, from either primary renal dysplasia or due to the presence of obstruction to urine flow or both of these factors. The initial damage occurs prenatally, and the timing of this directly relates to the severity of the renal involvement and damage, resulting in significant kidney disease present in 13–28 % of patients with posterior urethral valves (Holmdahl and Sullen 2005). It is unclear whether timing of valve ablation (ideally done as soon as the valves are known, in the newborn period) changes the degree of renal damage. These patients are at continued risk of incomplete bladder emptying, which may be related to recurrence of or incomplete ablation of these valves, secondary bladder neck obstruction, or side effects of anticholinergic medications.

All of these patients will need routine urodynamic studies and repeat ones for any reported changes. Again, the baseline at transition of care is essential, and patients and their parents may need reminding that preservation of upper tracts is the most essential goal of care. The most common time to see renal deterioration is at and during puberty; the reason and pathophysiology for this is unclear (Ardissino et al. 2012). Blood pressure monitoring, serum creatinine, and urinalyses need to be routinely performed throughout the life span as it is not known if the natural history of end-stage renal disease lasts throughout the life span (Glassberg et al. 2013).

Infertility and retrograde ejaculation in male patient can be an issue, but erectile dysfunction usually is not an issue. Any potential infertility issues should be referred for additional evaluation.

Nephrolithiasis is an increasing pediatric urology issue with the incidence increasing by 6–10 % per year and affecting 50 per 100,000 adolescents (Tasian and Copelovitch 2014). Many of these children have a syndrome or lab finding that makes them at high risk, and with adult stone specialists, this may be one of the easiest pediatric urology diseases to transition to adult providers. It becomes more complicated when stones are present in children with complex urological states (such as bladder exstrophy or myelomeningocele) or with metabolic diseases (such as growth delay due to renal issues or decreasing bone density due to reabsorption of urine through a bladder augmentation) with which adult providers may not be familiar (Lambert 2015).

Bladder Exstrophy

Bladder exstrophy and associated epispadias are very complex anomalies and are more and more often diagnosed prenatally, but if not, immediately at birth. These children undergo complex reconstructions that are usually staged; many of these patients require bladder augmentation and the creation of a catheterizable continent channel. Incontinence is a huge quality of life issue as is sexual function and cosmesis. This is due to the widened pubic symphysis creating shortened penile length and ejaculation issues and for women, sexual function, and pelvic organ prolapse. Pregnancy is possible with a higher incidence of preterm birth and a planned C-section at 37 weeks is recommended (Creighton and Wood 2013). Most of these patients are able to live a normal life span, but will continue to have the issues associated with complications of their childhood bladder surgeries such as bladder stones, UTIs, catheterization issues, and continence issues.

Disorders of Sexual Development

Disorders of sexual development and anorectal malformations are another complex group of congenital urogenital disorders. No matter what the specific disease process, these kids require endocrine, psychosocial, and urologic care throughout the life span, and a full discussion is beyond the scope of this book. Congenital adrenal hypoplasia is one of the most common genetic diseases in humans and 21-hydroxylase deficiency is the most common of these (Lambert 2011). Patients with this require long-term steroid and hormone replacement, initially to achieve adult height and pubertal development, but with changing goals in adulthood. Children with congenital adrenal hypoplasia are at risk for infertility and adrenal tumors and so routine renal ultrasounds are indicated. Gonadectomy may be indicated in late adolescence or early adulthood as the incidence of gonadal malignancy in adulthood is 14 % (Deans et al. 2012).

Dr. Rick Rink (2013) from Riley Hospital for Children provides the following list of concerns for transitions for patients with disorders of sexual development: sexual function, sexual identity, emotional well-being, concerns regarding intimacy, counseling patient on disclosure of their condition to others, informing the patient of their condition, gender dysphoria, vaginal stenosis, fertility, hormonal deficiencies, steroidal deficiencies, gonadal tumors, endocrine management, gynecological care, mucous-producing neovagina, tumors in neovagina, worsening virilization due to poor adherence to medical therapy, poor cosmesis, and bladder dysfunction.

Pediatric Urologic Cancer Survivors

Children who are genitourinary cancer survivors will have lifelong urologic needs. Adult survivors of genitourinary pediatric cancer (including Wilm's tumor, germ cell tumors, and rhabdomyosarcoma) are at risk for long-term complications and require serial follow-up and surveillance. Children are at risk for complications from chemotherapy and radiotherapy as well as complications and side effects from extirpative and reconstructive operations (Lambert 2015). These will depend on the tumor type and stage, treatment, and reconstructive procedures performed, but will affect multiple organ systems. With an 80 % cancer survival rate, the number of childhood cancer survivors is increasing, and National Cancer Institute Surveillance Epidemiology and End Results estimates 1 in every 250 young adults will be childhood cancer survivors (Howlader et al. 2011). Of non-progression, nonrecurrent causes of mortality, second malignancies are the leading cause of death among long-term childhood cancer survivors (Rink 2013).

Fertility is also a likely issue for these patients and something that pediatric providers need to address in any age-appropriate child (meaning at or approaching adolescence), as egg and sperm collection and storage are widely available, but these services are dependent on the developmental age of the child. Patients and their family must be offered information regarding these services and can be directed to organizations such as the American Society for Reproductive Medicine or Resolve in addition to information regarding facility or local services.

Congenital Kidney and Urinary Tract Anomalies

Vesicoureteral reflux, ureteropelvic junction obstruction, multicystic dysplastic kidney disease, ureterovesical junction obstruction, ectopic ureteral insertion, renal ectopia, duplicated collecting systems, ureteroceles, or a solitary kidney make up a broad diagnosis group of congenital kidney and urinary tract anomalies. These can vary greatly in severity and thus have wide-ranging impacts on adult life and consideration upon transition from pediatric to adult care. Children with chronic kidney disease require lifetime follow-up to prevent progression of the disease and monitor for early signs of renal deterioration (Mertens et al. 2008). The long-term effects of these varied congenital anomalies range in severity from none to end-stage renal disease. Many patients with these diagnoses need comanagement by urology and nephrology.

Hypospadias is a common complaint and surgical case in pediatric urology practices. The incidence is approximately 1 in 200 to 300 live male births (Lambert 2015). This condition encompasses a wide range of severity with the most mild being a mega meatus and the most severe with a perineal urethral meatus and/or penoscrotal transposition. The goals of correction are a normal urinary stream from an orthotopic urethral meatal position, prevention/correction of chordee, satisfactory cosmesis, and preservation of future ability to have intercourse. Unfortunately, at times, even a simple appearing repair can need grafting and multiple surgeries resulting in scarring, poor function, and poor cosmesis. All of these issues can be magnified during puberty with penile and scrotal growth. Some of the complications that can occur at any time are urethral stricture, chordee, persistent hypospadias, urethral diverticulum, cosmesis issues, voiding dysfunction, and sexual function issues (Rink 2013).

Varicoceles and cryptorchidism are two other pediatric urologic issues that require long-term education and adult follow-up; both can be repaired surgically and both have a potential for infertility in adulthood. Varicoceles in adolescent boys are repaired for indications including pain, testicular asymmetry, or abnormal semen parameters (which can be a challenge to obtain in pediatric patients).

The undescended testicle should be repaired and brought into the scrotum as soon as is reasonably safe; this is determined by discussion with pediatric anesthesia. This correction of an undescended testicle can take one or more surgeries, depending on the position of the testicle, so that the patient can more effectively perform testicular self-examination, to facilitate identification of a potential neoplasm. The incidence among men with an undescended testicle is approximately one in 1000 to one in 2500 (Misseri 2013). Although significantly higher than the risk among the general population (1:100,000), it does not warrant removal of all undescended testicles, and there are times when the neoplasm is actually on the contralateral side to the undescended testicle. As adults, these men must be reminded of their need for follow-up periodically with ultrasounds.

Summary

The goals of attaining preservation of kidneys and upper tracts, safe and effective urine storage and elimination, continence, sexual function, fertility, and genital cosmesis can only happen throughout the life span with planned and coordinated transitions from pediatric to adult urologic care. This takes time and is not simply saying "here are your records; your next appointment should be with an adult urologist." This approach is destined to fail pediatric patients for whom all on the pediatric urology team have worked diligently, usually throughout the patient's entire life to date, to achieve the abovementioned goals.

The obstacles that have been outlined include the need to shift patient/caregiver paradigms, locating and encouraging adult urologists with interest in these complex and challenging patients to take them into their practices, providing adult urologists' and other adult urology team providers' appropriate support from the pediatric team, coordinating care with other necessary specialists, and navigating the adult health-care world. These issues must be negotiated and overcome to provide exemplary care for complex pediatric urology patients as they transition to become complex adult urology patients.

Resources for the Nurse Practitioner
Kelleher, K., Deans, K. J., & Chisolm, D. J. (2015, April). Federal policy supporting improvements in transitioning from pediatric to adult surgery services. In *Seminars in pediatric surgery* (*Vol. 24*, No. 2, pp. 61–64). WB Saunders.

References

American Academy of Pediatrics, American Academy of Family Practice, American College of Physicians, Transitions Clinical Reporting Group, Cooley WC, Sagerman PJ (2011) Supporting the health care transition from adolescence to adulthood in the medical home. Pediatrics 128:182–199

Ardissino G et al (2012) Puberty is associated with increased deterioration of renal function in patients with CKD: data from the ItalKid project. Arch Dis Child 97(10):885–888. doi:10.1136/archdischild-2011-300685

Cardenas DD, Martinez-Barrizonte J, Castillo LC, Mendelson S (2010) Sexual function in young adults with spina bifida. Curr Bladder Dysfunct Rep 5(2):71–78

Children's Hospital of Wisconsin. Transition to adult care. http://www.chw.org/medical-care/transition-to-adult-care/. Accessed 10 Apr 2015

Creighton SM, Wood D (2013) Complex gynecological and urological problem in adolescents: challenges and transition. Postgrad Med J 89:34–38

Deans R, Creighton DM, Liao LM, Conway GS (2012) Timing of gonadectomy in adult women with complete androgen insensitivity CAIS: patient preferences and clinical evidence. Clin Endocrinol (Oxf) 76:894–899

Glassberg K, Van Batvia JP, Combs AJ (2013) Posterior urethral valves: transitional care into adulthood. Dialogues Pediatr Urol 34(4):5–20

Higuchi TT, Granberg CF, Fox JA, Husmann DA (2010) Augmentation cystoplasty and risk of neoplasia: fact, fiction and controversy. J Urol 184(6):2492–2496. doi:10.1016/j.juro.2010.08.038, Epub 2010 Oct 18

Holmdahl G, Sullen U (2005) Boys with posterior urethral valves: outcome concerning renal function, bladder function and paternity at ages 31 to 44 years. J Urol 174:1031

Howlader N, Noone AM, Wladron W et al (2011) SEER cancer statistics review 1975–2008. Bethesda: National Cancer Institute; Based on November 2011 SEER data submission, posted to the SEER website. Available from http://www.seercancergov/csr/1975-2008

http://www.abu.org/subspecialtyCert_PSCOverview.aspx. Accessed 13 July 2015

https://books.google.com/books?id=4PNICAAAQBAJ&pg=PA164&dq=%22bladder+stones%22+%26+%22augmentation+cystoplasty%22&hl=en&sa=X&ved=0CEsQ6AEwBGoVChMIv5rDt-bZxgIVgVuICh2HiQsp#v=onepage&q=%22bladder%20stones%22%20%26%20%22augmentation%20cystoplasty%22&f=false. Accessed 13 July 2015

http://www.springer.com/us/book/9783319140414 by Wood

Kelleher K, Deans KJ, Chisolm DJ (2015) Federal policy supporting improvements in transitioning from pediatric to adult surgery services. Semin Pediatr Surg 24(2):61–4. doi: 10.1053/j.sempedsurg.2015.01.001. Epub 2015 Jan 8

Lambert SM, Snyder HM, Canning DA (2011) The History of Hypospadias and Hypospadias Repairs. Urology 77(6):1277–1283

Lambert SM (2015) Transitional care in pediatric urology. Semin Pediatr Surg 24(2):73–78

Mertens AC, Liu Q, Neglia JP et al (2008) Cause-specific late mortality among 5-year survivors of childhood cancer: the Childhood Cancer Survivor Study. J Natl Cancer Inst 100:1368–1370

Metcalfe PD, Cain MP, Kaefer M et al (2006) What is the need for additional bladder surgery after bladder augmentation in childhood? J Urol 176:1801–1805

Misseri R (2013) Transition into adulthood: concerns and considerations for the pediatric urologist. Dialogues Pediatr Urol 34(4):2–3

Rink R (2013) DAD, transitions and my concerns. Dialogues Pediatr Urol 34(4):6–8

Sawyer SM, Roberts KV (1999) Sexual and reproductive health in young people with spina bifida. Dev Med Child Neurol 41(10):671–675

Smeulders N, Woodhouse CRJ (2001) Neoplasia in adult exstrophy patients. BJU Int 87:623–628

Spina Bifida Association. What is spina bifida. www.spinabifidaassociation.org. Accessed 13 April 2015

Tasian E, Copelovitch L (2014) Evaluation and medical management of kidney stones in children. J Urol 92:1329–1336

Trollmann R, Strehl E, Wenzel D, Dörr HG (1998) Arm span, serum IGF-I and IGFBP3 levels as screening parameters for the diagnosis of growth hormone deficiency in patients with myelomeningocele – preliminary data. Eur J Pediatr 157:451–455

Men's Urology: Vasectomy, Orchialgia, Testosterone Deficiency, Male Fertility, Peyronie's Disease and Penile Inflammation

2

Susanne A. Quallich

Contents

S.A. Quallich, ANP-BC, NP-C, CUNP, FAANP
Division of Andrology and Urologic Health, Department of Urology,
University of Michigan Health System, Ann Arbor, MI, USA
e-mail: quallich@umich.edu

© Springer International Publishing Switzerland 2016
M. Lajiness, S. Quallich (eds.), *The Nurse Practitioner in Urology*,
DOI 10.1007/978-3-319-28743-0_2

13

Objectives

1. Present an overview of men's health within the context of urology.
2. Explain the process for vasectomy.
3. Describe the state of the science for chronic unexplained orchialgia.
4. Establish criteria for screening men for low testosterone and determining who requires further evaluation.
5. Compare treatment strategies for testosterone deficiency-based patient need.
6. Examine male infertility as an area of health disparity.
7. Review current techniques used to evaluate male infertility and describe methods for preserving male fertility.
8. Discuss Peyronie's disease and its treatment.
9. Review diagnosis and management of inflammatory conditions of the penis.

Men's Health Overview

The Affordable Care Act (2010) will continue to expand the number of people seeking care, while tasking providers to maintain and improve the quality of that care. As more men enroll with health insurance plans, there will be a need for providers of all disciplines to become familiar with complaints that are unique to men and men's sexual and reproductive health needs. Men may seek evaluation in primary care clinics, but it is equally plausible that they will gravitate to urology providers, the closest parallel to a "gynecologist for men." Urology providers may have the unique opportunity to initiate evaluation and referrals as they enter the medical infrastructure, as many men may not have primary care clinicians, and avoid seeking care for social and cultural reasons. Men who are well informed as patients are more capable of monitoring their health, coping with their illness, and adhering to treatment – this is where the education role of the NP is vital.

In the context of urology, sexual health and erectile dysfunction complaints represent an obvious opportunity to evaluate for cardiometabolic disease (Chap. 4), especially in the "otherwise healthy" man. Concerns about possible low testosterone, possibly due to direct-to-consumer advertising, also prompt self-referral to urology clinics for evaluation. Emerging research points to testosterone deficiency and a possible role in multiple cardiovascular risk factors including obesity, diabetes, hypertension, and altered lipid profiles, again emphasizing the role of the urology provider as "first contact." This role is so vital that the American Urological Association developed guidelines to help its members identify screening needs across the lifespan (AUA 2014).

But men's health is more than simply identifying sexual and urologic issues. Healthcare shifts have focused on women's health, family health, and pediatric health, while it can seem that men's health is an afterthought. Providers must work to understand social and cultural determinants of men's health and work to creatively address any barriers. The urology clinic visit can be a "gateway" to discussion of screening for other risk factors, such as smoking, obesity, diet, and physical activity. Conceptualizing men's health in this way helps move us toward greater health equity between the genders and improving the overall health of not just men, but their families.

Vasectomy

Vasectomies are the most common nondiagnostic operation performed by urologists in the United States (AUA 2012); although other providers will also perform this procedure, approximately 75 % are done by trained urologists. It is an outpatient or clinic procedure, is covered to varying degrees by insurance, and involves far less cost and mortality than tubal ligation (the closest equivalent for female sterilization). It is usually performed under a local anesthetic, and sedation can be an option. Men or couples must understand that although vasectomy is very effective, it is not 100 % reliable in preventing pregnancy. The risk of pregnancy after vasectomy is approximately 1 in 2,000 for men who have postvasectomy azoospermia (AUA 2012).

Consultation and Evaluation

As with any invasive procedure, there should be a formal consultation, either with the patient himself or with the couple together. Minimal age for vasectomy is the legal age of consent in the location where the procedure will be performed. Emphasis should be placed on the intended permanent nature of this procedure, and the discussion will help ensure that appropriate expectations regarding the preoperative, operative, and postoperative consequences of this choice are understood. This consultation allows the provider to assess for any anxiety that may suggest sedation as an option for the procedure and allows for an examination that ensures the procedure can be safely and effectively performed in the outpatient setting.

Vasectomy does not increase one's risk for prostate cancer, coronary heart disease, stroke, hypertension, dementia, hypogonadism, or testicular cancer. Physical examination findings such as varicoceles do not prevent vasectomy form being an outpatient procedure.

Post-procedure instructions should be reviewed (Box 2.1), and men should be informed that there is a risk of developing chronic postvasectomy pain. Short-term discomfort may also be associated with formation of a sperm granuloma. Antibiotics are not usually necessary after this procedure.

Box 2.1 Sample Vasectomy Postoperative Instructions
1. You must have a companion to drive you home after your procedure.
2. Avoid strenuous exercise or activity for at least 7–10 days after your procedure, as long as there is no pain. This includes any heavy lifting and vigorous exercise. You may return to work the next day, as long as no strenuous activity is required.
3. You may shower after 24 h. Do not take a bath or use a hot tub for five (5) days.
4. You may apply ice or a cold pack to the scrotum as needed, for 10 min of every hour (a bag of frozen peas will mold to the area). This may help reduce any pain or swelling. It may also be helpful to wear supportive underwear, such as briefs.
5. Expect some mild pain, mild swelling of the scrotum, and possible slight fluid leak from the site of the puncture. A gauze pad may be applied to the scrotum if there is any leakage from the puncture site. Drainage may continue for several days and is normal.
6. Take extra-strength acetaminophen or ibuprofen as needed for any pain or discomfort; follow the package directions regarding dose. Stronger prescription pain medication is provided, but most men do not find that it is necessary.
7. Continue your normal diet.
8. Avoid sexual activity *for at least 7 days* after your procedure. You may resume having sex after a week, if comfortable enough.
9. Until you are told that you are sterile, it is essential that you use another form of birth control. No method is 100 % successful, and postvasectomy pregnancies have been documented, but are rare. After two (2) zero sperm counts, you may stop other methods of birth control. If any sperm are seen on the first two counts, additional checks will be necessary.
10. If you experience unusual or severe pain that is not relieved by pain medication, excessive bleeding or drainage, excessive swelling or redness, foul odor, or a fever over 101 ° F, please contact the clinic.

You will usually receive a phone call within 7–10 days after a specimen is dropped off, explaining the results. Please make sure that you provide an up-to-date phone number. If we *cannot* leave a message at that number, please let us know.

Follow-Up

A postvasectomy semen analysis (PVSA) is key to establishing the success of the procedure. While there is some controversy regarding the timing of PVSA, the most current guidelines recommend examination of the first sample 8–16 weeks after the procedure (AUA 2012). Specific guidelines will be provider dependent, and there may be a higher rate of first-sample compliance when men are given a specific appointment.

Chronic Unexplained Orchialgia

Chronic unexplained orchialgia (CUO) is "a subjective negative experience of adult men, perceived as intermittent or continuous pain of variable intensity, present at least 3 months, localizing to the testis(es) in the absence of objective organic findings, that interferes with quality of life" (pg. 8, Quallich and Arslanian-Engoren 2014). CUO is a male genital pain condition without an evidence-based treatment algorithm, one that stems from a urologic perspective (Levine and Hoeh 2015) but not a chronic pain perspective, and there is little high-quality research into the condition (Quallich and Arslanian-Engoren 2013). These factors contribute to men with CUO seeking repeated evaluation and treatment, like many other chronic pain populations. The treatment of any chronic nonmalignant pain can be challenging, and but caring for men with specific urologic or male genital pain complaints entails a through urologic evaluation to eliminate causes of acute scrotal pain (Chap. 3, Appendix).

Background

Chronic unexplained orchialgia has an unknown incidence, in part because there is no specific ICD code for it, and because several terms have been used historically to describe CUO. Reports of chronic genital pain conditions in men fail to evaluate their experience in a social, sexual, and self-esteem context, and there is no precedent for evaluating it as a multifactorial condition. No specific ethnic or genetic risk factors have been identified, and onset may be spontaneous or pain may linger after an infection or injury. The specific pattern of pain varies among men; some may report constant pain, while the pattern may be intermittent for others. This pain may make it difficult to work, continue recreational activities, and maintain intimate relationships.

Some authors have suggested that CUO is a regional extension of male chronic pelvic pain syndrome (Chap. 7), but actual evidence for this is sparse, as the reported symptoms in CUO do not typically involve voiding symptoms or pelvic floor dysfunction complaints.

Physical Examination and Diagnostic Testing

A thorough examination of the male genitals must be performed, with attempts to precisely locate the source of pain. A scrotal ultrasound should be ordered if the patient has not undergone this imaging in more than 6 months. Depending on risk factors and history, screening for sexually transmitted infections can be added, along with cultures for *Ureaplasma*. Individuals should always be asked about their personal history of vasectomy, as many men with CUO are subsequently diagnosed with postvasectomy pain syndrome.

A spermatic cord block may also be helpful in confirming the diagnosis. If symptoms seem consistent with an atypical radiculopathy (e.g., testicular pain and at the same time pain shoots down the leg), imaging of the low back (such as MRI) may be helpful.

Management

As men with CUO present like many other chronic pain populations, it is not unreasonable to proceed from a more noninvasive perspective: identify multidimensional (biopsychosocial) factors that may be contributing to the chronic pain and address these factors, resolve any facilitators of symptoms rather than simply treating them, engage the patient's self-care abilities, and carefully select procedures and medications. This may include NSAIDs, tricyclic antidepressants, or anxiolytics, paired with referrals for physical therapy or pelvic floor physical therapy. Psychology evaluation may also be helpful; some men may benefit from referral to a multidisciplinary pain management program.

Invasive options do have a place in management as well. Diagnostic procedures such as a spermatic cord block have a role in determining possible success with denervation procedures or orchiectomy. Long-term follow-up will be determined by specific causes and treatment plans.

Testosterone Deficiency Overview

Male hypogonadism is defined by the Endocrine Society (2010) as "a clinical syndrome that results from failure of the testis to produce physiological levels of testosterone (T) and sperm due to disruption of one or more levels of the hypothalamic-pituitary-testicular axis." The term "testosterone deficiency" (TD) has recently replaced the term hypogonadism due to its clarity and specificity. Testosterone is critical for the development of men and is the driving force behind adolescence in boys. Testosterone and its metabolites are responsible for the normal physiology of males including the muscle, bone, skin, sperm production, sexual function, brain and peripheral nerves, and production of red blood cells. It is the principal circulating androgen in males, it is synthesized primarily from Leydig cells in the testes, but a small percentage is synthesized in the adrenal glands.

Anatomy and Physiology

Testosterone synthesis in the Leydig of the testicles is stimulated by luteinizing hormone (LH) released from the anterior pituitary gland. The release of LH is driven by secretion of gonadotropin-releasing hormone (GnRH) from the hypothalamus. In turn, testosterone and its metabolism into estradiol inhibit GnRH and LH secretion via a negative feedback loop at the pituitary and hypothalamus. Testosterone acts by binding to the androgen receptor, and approximately 90 % of circulating testosterone is bound to protein carrier molecules. Free testosterone, a small fraction of a man's total testosterone, is unbound and biologically available. Testosterone is secreted in a diurnal rhythm, with peak secretion between 6 and 10 AM in the morning; this rhythm becomes blunted after age 40. Total testosterone declines approximately 1 % per year after age 40.

Table 2.1 Types of hypogonadism

	Total Testosterone	LH	FSH
Primary hypogonadism	Low	High	High
Secondary hypogonadism	Low	Low or low normal	Low or low normal
Mixed/combined hypogonadism	Low or low normal	Low or low normal	Low or low normal
Hypogonadism due to opiates	Low	Low	Low

Primary hypogonadism is the result of the testicular failure to produce normal serum testosterone levels, in an environment of adequate LH and follicle-stimulating hormone (FSH) stimulation (Table 2.1). Secondary hypogonadism is a low serum testosterone levels as a result of pituitary or hypothalamic dysfunction that results in a vote testicular production of testosterone. Mixed or combined hypogonadism is a reduced production of testosterone in a context of normal LH levels; this is most commonly associated with aging.

Epidemiology and Risk Factors

Varying definitions for testosterone deficiency in the literature have led to widely varying estimates of testosterone prevalence in adult men, ranging from 2 to 39 %. In clinical practice, strict reliance on laboratory ranges may lead to false negative results when evaluating individuals for TD; there is consensus that diagnosis of TD requires symptoms and low serum testosterone values.

A number of common conditions are associated with hypogonadism (Table 2.2), as are a number of medications (Table 2.3). Widespread screening for testosterone deficiency is not recommended, due to cost and a lack of consensus on treatment goals. However, these tables can help provide guidance for selection of men who may benefit from screening for hypogonadism.

History and Physical Examination

When considering TD, the focus history should look for sexual and nonsexual symptoms (Table 2.4). The most notable symptoms tend to be complaints of diminished libido and erectile dysfunction; in fact complaints of sexual a screen function issues can serve as a screen to determine which men may benefit from a more extensive evaluation. Patients should be asked if they went through puberty at approximately the same time as their classmates. Social history should include occupational exposure for chemicals and radiation, as well as a list of potential drugs of abuse such as marijuana. It is important to determine if there is a history of testicular injury or any surgery that may have compromised testicular function. Patients should be asked about the duration of their symptoms, whether their complaints are relatively new in onset or may be related to other chronic comorbidities such as renal failure or metabolic syndrome.

Table 2.2 Causes of testosterone deficiency

Primary male hypogonadism	Secondary male hypogonadism	Combined or mixed hypogonadism
Chromosome abnormalities (Klinefelter's)	Cirrhosis	Cirrhosis
Myotonic dystrophy	Metabolic syndrome/diabetes	Sickle cell disease
Orchitis (e.g., mumps)	Hemochromatosis	Aging
Cryptorchidism	Psychological stress	Narcotics for chronic pain management
Loss from trauma, tumor, torsion	Aging	Chemotherapy management
Chemotherapy	Kallman's syndrome	
Radiation to the genitals or pelvic area	Pituitary mass lesions, e.g., prolactinoma/other pituitary tumors	
HIV infection	Uremia	
Medication effects	Morbid obesity	
Anorchia	Cushing's syndrome diabetes	
	Narcotics for chronic pain management	
	Testicular cancer	
	Obstructive sleep apnea	
	Infectious disease (tuberculosis, tertiary syphilis)	

Table 2.3 Drugs associated with low testosterone

Anabolic steroids
Opioids
Marijuana
Phenothiazine antipsychotics
Progestins
Statins (high doses)
Steroids (e.g., high-dose glucocorticoids, spironolactone)
Thiazide diuretics
Ulcer drugs (e.g., cimetidine)
Antiarrhythmics (e.g., amiodarone)
Anticonvulsants (e.g., phenytoin)
Antifungals (e.g., ketoconazole)
Chemotherapeutic agents
Estrogens, progestins
Gonadotropin-releasing hormone (GnRH) agonists, antagonists

The physical examination is typically unrevealing except in cases of profound and long-standing hypogonadism. There may be some regression of secondary sexual characteristics, although this can be a challenging distinction in the setting of obesity. Scrotal examination should note the presence of both testicles, their size and consistency, as well as any potential testicular mass or varicocele. Small testes may provide a clue toward a genetic cause for TD, such as Klinefelter's disease. Gynecomastia may be a clue toward low testosterone; patients should be assessed for their Tanner stage as compared with their chronologic age to provide a measure of age-appropriate virilization.

Table 2.4 Summary of 2010 Clinical Practice Guidelines, Endocrine Society

Suggest testosterone deficiency in adult men	Associated with testosterone deficiency in adult men
Incomplete sexual development	Decreased energy, initiative, self-confidence
Reduced libido	Depressed/blunted mood
Reduced spontaneous erections	Dysthymia
Difficulty achieving orgasm Reduced intensity of orgasm	Poor concentration or memory
	Sleep disturbance
Gynecomastia	Increased sleepiness
Loss of body hair/reduced shaving	Mild anemia
Very small or shrinking testes (<5 mL)	Increased body fat/BMI
Low or zero sperm count	Decreased physical strength
Low trauma fracture	
Low bone density	
Decline in muscle bulk or strength	
Hot flashes/sweats	

Diagnostic Tests

Laboratory evaluation will assess total and bioavailable testosterone, free testosterone, LH, FSH, and prolactin levels; estradiol may be included if the patient has a high body mass index (BMI). For younger men, testosterone levels are most accurate in the morning (prior to 1100) due to circadian release of testosterone in the morning; this is blunted in older men. Additional laboratory evaluation may include PSA, thyroid studies, fasting lipid profile, liver function studies, screening for diabetes, and a complete blood count (CBC). The results of all these studies will determine the appropriateness of testosterone replacement therapy.

A scrotal ultrasound may be considered in the context of abnormal scrotal findings, such as small or absent testes. A pituitary MRI may be indicated, if men have a prolactin level more than twice the upper limit of normal or in men with severe hypogonadism. A karyotype analysis is appropriate in men who have small testes if there is a suspicion of Klinefelter's disease.

Management

The principal goal of androgen replacement therapy is to restore a physiologic pattern of the androgen exposure to all of the body's tissues, while avoiding supraphysiologic levels. Undue restoration of a normal testosterone level can have several effects on male physiology. This includes increased lean body mass, decreased fat mass, improved bone mineral density, improved libido, improved morning erections, and improved erectile function and a response to PDE5 medications. Restoring a eugonadal state can improve fasting glucose and insulin sensitivity, can improve total cholesterol results, and may improve depression. Many providers may be hesitant to pursue testosterone replacement, as the overall impact of testosterone on cardiovascular events is unknown. In response to this controversy regarding the cardiovascular safety of testosterone supplementation, in September 2014, the FDA determined that there was insufficient evidence to support an association between testosterone supplementation and increased cardiovascular events.

Prior to beginning therapy, men should have a PSA, hemoglobin and hematocrit, and liver function testing within the preceding 6 months. Men also need a baseline digital rectal examination documented.

The best indicator of the success of testosterone replacement therapy is the patient report of improvement of symptoms such as libido and fatigue. Men may have reports of urinary function changes and exacerbation of lower urinary tract symptoms within the first 6 months after starting therapy. Prior to the initiation of any testosterone replacement therapy, the provider and patient should have a thorough discussion of the individual goals of management, risks, and potential side effects. Restoring normal testosterone levels in a hypogonadal male does not predict risk of subsequent prostate cancer.

Behavioral and Conservative Management

TD in the setting of obesity is often the result of decreased androgens due to the aromatization of testosterone to estradiol. Weight loss and moderate intensity exercise can prove testosterone levels. After a weight loss of 15–20 pounds, testosterone levels can be reevaluated for progress toward normalization.

Medical Management

Men prefer testosterone products that maintain stable blood levels and have smoother clinical effects. There are multiple therapies available for testosterone replacement (Table 2.5). Oral therapies are not available in the United States at this time and have a history of increased risk for hepatocellular carcinoma. All currently available therapies are effective and result in impairment of spermatogenesis. Alternative therapies can include aromatase inhibitors or selective estrogen receptor modulators (SERMs). Testosterone replacement products are becoming subject to extensive prior authorization procedures from insurance companies. As a result, these medications are becoming increasingly difficult for men to obtain, both in terms of cost and in meeting insurance company eligibility criteria, especially if they are newly diagnosed with testosterone deficiency.

The management of comorbidities such as obesity or diabetes is vital to the promotion of the success of both testosterone deficiency and comorbidity management. To date, there have been no reports of thromboembolic events associated with men on testosterone replacement.

All transdermal testosterone therapies have similar pharmacokinetic profiles and achieve normal physiologic concentrations of testosterone in approximately 2–3 weeks. Patients should be cautioned against transfer to other people via skin to skin contact. Products must be applied to clean dry skin into which showering or swimming for 2–4 h after administration.

Injection therapy creates supraphysiologic doses and patients may notice the variations in their testosterone levels. Peak levels are achieved in the 8–96 h following the injection. These are usually the least expensive of the testosterone or placement options.

Table 2.5 Testosterone replacement products

Product	Dose	Considerations
Testosterone enanthate Testosterone cypionate	100 mg weekly or 200 mg every 14 days injected into the gluteal muscle	Check level after ~8 weeks on therapy at midway between injections Testosterone target is midrange of facility values or patient reports of symptom improvement Men can be taught to self-administer these injections Caution patients against "stacking" doses at home (injecting more frequently than prescribed) Supraphysiologic levels shortly after injection
Testosterone undecanoate (Aveed®)	750 mg initially 750 mg repeated at 4 weeks then q10 weeks Injected into the gluteal muscle	Injection is performed in the office Longer duration of action For specifics, refer to the procedures Chap. 20
Testosterone propionate (Testopel®)	4–12 pellets every 3–6 months Less flexible dosing	Requires a short procedure in the office to implant pellets under the skin For specifics, refer to the procedures Chap. 20 Midrange levels should be seen after 4–10 weeks
Testosterone gel Androgel®, Axiron®, Fortesta®, Testim®	50–120 mg applied Qam depending on product	Application sites vary by product All offer good absorption with low incidence of skin reaction Primary risk is potential for secondary exposure via skin to skin contact
Testosterone buccal system (Striant®)	Placed on the gum above the incisor Delivers 30 mg of testosterone	Instruct on rotation of application site every 12 h Men may complain of difficulties eating while using this product Gum irritation is a common side effect
Transdermal patch	2–6 mg patch Men should be instructed to apply the patch to the back, abdomen, upper arms, or thighs	Little risk of transfer of testosterone product Common to have irritation due to adhesive Can treat irritation with low-dose steroid cream, but this may interfere with absorption of testosterone product Check morning testosterone after 2 weeks

Subcutaneous pellets provide physiologic testosterone levels for approximately 3 months and should be considered after men have demonstrated favorable response and side effect profile on other shorter-acting products.

Aromatase inhibitors prevent the peripheral conversion of testosterone to estradiol and can result in significant improvements in testosterone. Selective estrogen receptor modulators (SERMs) such as clomiphene citrate are used off-label to increase testosterone in men who wish to preserve sperm production.

Testosterone replacement is contraindicated if there is evidence for prostate cancer, any abnormality suspicious for prostate cancer, or in cases of male breast cancer. Elevated PSA is not an absolute contraindication to testosterone replacement therapy; however, this should be managed individually, based on the need for prostate biopsies and ongoing PSA surveillance.

Ongoing Management

There is no consensus regarding definitive recommendations for laboratory testing of men on testosterone replacement therapy. However, men undergoing testosterone replacement therapy need to be monitored minimum of every 6 months once they are stable on a particular product. There should be an initial interval testing at 3–4 months after starting any replacement therapy, to evaluate for increases to their total testosterone level and symptom improvement. Ongoing management should include digital rectal exam and PSA testing every 6 months; other laboratory evaluations are up to the discretion of the provider, in the context of other existing comorbidities.

If after 6 months the patient does not report any improvement to his symptoms, consideration should be given to discontinuing testosterone supplementation.

Male Fertility Overview

Infertility is a disease of the reproductive system that affects about 6.1 million people in the United States or about 10 % of the reproductive age population. It affects men and women, and most cases are treated with conventional therapies such as medical management or surgery. Babies born by in vitro fertilization represent 1.5 % of the children born in the United States, as 2015. In 50 % of infertility cases, the male is contributing to the problem, but the majority of male infertility is idiopathic.

Male infertility is constructed as a medical condition with psychological consequences, and many disciplines have contributed to the study of nonmedical aspects of infertility. Masculine norms (such as control, stoicism, or strength) impact the emotional well-being of men who do not live up to either reproductive or sexual cultural ideals. Little attention has been directed toward men's experience of infertility in differing social, cultural, and political contexts. Infertility challenges one's life expectations, and couples report disruptions in both their personal life and emotional and sexual relationships.

There is a substantial amount of published literature that focuses on the impact of infertility on sexual and marital relationships, and in women's reproductive lives, which have been extensively explored by social science research in the last 25 years. However, little research has been directed toward examination of the male infertility experience; available research is compounded by small sample sizes, uncontrolled study designs, and a lack of validated instruments. This limited body of social research marginalizes the experience of men and has left providers with little knowledge of the emotional repercussions of a diagnosis of male infertility. The few studies that have been completed confirm that infertility is experienced as a threat to masculinity.

Male infertility remains a hidden issue within the context of overall fertility care. Outcomes of fertility treatments are tracked only at conception or live birth, making a clear picture of the epidemiology of male fertility unclear. Study of male fertility issues is further hindered by the fact that male fertility is not a reportable disease, is almost exclusively treated outpatient, and is almost always paid for out of pocket. For in vitro fertilization cases, the Centers for Disease Control tracks only whether or not there was a male fertility factor present.

The Affordable Care Act does not mention any mandate for infertility evaluation and treatment, leaving the issue to the individual states. Currently only 16 states address coverage for infertility, and only six of these mandate male factor evaluation and treatment. This creates a disparity in coverage for risks identifying contributing male health issues; it means that men are denied the opportunity to consider treatment for reversible causes. It means that men are denied the opportunity for cost-effective interventions that may decrease the sophistication of any assisted reproductive technology required.

An infertility evaluation should be considered when there is a history of unprotected intercourse for at least 12 months without a positive pregnancy test or if intercourse has been timed with ovulation. This length of time can be shortened if the female partner is age 35 or older or if the couple is simply worried about their fertility status. There are other reasons to consider an evaluation, such as female infertility issues or a history of male risk factors for infertility, such as cryptorchidism or a history of cancer treatment.

History and Physical Examination

A targeted history for potential fertility issues in male includes general reproductive history including a history of previous paternity, any past medical history or surgical history that could affect the structure or function of the male genitalia, occupational exposure to temperature extremes, and environmental toxins. Relevant surgical history includes any procedure that can alter the structure or function of the male genitalia, including retroperitoneal surgery or hernia repair. The sexual history and a history of female fertility evaluation are also necessary components.

Physical examination includes a general assessment with special focus on the genitalia and the presence and consistency of the vas deferens. Men should be examined for unilateral or bilateral varicoceles (have patients perform Valsalva maneuver to reverse flow into the pampiniform plexus while standing to provoke palpable distention of the vessels) and evidence of appropriate virilization including hair distribution.

Management

The goal of the male fertility evaluation is to identify any potentially reversible, treatable causes (Tables 2.6 and 2.7). The goal is also to provide a treatment that may raise the overall semen quality into a range where less sophisticated assisted reproductive technologies may be appropriate. Referral to a male infertility specialist is recommended, but some tests can be ordered in advance: semen analysis, morning testosterone level, LH, FSH, and prolactin.

Table 2.6 Evaluation for male factor infertility

Test	Discussion
Semen analysis	Men will be asked to provide a semen sample after a period of abstinence of 2–5 days This can include a urine sample in the case of suspected retrograde ejaculation Values that are evaluated are the volume of the ejaculate, sperm motility, total sperm count, and sperm morphology (shape)
Hormone studies	Total testosterone, luteinizing hormone (LH), follicle-stimulating hormone (FSH), prolactin levels Estradiol may be included if the patient has a high body mass index (BMI)
Estimation of testicular size/volume	Aid in establishing testicular function
Genetic testing	Karyotype analysis and Y-chromosome microdeletion testing may be included if the sperm counts are very low or zero Screening for cystic fibrosis may also be included if the vas deferens is not noted on physical examination
Other	Other tests, such as a scrotal ultrasound, can be included based on an individual's presentation and history

Table 2.7 Selected contributors to male factor infertility

Pre-testicular	Testicular	Post-testicular
Anabolic steroid use Diabetes with anejaculation Idiopathic hypogonadotropic hypogonadism Kallman's syndrome Obesity Pituitary or hypothalamic dysfunction Spinal cord injury Medications (antihypertensives psychotherapeutic agents, hormonal agents, antibiotics, cimetidine, cyclosporine, colchicine, allopurinol, sulfasalazine)	Cryptorchidism Mumps orchitis Klinefelter's syndrome Previous chemotherapy or radiation treatment Varicocele	Antisperm antibodies Congenital bilateral absence of the vas deferens (cystic fibrosis and its variants) Erectile dysfunction Failed vasectomy reversal Inguinal hernia repair Retrograde ejaculation Vasectomy Pediatric hernia repair

Behavioral and Conservative Management

Because obesity is associated with male factor infertility, weight loss and exercise are the primary recommendations for men who are overweight and obese. This is in part due to decreased serum testosterone levels seen with obese men, although the precise mechanism by which obesity influences male fertility is unknown.

Men should also be instructed to limit their exposure to known environmental toxins that affect semen quality such as pesticides, radiation, heavy metals, bio-persistent chemicals, smoking, marijuana, and other drugs of abuse.

Male fertility may be improved by the use of antioxidants. A 2014 Cochrane review looked at randomized controlled trials that use antioxidants and concluded that only low-quality evidence supports the use of antioxidants, which may improve the birth rate by improving sperm function. However, no over-the-counter supplement has been conclusively proven to prove male fertility.

Medical Management

Medical management for male infertility can be successful if a specific contributing factor is identified (Table 2.7). This can include removing environmental toxins, such as recommending smoking cessation, cessation of recreational drug use such as marijuana, and cessation of alcohol intake. Medical management can address endocrine abnormalities and restore the patient to normal hormone levels. Medical management can include such options as clomiphene citrate, antibiotics, FSH, human chorionic gonadotropin (hCG), or pseudoephedrine; patients should be advised that it may take a few weeks to obtain prior authorization from their insurance for some of these medications. After a period of time, often 6 months or more, there can be improvements in overall semen parameters.

Surgical Management

Surgical management options include testicular or epididymal biopsy, microsurgical testicular sperm extraction (microTESE), vasectomy reversal, epididymal or testicular aspiration for IVF, and transurethral resection (TUR) of the ejaculatory duct in cases of blockage.

Long-Term Follow-Up

Because sperm take approximately 90 days to grow and mature, follow-up for male fertility treatment occurs every 3 months. At this point, men can be expected to need a semen sample for analysis and to undergo repeat physical examination. The management of additional comorbid conditions should be encouraged, such as obesity, erectile dysfunction, ejaculatory dysfunction, and any depression or anxiety issues that may be impacting fertility management.

Peyronie's Disease Overview

Peyronie's disease (PD), first described in 1743 by French surgeon François de la Peyronie, is an acquired disorder of the tunica albuginea (TA) of the corpora cavernosa of the penis that often involves a fibrotic, palpable, inelastic tunical plaque.

There is an estimated prevalence of ~9 %, although it is suspected that this may be an underestimate, and definition among studies varies. This condition can involve the penile corpora, and some men will complain of poor erectile quality distal to the plaque, penile shortening, or narrowing of the penile shaft.

The 2015 American Urological Association guidelines for Peyronie's disease emphasize that providers should "evaluate and treat a man with Peyronie's disease only when [he/she] has the experience and diagnostic tools to appropriately evaluate, counsel, and treat the condition." An individual's symptoms and course for PD can vary, and some men experience improvement with time.

Active Peyronie's disease involves changing symptoms and progression of curvature, and men are likely to report pain. There may or may not be a notable plaque, and erectile function may not be affected. *Stable Peyronie's disease* describes symptoms that are stable and have not changed for some time. There is likely to be a palpable plaque, reports of penile curvature or other deformities, and possible erectile dysfunction due to restriction of the elastic tissue of the penis. Men usually report some degree of distress, due to appearance, penile shortening, or ED.

Risk Factors

Research has not uncovered risk factors for PD, other than a history of trauma or Dupuytren's disease, and there is in uncertain genetic component. Most cases of PD have a history of spontaneous presentation.

History

PD can begin spontaneously as localized inflammation or as the result of penile trauma and may develop into a hardened, sometimes calcified scar that can incorporate varying degrees of collagen and calcium. It can present with pain, spontaneous onset curvature or "waisting" of the erect penile shaft, or erectile dysfunction, and these changes may be significant enough to cause pain and distress during sexual activity for the man and/or his partner. Men should be asked about a history of penile injury and whether any pain is always present or occurs only with erection. Sexual function should be established to distinguish the effects of PD from routine ED, to help guide therapy.

Physical Examination

With the penile shaft on a gentle stretch, it may be possible to palpate a distinct plaque along the shaft. PD can also present as an "i-beam" with the plaque presenting between the corpora at some point along the shaft. The plaque may be tender during the early phases of the disease, or there may be reports of pain only with erection. Men may provide a picture of their erect penis to establish its presentation, and providers may ask for photographic documentation as well. Evaluate for areas of tenderness.

Diagnostic Testing

No specific tests are necessary for evaluation, although penile length measurements and measurement of the curvature can be taken as a marker to measure treatment success, and photographs provided by patients are often sufficient. Some providers may choose to administer an intracorporeal injection to produce an artificial erection to better establish the degree of curvature and deformity. This can be accompanied by a penile Doppler study.

Management

Peyronie's disease is not simply penile curvature, but a collection of both physical and psychosocial symptoms that affect sexual function. Some men will respond to reassurance and choose not to pursue any additional intervention. For some men, treatment for any erectile function issue may be satisfactory.

Oral Therapies

If pain is present, NSAID medications can be helpful in increasing overall comfort levels and may improve ability for sexual activity.

The AUA 2015 PD guidelines advise against most other oral therapies that have been historically recommended for PD: vitamin E, tamoxifen, procarbazine, omega-3 fatty acids, or a combination of vitamin E with L-carnitine. Studies looking at these options have been flawed in design or present low-grade evidence. These therapies involved cost to the patient and can delay treatment with therapeutic options that are effective.

Colchicine, potassium aminobenzoate, and pentoxifylline have shown some success in treating curvature, but previous studies have had insufficient rigor for these medications to be recommended as first-line treatments.

Intralesional Therapy

Current intralesional treatment for Peyronie's disease centers on the use of collagenase clostridium histolyticum (Xiaflex®) and penile modeling, which is indicated in men with stable PD and curvature >30° and intact erectile function (Gelbard et al. 2013). This product was not evaluated for use in men with an hourglass deformity, ventral curvature, calcified plaque, or plaque located proximal to the base of the penis. Prescription guidelines and the AUA guidelines emphasize that men must be aggressively counseled about the risks of this medication and counseled to help ensure their treatment expectations are realistic.

Other potential intralesional treatment includes interferon α-2b interferon or verapamil. The same emphasis on pretreatment counseling applies, although the strength of evidence is weaker.

Other Nonsurgical Treatments

Topical therapies, such as magnesium or verapamil, have improved curvature when compared with placebo (AUA Guidelines 2015) but studies have been small. Providers are advised against offering extracorporeal shock wave therapy, electromotive therapy with verapamil, or radiotherapy as treatment options, due to the low-level evidence or absent evidence for success. Penile traction devices may be helpful for some men, but at this point the evidence for this is weak, and men will have to pay out of pocket for the device.

Surgical Treatments

Men with stable PD (no changes for >12 months), who are not candidates for other therapies, may wish to consider surgery. Several options are available with the goal of preserving penile length and correcting curvature and depend on the specific location of the plaque and presence of comorbid ED. Indications for surgery are deformity that impairs sexual relations, stable deformity without pain, extensive plaque calcification, or failed nonsurgical treatment (Levine and Burnett 2013). Men with ED may be offered a penile implant as a way to address both the PD and ED during the same surgery.

Surgical outcomes are good, and the surgery itself is low risk. Men should again be counseled about realistic expectations, and short term they may report some numbness and tingling at the operative site.

Inflammatory Conditions of the Penis

Condition	History	Signs and symptoms	Evaluation	Therapeutic interventions
Phimosis	Seen only in males who are uncircumcised History of progressive difficulty retracting the foreskin History of poor personal hygiene and/or a recent groin skin infection Creates risk for chronic inflammation and squamous cell cancer of the penis	Foreskin may show signs of chronic irritation: erythema, fissuring, tightening of the opening of the foreskin Possible urinary obstruction or "ballooning" of the foreskin when voiding as it traps urine Pain Balanitis or balanoposthitis	History and presentation sufficient to confirm diagnosis	Consider circumcision or dorsal slit May require catheter if urinary function has been compromised

Condition	History	Signs and symptoms	Evaluation	Therapeutic interventions
Balanitis	Greatest risk: uncontrolled diabetes mellitus Seen in uncircumcised males Inflammation of the glans Commonly caused by *Candida albicans*	Symptoms can include edema, erythema, and pain of the glans Dysuria Urethral discharge Scaling of skin Possible history of discharge between the foreskin and glans Phimosis Meatal stenosis Rash to the genitals	Consider screening for diabetes, especially with higher BMI Culture for STDs and for other viral and fungal organisms KOH (potassium hydroxide) and Tzanck preparations can be included If ulcers are present, screen for herpes and syphilis Biopsy may be indicated in refractory cases (no response to treatment after 6 weeks)	Empiric treatment without cultures is common NSAIDs may improve comfort level If patient is diabetic, his diabetes must be controlled in order to help eradicate any infection and prevent recurrence Retract foreskin and clean daily with warm saline and hypoallergenic soap Depending on severity, you can treat with oral antifungal +/− topical antifungal alone or combined topical antifungal and low-strength steroid Topical antibiotics may have a role in suspected anaerobic infection Consider circumcision or dorsal slit in refractory cases
Balanoposthitis	Greatest risk: uncontrolled diabetes mellitus Seen in uncircumcised males Inflammation of both the glans and foreskin	Similar to balanitis Can include an edematous and painful foreskin that may not retract	Same as for balanitis	Same as for balanitis

(continued)

Condition	History	Signs and symptoms	Evaluation	Therapeutic interventions
Balanitis xerotica obliterans (BXO) or lichen sclerosis	Common in middle-aged men Result of chronic infection or inflammation or trauma Uncircumcised and diabetic males have an increased risk A personal history of long-standing BXO creates higher risk for squamous cell carcinoma of the penis Can also be seen on the external genitalia of females	Painful condition associated with flat patches of white, thinned skin (mosaic pattern) Localized penile discomfort Painful erections Urinary obstruction Meatus may become edematous, indurated Possible erosions, fissures Often results in meatal stenosis and urethral strictures Foreskin may adhere to the glans	Diagnosis can be made only via tissue biopsy	If asymptomatic, no treatment Manage associated symptoms Low-strength steroid can improve comfort level Yearly follow-up due to risk for malignancy

Clinical Pearls

- Guidelines for vasectomy counseling do not *require* the female partner's presence.
- Vasectomy does not increase risk for other diseases, such as prostate cancer or dementia.
- Chronic orchialgia can be the result of an undiagnosed varicocele, postvasectomy pain syndrome, or potential radicular issue. The management of chronic pain condition may be helpful.
- Consider screening for hypogonadism in men on long-term (>3 months) opioid therapy.
- When considering hypogonadism, the most notable symptoms are diminished libido and sexual function complaints.
- When scheduling initial lab draws to screen for hypogonadism, consider the work schedule of the individual: night shift/swing shift workers should have levels during their "morning" when they wake after their sleep cycle.
- Testosterone replacement therapy has not been shown to increase risk for prostate cancer, and no thromboembolic events have been reported.
- Testosterone replacement requires a partnership between provider and patient, for consistent monitoring and physical examinations.

- Hypogonadism in young men should prompt consideration for genetic testing and should never be treated with testosterone replacement until an explanation for the low levels is established. Premature initiation of testosterone replacement risks potentially irreversible cessation of sperm production.
- Male infertility is a hidden issue within the context of overall fertility care, and evaluation can be initiated if the male or couple is concerned about their fertility status. Most medical therapies for men are empiric.
- While many nonsurgical options for treatment of Peyronie's disease have been suggested, most have very little evidence to support their use.
- When faced with inflammation of the penis, always consider screening for undiagnosed or poorly controlled diabetes.

Resources for the Nurse Practitioner
American Urological Association: The Optimal Evaluation of the Infertile Male: AUA Best Practice Statement http://www.auanet.org/common/pdf/education/clinical-guidance/Male-Infertility-d.pdf
RESOLVE: The National Infertility Association: www.resolve.org
American Society for Reproductive Medicine: http://www.reproductivefacts.org
Men's Health Month: www.menshealthmonth.org/
American Academy of Family Physicians curriculum for Men's Health http://www.aafp.org/dam/AAFP/documents/medical education residency/program_directors/Reprint257_Men.pdf
Centers for Disease Control statistics on Men's Health http://www.cdc.gov/nchs/fastats/mens-health.html

Resources for the Patient
The Urology Care Foundation: www.urologyhealth.org
RESOLVE: The National Infertility Association: www.resolve.org
American Society for Reproductive Medicine: www.reproductivefacts.org
Men's Health Network (MHN): www.menshealthnetwork.org
Men's Health Month: www.menshealthmonth.org
Association of Peyronie's Disease Advocates (APDA): http://www.peyroniesassociation.org

References

111th United States Congress (2010) Compilation of patient protection and affordable care act. http://housedocs.house.gov/energycommerce/ppacacon.pdf
American Urological Association (AUA) Guideline (2012) Vasectomy: AUA guideline. AUA Board of Directors. http://www.auanet.org/common/pdf/education/clinical-guidance/Vasectomy.pdf

American Urological Association (AUA) Guideline (2014) AUA men's health checklist. AUA Board of Directors. https://www.auanet.org/common/pdf/education/clinical-guidance/Mens-Health-Checklist.pdf

American Urological Association (AUA) Guideline (2015) Peyronie's disease: AUA Guideline. AUA Board of Directors. http://www.auanet.org/common/pdf/education/clinical-guidance/Peyronies-Disease.pdf

Gelbard M, Goldstein I, Hellstrom WJ et al (2013) Clinical efficacy, safety and tolerability of collagenase clostridium histolyticum for the treatment of Peyronie disease in 2 large double-blind, randomized, placebo controlled phase 3 studies. J Urol 190:1199

Levine LA, Burnett AL (2013) Standard operating procedures for Peyronie's disease. J Sex Med 10(1):230–244

Levine LA, Hoeh MP (2015) Evaluation and management of chronic scrotal content pain. Curr Urol Rep 16(6):1–8

Quallich SA, Arslanian-Engoren C (2013) Chronic testicular pain in adult men: an integrative literature review. Am J Mens Health 7(5):402–413. doi:10.1177/1557988313476732

Quallich SA, Arslanian-Engoren C (2014) Chronic unexplained orchialgia: a concept analysis. J Adv Nurs 70(8):1717–1726. doi:10.1111/jan.12340

Further Reading

Berookhim BM, Choi J, Alex B et al (2014) Deformity stabilization and improvement in men with untreated Peyronie's disease. BJU Int 113:133

Bhasin S, Basaria S (2011) Diagnosis and treatment of hypogonadism in men. Best Pract Res Clin Endocrinol Metab 25(2):251–270

Buvat J, Maggi M, Guay A, Torres LO (2013) Testosterone deficiency in men: systematic review and standard operating procedures for diagnosis and treatment. J Sex Med 10(1):245–284

Casabé A, Bechara A, Cheliz G, De Bonis W, Rey H (2011) Risk factors of Peyronie's disease. What does our clinical experience show? J Sex Med 8(2):518–523

Corona G, Rastrelli G, Monami M, Guay A, Buvat J, Sforza A, Forti G, Mannucci E, Maggi M (2011a) Hypogonadism as a risk factor for cardiovascular mortality in men: a meta-analytic study. Eur J Endocrinol 165(5):687–701

Corona G, Rastrelli G, Morelli A, Vignozzi L, Mannucci E, Maggi M (2011b) Hypogonadism and metabolic syndrome. J Endocrinol Invest 34(7):557

Elterman L (2012) New insights into the medical management of idiopathic male infertility—What works, what does not and does it matter? J Urol 188(2):355–357

Gelbard MK, Dorey F, James K (1990) The natural history of Peyronie's disease. J Urol 144:1376

Ko EY, Siddiqi K, Brannigan RE, Sabanegh ES (2012) Empirical medical therapy for idiopathic male infertility: a survey of the American Urological Association. J Urol 187(3):973–978

Moskovic DJ, Araujo AB, Lipshultz LI, Khera M (2013) The 20-year public health impact and direct cost of testosterone deficiency in US men. J Sex Med 10(2):562–569

Nelson CJ, Mulhall JP (2013) Psychological impact of Peyronie's disease: a review. J Sex Med 10:653

Rosen R, Catania J, Lue T et al (2008) Impact of Peyronie's disease on sexual and psychosocial functioning: qualitative findings in patients and controls. J Sex Med 5:1977

Sharlip ID, Belker AM, Honig S, Labrecque M, Marmar JL, Ross LS, Sandlow JI, Sokal DC, American Urological Association (2012) Vasectomy: AUA guideline. J Urol 188(6 Suppl):2482–2491

Stember DS, Nagler HM (2012) Update on vasectomy protocol. Curr Urol Rep 13(6):467–473

Wu JA, Eisenberg ML (2012) Male infertility. In: Essential urology. Humana Press, New York, pp 229–241

Evaluation and Management of Common Scrotal Conditions

3

Katherine Marchese

Contents

K. Marchese, MSN, ANP-BC, CUNP
Department of Urology, RUSH University Medical Center,
Chicago, IL, USA
e-mail: kathymarchese@gmail.com

© Springer International Publishing Switzerland 2016
M. Lajiness, S. Quallich (eds.), *The Nurse Practitioner in Urology*,
DOI 10.1007/978-3-319-28743-0_3

Objectives
1. Identify three conditions associated with acute scrotal pain.
2. Review the anatomy associated with hydrocele formation.
3. Discuss two percutaneous treatment options for varicoceles.
4. Outline the differences between a retractile testis and an undescended testis.

Introduction

In this chapter, a variety of common scrotal disorders will be discussed. Many of them are benign and require minimal evaluation and follow-up. Others present as emergent disorders and need immediate evaluation and treatment. Therefore, history taking needs to be comprehensive, structured, and relevant to the patients' stated chief complaint and current symptoms. The chief complaint points to the direction of your exam; the history of the present illness is where the NP collects pertinent information of where and what the symptoms are, the onset, and duration. It is important to listen to the patient and allow him to explain in his own terms. Obtaining the medical and surgical past history helps to focus on the possible differential diagnoses. The next step in evaluation of any scrotal disorder is the physical exam.

Review of the Components of a Scrotal Exam

Remember that the medical and surgical history just obtained helps to guide the examination of the scrotum (Table 3.1). Focus on the components of the scrotal exam that relate to the history given. Males, both adolescents and adults, experience anxiety and embarrassment about this genital exam. The practitioner can help to reduce this anxiety by teaching and explaining each step of the exam as it is being done. As the exam progresses, explain exactly what you are looking at and what you are seeing. This is also a good time to teach a patient how and when to do a testicular self-exam.

The best complement you can receive is when the patient says thank you and tells you that he has never heard that information before. Remember you will likely see this patient again and this exam done properly helps to promote your therapeutic relationship with him.

Acute Scrotum (Acute Scrotal Pain)

Overview

Acute scrotal pain is defined as the sudden onset of pain, swelling, and/or tenderness in the scrotum with associated pain in the pelvis or abdomen. It requires a quick, efficient, and thorough assessment that includes an in-depth history and physical examination. Based on this immediate evaluation, further testing may be recommended or the patient may be scheduled for emergent surgery. Differential diagnosis for the adult with acute onset of scrotal pain includes testicular torsion, appendix torsion, epididymo-orchitis, idiopathic acute scrotal edema, Fournier's gangrene, testicular trauma, testicular tumor, or a strangulated inguinal hernia. These scrotal conditions range from benign and short term to complex, life-altering, malignant medical problems. The nurse practitioner

Table 3.1 Scrotal examination review

Action	Structure	Comments
Inspection	Scrotal sac	Patient may be in a standing position or a lying down position and sometimes both positions are necessary
		Inspect the scrotum for overall size, shape, skin characteristics, and hair distribution
		May appear asymmetric with the left hemi-scrotum and left testes hanging lower than the right side
		Look for any visibly dilated veins; assess using the Dubin and Ametar's varicocele grading system
		Darker pigmentation is a normal variant
Palpation	Testicles	Using the thumb, middle, and index fingers, gently slide your fingers over the surface of each testicle, first one side then the other
		The size, preferably using an orchidometer, and consistency of each testis should be recorded. Normal testicular size is 4 cm in length and ≳5 cm in width, approximately 20 cc's
		Gentle compression should not produce any discomfort
		The exam should demonstrate a smooth appearance with no lumps
		Any alteration in size, orientation, location, or texture should warrant further evaluation
	Epididymis	Located on the posterolateral aspect of each testes, the epididymal head, body, and tail should be palpated gently
		Assess for any area of increased size, tenderness, or induration
		Findings should demonstrate a smooth, non-tender surface with some enlargement at the head of the epididymis
	Spermatic cord	Palpated at the opening of the inguinal canal and from the testes up to the inguinal canal
		Contents of the spermatic cord include arteries, nerves, and vas deferens. Thickness of the cord may vary if lipomas are present and do not resolve when the patient lies down
		During visual inspection and palpation, the presence/absence of dilated veins should be assessed and graded with the patient in a supine and standing position. A Valsalva maneuver will help with grading
		The term "bag of worms" is used to describe large varicoceles
	Vas deferens	Width of a pencil lead
		Should feel smooth, cord-like without lumps or beads
		Absence of the vas is an important finding in an azoospermic male
Reflex assessment	Cremasteric reflex	Brush the inner thigh with a finger in a light, upward movement
		Slight elevation of the testicle and scrotum on the ipsilateral side should be seen

must be able to accurately triage these patients, plan a targeted workup, and implement the optimal treatment plan. The prime objective for the practitioner is to identify a true urologic emergency that, if not treated promptly, could result in the loss of a testis, testicular atrophy, infertility, and altered self-image. The four most common and serious causes of acute onset scrotal pain will be discussed in this section.

History

The initial history taken for acute scrotal pain can help the practitioner delineate the potential causes of the acute pain and provide a focus for the assessment and correct diagnosis.

1. What was the nature of the onset of pain (sudden, insidious), location, duration, and severity?
2. What makes the symptoms worsen and what helps them improve?
3. Have there been prior episodes and how did they resolve?
4. Is there edema present? What are the location, duration, and degree?
5. Are there any associated symptoms such as nausea, vomiting, fever, chills, and urinary symptoms?
6. Is there a history of urinary tract infections, sexually transmitted infections, epididymitis, orchitis, or prostatitis?
7. Have there been any urologic traumas, procedures, instrumentations, or known urologic anomalies?

Testicular Torsion

Overview

Testicular torsion is defined as the twisting of the spermatic cord and testis and is considered a true urologic emergency that must be evaluated and treated in less than 6 h for the best outcome. The torsion is related to inadequate fixation of the testis to the tunica vaginalis; this anomaly is called the bell clapper deformity. The twisting of the cord results in decreased arterial flow, venous outflow obstruction, and ischemic testicular tissue. This deformity is seen in intravaginal torsion. Intravaginal torsion of the testis and spermatic cord is the most common variant of testicular torsion.

The extravaginal testicular torsion is seen only in neonates. As indicated by its name, the twisting of the testis and gubernaculum occurs outside of the tunica vaginalis usually at the external inguinal ring. The entire cord and testis can become twisted resulting in ischemic testicular tissue noted at birth. The affected testis is usually not salvageable, appears atrophic, and does not require an emergent orchiectomy. At some point, a contralateral scrotal exploration and orchiopexy should be done. The infants may present as slightly restless and no acute pain and have a firm, non-tender, discolored scrotum.

Testicular torsion can also be intermittent in nature and resolve on its own within an hour or two. It can present with sudden acute onset of pain, and by the time an examination happens, there are no signs or symptoms. This chronic intermittent torsion over time can still result in ischemic changes in the testis.

Incidence

The incidence of testicular torsion in males under the age of 25 is 1:4000 and is the most common cause of testicular loss (Kapoor 2008; Wampler and Llanes 2010). The incidence is bimodal with two peaks. The initial peak is in the neonate and the secondary peak is in the puberty period. Torsions in males under the age of 21 account for 61 % of all torsions (Kapoor 2008). Torsions in the elderly male are rare but have been found in males as old as 69 years old. Males with a history of cryptorchidism have a tenfold greater risk for torsion.

Pertinent Anatomy and Physiology

The bell clapper deformity, seen in about 12 % of all males (Beni-Israel et al. 2010), is a congenital anomaly that increases the risk for intravaginal testicular torsion. The bell clapper deformity is responsible for almost 90 % of all cases. In this anomaly, the tunica vaginalis cloaks the entire testis and epididymis, preventing the tethering of the testis to the posterior scrotal wall allowing a twisting movement of spermatic cord. The testis floats freely within the tunica vaginalis, suspended by the spermatic cord. This anomaly is bilateral 80 % of the time.

History

The general history discussed in the previous section provides the components needed to begin the evaluation. Given the presence of medical information on the Internet, it is possible for the history to include episodes of manual self-detorsion by the patient, after diagnosing his condition with the help of search engines.

Signs and Symptoms

The classic presentation of testicular torsion is sudden, severe, usually unilateral hemi-scrotal pain, possibly accompanied by nausea and vomiting. Abdominal pain may be the presenting symptom and should also raise the specter of suspicion for torsion. Scrotal edema, fever, and changes in urinary symptoms such as dysuria, frequency, and urgency may develop. Most torsions are left-sided.

Risk Factors

No specific risk factors have been identified but researchers have found a higher incidence of testicular torsion with certain anatomical anomalies. Males with a long mesorchium, bell clapper syndrome, or a history of cryptorchidism are linked to higher incidence of torsion. Term infants who underwent a prolonged, difficult labor were also at increased incidence. A possible link has been established with recent trauma and extreme physical workouts especially bicycling.

Physical Exam

Inspection: Observe the demeanor in the patient. Patients with torsion are anxious, have a difficult time sitting in one position, and look very uncomfortable. Observe the gait. If the gait is normal, torsion is unlikely.

During the exam, the practitioner should compare and contrast both testicles for size, symmetry, and consistency although the extreme pain and edema experienced by the patient may preclude a thorough examination. Begin the exam with the normal testis. The affected testis and spermatic cord would be tender, possibly edematous, and warm. If the lower portion of the testis is painful, consider torsion of the testis. If the upper part of the testis is painful, consider torsion of the appendix and look for the "blue dot" sign. The torsed testis may present in a horizontal line and appear retracted or high riding due to the shortened spermatic cord. The degree of torsion can range between $180°$ and $720°$.

A hydrocele may be present. The cremasteric reflex may be absent. This finding has a sensitivity of 88.2 % and a specificity of 86.2 % (Kapoor 2008). Prehn's sign is negative but is not considered a definitive diagnostic sign for torsion but may help to rule out epididymitis. The epididymis may present in an anterior position. The ipsilateral skin may appear indurated or erythematous. After 12–24 h, the edema and inflammation make it difficult to identify any anatomical structures in the scrotum.

Diagnostic Tests

Laboratory evaluation is not recommended for the diagnostic evaluation of testicular torsion but may help to identify an alternate differential diagnosis. A complete blood count (CBC) would be normal in the early phase of a torsion, but the white blood count (WBC) would be elevated in an infectious process. After 12–24 hours the WBC would become elevated due to the inflammatory response. A urinalysis (UA) would also be normal in torsion but pyuria might indicate a differential diagnosis of epididymitis or prostatitis.

If the history, symptoms, and physical findings are suggestive of torsion, ultrasonography should not be recommended if it would delay the emergent need for scrotal exploration. A delay may result in further ischemia to the testicular tissue and adversely affect the salvage rates.

Color Doppler ultrasonography, the most commonly used imaging modality, has a high sensitivity and specificity for testicular torsion with only a 1 % false-negative rate. A negative result alone should not rule out the need for surgical exploration. The Doppler flow study will assess the arterial flow patterns. If no flow pattern is noted, torsion is likely. Further, this imaging modality can identify testicular trauma, epididymitis, or an inguinal hernia that has prolapsed into the scrotum.

Management

The gold standard for suspected testicular torsion is scrotal exploration with intra-operative detorsion of the testis, possible orchiectomy, and orchiopexy. Torsion is considered to be a urologic emergency that requires immediate surgical intervention. Delays to allow for further imaging or manual detorsion can result in lower salvage rates.

Manual detorsion can be attempted but this procedure should not delay preparations for the surgical intervention. The manual detorsion procedure is contraindicated if the onset of symptoms has been greater than 6 hours because of the strong likelihood of tissue ischemia and necrosis. Detorsion is very painful to the patient because the procedure needs to be done without local or general anesthesia. A mild analgesic may be given.

In torsion, the testis usually rotates medially toward the thigh but up to 33 % will rotate laterally. Therefore, when attempting detorsion, the testis and cord are rotated medially and based on the degree of twisting may need to be untwisted multiple times. Detorsion can be successful in 70 % of attempts but scrotal exploration and orchiopexy are still required.

Sudden resolution of pain and return of the testis to the normal physiological location with good vascular reperfusion are the criteria for a successful manual detorsion. A Doppler study is usually done prior to the procedure and then post-procedure to document improved arterial flow to the tissue.

Surgical Options

The diagnosis of testicular torsion is an indication for an emergent scrotal exploration with best results achieved if done within 6 h of the initial onset of symptoms.

Criteria for surgery is simply a clinical decision based mostly on history and physical exam that a testicular torsion is present and needs immediate surgical exploration.

The usual incisional approach for the scrotal exploration is trans-scrotal. After the detorsion of the affected testis and spermatic cord is completed, the testis is assessed for viability. If the testis is viable, an ipsilateral orchiopexy should be performed. An orchiopexy involves suturing the tunical albuginea to the dartos muscle in three points with nonabsorbable sutures. An orchiectomy is required if a clearly necrotic testis is uncovered. An orchiectomy will minimize the potential for possible injury to the contralateral testis related to postoperative swelling, inflammation, and infection. The contralateral, unaffected testis should also undergo an orchiopexy.

Delayed injury to the testis can be secondary to "testicular compartment syndrome." This is defined as increased pressure in the testis from the swollen inflamed testicular tissue. The structure of the tunica albuginea further increases this pressure and increases the potential for a later onset of testicular ischemia. A testicular fasciotomy with a small tunica vaginalis patch has been used to reduce the pressure and reduce the tissue injury.

In addition, some surgeons recommend concurrent removal of the testicular and epididymal appendices to prevent their possible torsion in the future.

Preoperative Considerations

The patient and the parents of a minor should always be counseled on the potential for an orchiectomy based on the ischemia found intraoperatively. Orchiectomy rates vary from 39 to 71 % based on the age of the patient and time from first symptom to surgical exploration (Sharp et al. 2013). The potential for immediate placement of a testicular prosthesis should also be presented. The bell clapper deformity, known to be bilateral in 80 % of the patients, indicates a need to discuss a preemptive orchiopexy on the contralateral side.

Postoperative Management

This procedure may be done outpatient or may require an overnight stay in the hospital. Scrotal support, scrotal elevation, ice packs, and heat application will help to alleviate the swelling and discomfort. The scrotum and groin area may be bruised and swollen for 1–3 weeks. No heavy lifting or sports activities for approximately 4 weeks. No baths or showers until the practitioner gives clearance. Antibiotics, stool softeners, anti-inflammatory medication, and narcotics may be prescribed. No straining with bowel movements.

Complications/Risks

Postoperative complications can include hemorrhage, hematoma formation, infections, and pain. Recurrence of the torsion can occur.

Complications related to the torsion and related surgery can include testicular damage, testicular atrophy, contralateral testis injury, infertility, and a change in self-image related to an orchiectomy. Semen parameters following these procedures may be altered.

Long-Term Considerations

After recovering from surgery, there are no activity restrictions. Men should be advised that a male fertility evaluation may be appropriate if they are having trouble conceiving.

Torsion of the Testicular Appendage

Overview

The most important thing to know about the torsion of the testicular appendage is that it does not lead to loss of testicular function. This torsion is defined as a twisting of a vestigial testis appendage that has no function.

Incidence

This type of torsion is rare in adults. Children between the ages of 7–14 account for 80 % of all torsion of the testicular appendage.

Pertinent Anatomy and Physiology

The testicular appendage is a remnant of the embryonic duct also called the Mullerian duct. Not all males will have a testicular appendix; it is seen in about 92 % of all males. The appendix may be found on only one side. It is located on the upper pole of the testis, fitting between the testis and epididymal head. On an ultrasound image, it presents as an oval, sessile structure about 1–7 mm in length.

History

The initial history taken for acute scrotal pain is the same history used for torsion of the testicular appendage. It can help the practitioner delineate the potential causes of the pain or acute swelling and provide a focus for the assessment and correct diagnosis:

1. What was the nature of the onset of pain, location, duration, and severity?
2. What makes the symptoms worse and what helps them improve?
3. Have there been prior episodes of pain and how did they resolve?
4. Is there edema present?
5. Are there any associated symptoms such as nausea, vomiting, fever, chills, and urinary symptoms?

6. Is there a history of urinary tract infections, sexually transmitted infections, epididymitis, orchitis, or prostatitis?
7. Have there been any urologic procedures, instrumentations, or known urologic anomalies?

Signs and Symptoms

The symptoms of scrotal pain have a more gradual onset than the pain associated with testicular torsion. The pain is one sided and can range from mild to severe and worsen with activity. The focus of the pain is on the superior aspect of the testis and a palpable nodule may be appreciated in that area. The "diagnostic sign" is the presence of a blue dot on the paratesticular nodule but it is seen in only about one third of the cases. The cremasteric reflex remains present. The appendix torsion is not normally associated with nausea and vomiting. Reactive hydrocele, scrotal edema, and erythema may be present.

The symptoms of testicular appendage torsion mimic the symptoms of testicular torsion. The presentation of these symptoms helps to differentiate it from testicular torsion. In testicular torsion, the pain is more acute onset, more diffuse, and not isolated to the superior aspect. There is no "blue dot."

Risk Factors

A torsion is more likely to occur if the appendix is pedunculated.

Physical Exam

During the focused exam, the affected testis will be in the normal location. There may be focal tenderness at the superior aspect of the testis. The affected testicle should be pulled forward and out, stretching the scrotal skin. The "blue dot" may be seen on the superior aspect in this position; this "blue dot" is the necrotic appendix. Scrotal edema, erythema, and reactive hydrocele may be present.

Diagnostic Tests

Laboratory evaluation is not needed to diagnose this condition but a complete blood count (CBC), urinalysis (UA), and urine culture may be obtained to rule out an infectious process.

As with most of the other scrotal disorders, the color Doppler ultrasound is an invaluable diagnostic tool. Results of the study document the structures in the scrotum, the presence of a testicular mass, and signs of inflammation and most importantly demonstrate normal testicular blood flow. Images on the ultrasound show a small hypo- or hyperechogenic structure adjacent to the testis, frequently accompanied by the reactive hydrocele.

Management

If torsion of the testicular appendage occurs, it can lead to infection and necrosis of the appendix tissue. This tissue will become calcified and reabsorbed in 10–14 days with no complications. Conservative treatment options include observation, elevation of the scrotum, use of a scrotal support, and use of appropriate pain medication. NSAIDS would be first line but some patients may require a narcotic pain medication. Strenuous activity is discouraged until the symptoms abate. Application of heat and alternating with ice bags are comfort measures that may lessen the discomfort. The pain can persist up to several weeks. Long-term prognosis is good with no long-term complications or alterations in normal testicular function.

Exploration of the scrotum should only be done emergently if there is an uncertain diagnosis about testicular torsion. The decision for delayed exploration of the scrotum is only done for poor tolerance of the pain, prolonged pain, concerns about an infectious process/abscess formation, or anxiety by the patient or parent. As discussed in earlier sections, the potential complications of scrotal exploration are severe, and the patients and parents need to be educated about the long-term complications.

Epididymo-Orchitis

Overview

Epididymitis and orchitis often occur concomitantly; rarely is orchitis seen as a single entity and, if seen, is associated with mumps. This chapter will discuss the entities of epididymitis and orchitis together.

Epididymo-orchitis (EO) is one of the most common causes of acute scrotum with different studies citing an incidence of between 10 and 71 %. This is much higher than originally thought and may be a result of better imaging modalities identifying the correct diagnosis. It is defined as an inflammation of the epididymis and testis, often accompanied by an infectious process, resulting from an ascending infection from the urinary tract.

Epididymo-orchitis is classified as acute or chronic. In the acute phase, the symptoms are present for up to 6 weeks. Most patients present to the emergency room or their primary care physician after 5 days of symptoms. Acute epididymo-orchitis may be further characterized as infectious or inflammatory in origin.

Acute *infectious* epididymo-orchitis (MO) is caused by a bacterial, viral, fungal (coccidioidomycosis and blastomycosis), or parasitic organism (*Schistosoma mansoni*). In the age group of males between 14 and 35, the common bacterial etiology is sexually transmitted infections, most frequently *N. gonorrhea* and *C. trachomatis*. Most cases of EO occur in this age group. Nonsexual transmission is most commonly seen in males less than 18 and older than 35. It is related to obstruction, urethral instrumentation, or a surgical procedure and is primarily *E. coli*.

Acute *inflammatory* epididymo-orchitis (MO) is caused by an inflammatory or systemic disease, an obstructive condition, or a medication. Included in this group could be benign prostatic hyperplasia (BPH), recent urologic instrumentation, urethral stricture, or prostate cancer. The use of amiodarone, an antiarrhythmic, can cause an inflammatory EO because the medication accumulates in the head of the epididymis causing an inflammatory response and symptoms.

In the chronic phase, the symptoms are present for more than 3 months; men usually present with a more gradual onset and usually localized to the scrotum. Typically the swelling, tenderness, and erythema are mild or not present. They may respond to treatment but still present with ongoing symptoms, including scrotal pain for months and even years.

Isolated orchitis is considered rare and is usually associated with a mumps viral infection in prepubertal and pubertal males who were not vaccinated or did not complete the vaccination cycle. Mumps orchitis may be unilateral or bilateral. Mumps orchitis is the most common complication of the mumps infection and has been linked to testicular atrophy in up to 50 % of the affected testis. There is also a potential link to infertility or altered spermatogenesis.

Incidence

Each year there are over 600,000 cases of EO with the highest incidence in men between the ages of 18 and 35 (Trojian et al. 2009). The incidence is bimodal with the first group consisting of males between the age of 16 and 30. The second group is males between the ages of 51–70. Over 27 % of patients will have a recurrence of EO.

Pertinent Anatomy and Physiology

The etiology of EO may be related to the retrograde flow of urine from the prostatic urethra, through the ejaculatory duct and up into the vas deferens and epididymis. The oblique angle that the prostatic ducts enter the urethra in theory should prevent this reflux. Males with an enlarged prostate, obstruction in the urethra, or a congenital anomaly are at risk for this reflux. But in males with bladder outlet obstruction, urethral stricture, BPH, the straining to void (Valsalva) overrides the integrity of the anti-reflux potential. Similarly men who have urologic procedures that alter the angle of the duct or damage the integrity of the prostatic duct also increase their risk of reflux. Straining while doing strenuous exercise can also override this anti-reflux mechanism.

History

As with other conditions under the section of acute scrotum, testicular torsion must be considered first. The initial history taken for acute scrotal pain is the same history used for epididymo-orchitis with a few additions. This history can help the practitioner delineate the potential causes of the pain or acute swelling and provide a focus for the assessment and correct diagnosis. What was the nature of the onset of pain, location, duration, and severity? What makes the symptoms worse and what helps them improve? Have there been prior episodes of pain and how did they resolve? Is there edema present? Are there any associated symptoms such as nausea, vomiting, headaches, fever, chills, general malaise, and urinary symptoms? Is there a history of urinary tract infections, sexually transmitted infections, epididymitis, orchitis, or prostatitis? Have there been any urologic procedures, instrumentations or known urologic anomalies? Have there been any viral illnesses within the past 2–6 weeks? Is there any swelling in the parotid glands? Have you been immunized with the MMR vaccine?

Signs and Symptoms

It may be difficult to differentiate between EO and testicular torsion (Table 3.2) and, in fact, torsion is often misdiagnosed as epididymo-orchitis. In EO, the onset of pain and swelling is more gradual than in a torsion and is expected to be localized posterior to the testis with possible radiation into the groin or flank. The epididymis may be swollen to ten times its normal size, with an accompanying reactive hydrocele and

Table 3.2 Distinguishing acute epididymitis from testicular torsion

	Acute epididymitis	Testicular torsion
Onset	Gradual; can escalate quickly	Sudden Pain often begins during physical activity but can occur during sleep as well
Pain character	Mild to severe testicular or scrotal pain that is usually unilateral	Severe, unilateral scrotal pain and tenderness followed by scrotal swelling and erythema
Cause	Infectious (usually *Chlamydia trachomatis* and *Neisseria gonorrhoeae*)	Unknown
Common age group	Postpubertal (sexually active) males	Most common in boys between the ages of 12 and 18 years (but can occur at any age)
Ureteral discharge	Yes	No
Scrotal elevation	May decrease pain	Often causes intense pain
Treatment	Antibiotics, supportive symptomatic management	Surgery

significant scrotal asymmetry. The testicular/epididymal pain is primarily unilateral. Symptoms of fever, chills, headaches, tachycardia, frequency, urgency, hematuria, and dysuria may be present. Symptoms of hematospermia, painful ejaculation, and prostatitis may also be seen. If a mumps diagnosis is in the differential, the scrotal pain and swelling develops days to weeks after the parotiditis

Risk Factors

At-risk sexual behaviors increase the risk of epididymo-orchitis. Excessive physical activity, bicycle riding, and prolonged sitting increase the risk especially in males under 35. A history of prostatitis, urinary tract infections, recent urologic trauma, instrumentation, or surgery also increases the risk of EO. Uncircumcised males are at increased risk for genitourinary infections which also puts them at risk for EO. Risks are also increased for men with an enlarged prostate or blocked ejaculatory ducts that produces obstruction.

Physical Exam

Vital signs may demonstrate a fever or elevated pulse as an indication of an infection. Palpate for the parotid gland from the area in front of the ears down to below the jawbone. Record any nodule, swelling, or pain that may be present. This is indicative of mumps. Palpate the costovertebral angle for tenderness which could indicate a pyelonephritis. Suprapubic tenderness could indicate cystitis. The lower abdomen should be assessed for any indication of a hernia or enlarged inguinal nodes.

Inspect the penis, perineum, and anal area for signs of any rash, lesion, and open sores that could indicate a sexually transmitted infection. Inspect the meatus before and after a digital rectal exam and assess any urethral discharge.

Inspect the scrotum for erythema and scrotal edema. Normal cremasteric reflex should be present. Palpate the scrotum for a reactive hydrocele, testicular tenderness, epididymal tenderness, cord tenderness, and any unusual enlargement. As the swelling increases, it may become impossible to palpate the epididymis separate from the testis. The scrotum should also be examined for an indirect inguinal hernia. If indicated a stethoscope could be used over the scrotum to assess for potential bowel sounds. The testicle should be in the normal position. The above findings may be unilateral or bilateral. In most cases of EO, there will be a normal Prehn's sign.

A prostate exam may indicate a tender prostate asymmetrical with increased warmth, induration, and a change in consistency.

Diagnostic Tests

Laboratory evaluation should include a urinalysis and a subsequent culture if indicated. If an infection is present, the leucocytes, nitrites, and blood will be positive. First voided morning specimen should be sent to evaluate for a possible sexually transmitted infection. A UA would be positive for acute EO but is usually negative in chronic EO. A complete blood count (CBC) should be drawn and checked for leukocytosis. Some facilities would also order a C-reactive protein (CRP) and a sedimentation rate to further assess the inflammatory state versus a testicular torsion. If during the physical exam a urethral discharge is noted, a culture should be sent.

The imaging study of choice would be color Doppler ultrasonography. It has a high sensitivity (70 %) and specificity (88 %) for epididymo-orchitis (Trojian et al. 2009). The Doppler flow study will assess the arterial flow patterns. If no flow pattern is noted, a torsion is likely. Further, this imaging modality can identify testicular trauma, epididymitis, or an inguinal hernia that has prolapsed into the scrotum. Epididymo-orchitis would be suspected if the epididymis is enlarged, thickened, and demonstrating an increase in the Doppler wave pulsations.

Management

Once the diagnosis of epididymo-orchitis has been made, antibiotics may be ordered based on the specific causative agent. If the etiology of the infection is a STI, both the patient and the partner need to be treated and counseling given about the use of condoms and other safe sex practices. Current CDC guidelines should be reviewed because of increasing drug resistance patterns. If the drug amiodarone is the cause of EO, simple dose reduction will resolve the symptoms.

Conservative medical care includes scrotal elevation, scrotal support, application of ice or heat, and the use of nonsteroidal anti-inflammatory (NSAIDS) agents. Bed rest during the acute phase is recommended. Improvement in symptoms should be seen within 2–4 days. Patients should be told to return to clinic if no improvement is noted. Short-term narcotic usage may be indicated during the acute phase but is not recommended long term. A nerve block into the spermatic cord using a long-acting local anesthetic may be tried. This may control the pain and indicate if permanent pain relief would be achieved if the nerves to that area were cut.

If chronic pain develops, the patient should be referred to the pain clinic for a nerve block. Some patients may respond to oral antiepileptic drugs such as Gabapentin or a tricyclic antidepressant amitriptyline or improvement in chronic pain symptoms. A recent adjunct to treatment for chronic scrotal pain is pelvic floor muscle rehabilitation. Some centers will have special physical therapists or nurses who are specifically trained to treat chronic pain without medications, focusing on the relaxation of the pelvic floor nerves and muscles.

Complications of acute epididymis-orchitis are abscess formation, chronic pain, testicular atrophy, testicular tissue damage, and the potential for infertility or decreased spermatogenesis. In the rare case where the conservative measures do not resolve the infection, the patient may be admitted to the hospital for IV antibiotics. Scrotal abscesses, unresponsive to IV or oral antibiotics, may develop and require an incision and drainage of the wound. The wound would be allowed to heal by secondary intention and would require daily wound care and dressing changes.

The surgical options of scrotal exploration should be considered only if there is a concern for testicular torsion, if chronic pain is not alleviated by any of the therapies, or if a scrotal abscess has not responded to antibiotics.

An epididymectomy with a small incision and removal of the affected epididymis can be done as an outpatient. Complications can include recurrent chronic scrotal pain, recurrent infections, wound infections, and most importantly testicular damage resulting in atrophy, infertility, and altered self-image if the testis is removed.

An orchiectomy, also an outpatient procedure, can be done if testicular injury has resulted in testicular death or if recurrent infections and abscess formations continue.

Long-Term Management

Men should be advised to avoid unprotected intercourse until their symptoms have resolved. Once the infection has resolved, further studies such as a uroflow and bladder scan to evaluate for retention should be considered if obstruction was the etiology of EO; a retrograde urethrogram and possible cystogram may be indicated.

Testicular Descent Problems (Maldescensus)

Cryptorchidism Overview

Cryptorchidism is a constellation of congenital or acquired anomalies in which the testis, unilateral or bilateral, does not descend completely and remain in the scrotum. Unilateral undescended testes are seen in almost two-thirds (Hensle and Deibert 2012). The classifications of cryptorchidism include palpable and non-palpable types. Palpable is further delineated into retractile, ectopic, and undescended. Non-palpable is subdivided into canalicular, intra-abdominal, and absent. The cryptorchid testis can be palpable in 70–80 % of the cases or unpalpable in 20–30 % (Wampler and Llanes 2010).

Palpable

The undescended testis is defined as failure of a testis to descend into the normal scrotal position. The spermatic cord may be shorter than normal, thus limiting the natural progress into the scrotum. There is also the possibility that the ipsilateral scrotum may be underdeveloped.

Retractile testis is considered by some to be a normal variant and can be unilateral or bilateral. The retractile testis are usually fully descended at puberty but may move out of the scrotum and return spontaneously or with manipulation be brought to the base of the scrotum and remain in the scrotum for a finite period. The peak incidence of retractile testis is age 5 or 6. The site of the retractile testis can range from inguinal to low scrotum. The movement occurs with the strong cremasteric reflex. The affected testis is noted to have increased risk of impaired testicular growth, altered functioning, and increased infertility that is linked to the site with inguinal location being more affected. Annual or biannual examinations are recommended until puberty because as the male matures the cremasteric muscle weakens, the testicular size increases, and the force of gravity work together to keep the testis in the scrotal position.

The ectopic testes are located in regions that are not part of the normal pathway for descent into the scrotum. There are five common sites that are associated with ectopic testis. They include perineum, femoral canal, superficial inguinal pouch, suprapubic area, and contralateral scrotal pouch. The most common site of the ectopic testis is in the superficial inguinal pouch. The ectopic testis has normal development and normal spermatogenesis. Because of their location, they are prone to injury. They do not have increased risk of malignancy or infertility.

Unpalpable

The canalicular testis is located above the normal position in the scrotum in between the internal and external inguinal rings. Its descent into the scrotum is restricted by tension exerted by the external musculature of the body wall.

Classifications of Cryptorchidism

Palpable	Unpalpable
1. Retractile	1. Canalicular
2. Ectopic	2. Intra-abdominal
3. Undescended (groin or abdominal)	3. Absent

The intra-abdominal testes, as its name implies, are located in the abdominal cavity proximal to the internal inguinal ring. Its position makes difficult for examination and has increased risk of becoming cancerous.

The absent testis literally means no testis is present. This can be unilateral or bilateral. It is believed to be associated with in utero torsion, vascular insult, or agenesis.

Incidence

Cryptorchidism is seen in approximately 2–4 % of full-term male infants (Hutson et al. 2010) but as high as 30 % in premature male infants (Hensle and Deibert 2012). Approximately 20 % of undescended testes are non-palpable (Abaci et al. 2013).

Pertinent Anatomy and Physiology

The normal descent of the testis is usually complete by gestational week 32. The normal descent can be divided into 3 phases. The transabdominal phase begins by week 10–15 and is complete by week 22–25. This movement is assisted with the insulin-like hormone INSL3. The trans-inguinal phase occurs between weeks 25–30 in which the testis is moving down the inguinal canal. The final phase, the scrotal phase occurs in week 30–35 and is influenced by androgen production.

Signs and Symptoms

The predominant sign is an empty scrotum. The undescended testis may be unilateral or bilateral with 70 % of the undescended testis noted on the right (Abaci et al. 2013) .

Risk Factors

Associated risk factors for cryptorchidism include preterm babies, low birth weight babies <900 g, twins, or a family history of cryptorchidism. Maternal issues such as gestational diabetes, alcohol, or tobacco use during pregnancy, preeclampsia, breech presentation, cesarean section, or a complicated delivery may increase the likelihood of cryptorchidism. Less understood mechanisms include hormonal imbalance, environmental factors, and genetics. Infants with a neural tube defect, prune belly syndrome, bladder exstrophy, trisomy 13 and 18, posterior urethral valves, or other abdominal wall defects also have a higher incidence of cryptorchidism. Hormonal imbalance as seen with the hypothalamic-pituitary-testicular axis disruption is also associated with cryptorchidism. An in-depth explanation of the various embryologic, hormonal, and mechanical causes is beyond the scope of this chapter.

Physical Exam

The testis should be examined and palpated at every infant well-being exam to assess for the position, mobility, size, and consistency. The focused examination to locate the undescended testis is done with the patient in a supine and cross-legged position. The external inguinal ring should be palpated, tracing the path of the inguinal canal. The ectopic testis may be palpated in the front of the pubis, in the perineum, or even in the medial aspect of the upper thigh.

During the exam, other abnormal findings may include a hypospadias or a hydrocele. Approximately 17–30 % of males born with hypospadias will have undescended testes (Hensle and Deibert 2012). The examiner should also be assessing for a micropenis, ambiguous genitalia, and inguinal hernias. Epididymal anomalies may be seen in 36–79 % and may impact fertility.

Specific Maneuvers

During the assessment of the testis, the examiner places the nondominant hand at the anterior superior iliac spine and slides his hand medially toward the groin. The use of a lubricant can assist this movement. The dominant hand is poised to capture and hold the testis and try to pull it into the scrotum. If the testis remains in the scrotum for 1 min after being released, it is termed a retractile testis. If it immediately ascends after release, it is termed an undescended testis.

Diagnostic Tests

The diagnosis is made primarily by the physical exam. Laboratory evaluation could include FSH, LH, and testosterone levels especially if bilateral undescended testis is suspected. Further testing could include Muellerian-inhibiting substance (MIS) or anti-Mullerian hormone (AMH) levels. The results of these labs can indicate the presence or absence of the testis.

Imaging studies are not usually required in the initial workup. The current AUA guidelines do not recommend the use of imaging as a component of a routine evaluation of undescended testes because it does not provide any new information that would guide the treatment choice. However, if bilateral undescended testes (UDT) are seen in a patient with ambiguous genitalia, an ultrasound would be able to assess for the Mullerian structures, including a uterus and cervix.

An ultrasound will identify the testis in the inguinal canal but has a low sensitivity for locating an intra-abdominal testis, only 12–45 % (Wampler and Llanes 2010). Similar findings are noted with CT or MRI. Because the MRI would require sedation for the infant, it is seldom used. Due to the high number of false-negatives, imaging studies results should not be used to avoid the surgical approach for localization and fixation of the impalpable testis.

A laparoscopic surgery may be recommended as part of an initial workup if the testes in unpalpable.

Management

Medical

Medical treatment for undescended testis is controversial and is not currently recommended in the AUA guidelines. Hormones are used in some countries as a corrective measure for the disruption of the hypothalamic-pituitary-testis axis disruption. Hormones may help to promote the natural descent of the testis into the scrotum. The most commonly used therapy is hCG (human chorionic gonadotropin) with doses ranging from 250 IU to 1000 IU based on age. Patients are dosed twice each week, usually for 5 weeks, and may start therapy when less than 1 year old.

Other therapies include the use of testosterone or combining hCG with a GnRH (gonadotropin-releasing hormone).

The goals of this therapy would be to encourage normal androgen-related responses including penile growth and onset of pubic hair development. Side effects could include painful erections and behavioral changes.

The AUA guidelines recommend that a patient with undescended testis, congenital or acquired, not in the scrotal position at 6 months should be referred to a pediatric urologist for follow-up. This patient may be a candidate for an orchiopexy.

Surgical

Treatment for the undescended testis whether palpable or unpalpable is an exam under anesthesia and localization of the testis followed by an orchiopexy. At this time the integrity of the testicular vessels and viability of the testis should be evaluated. An orchiectomy may be considered. Goals of surgery include prevention of further testicular damage, resumption of testicular growth, improvement in fertility, and reduction of the risk for testicular malignancy. The recommended age for the orchiopexy is between 12 and 18 months (Lee and Houk 2013). The surgical approach may be open or performed laparoscopic. Short-term complications of orchiopexy include hematoma, infection, wound breakdown, and pain. Long-term complications include testicular damage, testicular atrophy, and damage to the vas deferens or epididymis.

Some physicians will suggest a testicular biopsy during the orchiopexy if genital disorders are present.

Treatment options for the retractile testis are still controversial. The retractile testis in the prepubertal males may be followed with annual or biannual evaluation, postponing surgical repair until puberty. If the testis is still highly mobile, an orchiopexy is warranted. Criteria for surgery for a retractile testis include no spontaneous return of the testis in a postpubertal male, the presence of a smaller and softer testis, or symptoms of rapid retraction and persistence of tightness of the spermatic cord.

Long-Term Complications of Cryptorchidism

Complications of cryptorchidism include infertility, increased risk of testicular cancer, testicular torsion, atrophy, trauma, and inguinal hernia. The incidence of infertility increases by more than 30 % with bilateral cryptorchidism. There is also a significant psychological component related to abnormal scrotal structures, causing embarrassment and altered self-esteem.

Teaching Points

Parent of the child should be given information regarding the potential long-term risks and complications of cryptorchidism and monorchidism with a special focus on infertility and potential for cancer. Further, these boys as they mature should be reeducated regarding these risks.

Acute Idiopathic Scrotal Edema

Overview

Acute idiopathic scrotal edema (AISE) is part of the constellation of diagnoses that require immediate assessment because of the concern for testicular torsion, torsion of the appendix testis, or epididymo-orchitis. It is often a diagnosis of exclusion. Rapid, thorough evaluation is necessary to avoid an unnecessary scrotal exploration. This condition is usually self-limiting.

While the exact etiology of AISE is unknown, it is possible that it is related to a condition called angioneurotic edema. Angioneurotic edema presents as hypersensitivity, possibly allergic or nonallergic, to some unknown food, medication, or environmental exposure. This exposure results in the subcutaneous tissue swelling seen in the scrotum.

Incidence

Acute idiopathic scrotal edema is the fourth most common cause of acute scrotum in males under 20 years of age. It is less common than testicular torsion, torsion of testicular appendages, and epididymo-orchitis. The overall incidence rates vary from 20 to 69 %. Acute idiopathic scrotal edema is typically seen in the prepubertal male less than 10 years old but has been noted in adults.

History

The initial history taken for acute scrotal pain (described in section "Testicular appendage") is the same history used for AISE. It can help the practitioner delineate the potential causes of the pain or acute swelling and provide a focus for the assessment and correct diagnosis. In addition, the medical history should include a personal and familial history of similar episodes, current medications, exposure to known allergens (food, medication, or environmental), a sudden change in physical stimuli (heat, cold, exercise), and the timing of the exposure to the current episode.

Signs and Symptoms

Patients may present with rapid onset of painless scrotal edema that extends into the perineum and penis. However, some patients will present with pain in the scrotal or inguinal area. Superficial skin tenderness has also been noted. The edema may be unilateral (90 %) or bilateral. Diffuse erythema is present and may extend into the perineum and inguinal area. The testis is non-tender. A hydrocele may be present. Fever, urinary symptoms, or urethral discharge are not usually seen. The swelling resolves quickly over a period of 3–4 days.

Risk Factors

Since the etiology is unclear, it is difficult to predict risk factors. But if future studies support the theory about angioneurotic edema, exposure to the known allergens would be a significant risk factor.

Physical Exam

Inspection of the scrotum would demonstrate diffuse erythema on the scrotum with possible radiation to the inguinal area, perineum, and penis. Scrotal edema with similar radiation may be seen and may be unilateral or bilateral. Palpation would elicit possible scrotal skin tenderness, scrotal edema, and a hydrocele.

Diagnostic Tests

Laboratory evaluation is not indicated as a diagnostic tool for AISE, but a urinalysis (UA), urine culture, and complete blood count (CBC) could be ordered to rule out other pathologies.

Color Doppler ultrasound is the imaging modality of choice. Ultrasound images demonstrate a thickened, edematous scrotal wall with normal appearing testis and epididymis. The "Fountain Sign," a unique finding on a transverse image of the Doppler study, demonstrates an unusual pattern of hypervascularity in the scrotal wall that is suggestive of AISE. The ultrasound may also document a reactive hydrocele and enlarged lymph nodes. The use of the color Doppler ultrasound is associated with a reduction in unnecessary scrotal explorations.

Management

Since AISE is benign and usually self-limiting, there is no specific treatment algorithm. Conservative management is the initial approach and symptoms usually resolve in less than 5 days. The use of nonsteroidal anti-inflammatory drugs is the first choice. Some practitioners may choose to add an antibiotic. Comfort measures such as scrotal support, elevation, heating pads, and application of ice are included in the conservative management.

Surgical exploration of the scrotum should be avoided unless serious concern exists. Scrotal exploration may be considered if there was no response to the conservative measures discussed above. Other reasons to consider surgery would be extended duration and severity of pain, no resolution of the swelling and associated quality of life issues, or to alleviate the anxiety/fear of the patient or parent. Complications of the surgery should be carefully reviewed and include potential damage to testicular, epididymal, and vas deferens tissue. Potential long-term complications include testicular atrophy, infertility, and infections.

Spermatocele

Overview

A spermatocele is a fluid-filled cyst, most commonly seen in the caput of the epididymis but may also be located in the rete testis or vas deferens. The fluid is clear or opaque and may contain viable and nonviable sperm. Spermatoceles, sometimes located in the epididymis, may alternately be called epididymal cysts when smaller. The exact cause of the spermatocele formation is unclear, but some studies link it to a blockage in the tubules of the epididymis complicated by recent urological procedure, instrumentation, trauma, or inflammation. They are normally benign.

Incidence

Spermatoceles, rarely seen in children, increase with aging with the peak incidence in males between 40 and 50. They may be found as an incidental finding during an annual examination. Approximately 30 % of males having a scrotal ultrasound will have an incidental finding of a spermatocele.

History

A patient or his partner is usually the one to discover the mass, although it can be noted because it can be quite tender or painful. This usually prompts a visit to the primary care provider. The detailed history should include onset, location, and any information regarding a change in size of the mass. Information about recent infections, trauma, or surgical procedures should be recorded. The patient should be asked about exposure to diethylstilbestrol (DES).

Signs and Symptoms

Often a spermatocele does not cause symptoms. A small lump or mass may be felt on the superior aspect of the testis, usually painless. Rarely, it will be accompanied by scrotal enlargement on the ipsilateral side, pain, redness, or sense of pressure. Spermatoceles by themselves do not affect fertility, but the corrective surgical procedure listed below can impair fertility by damaging the epididymal and vas deferens tissue.

Risk Factors

No significant risk factors for developing a spermatocele have been identified except for increasing age. While no clear link exists between Von Hippel-Lindau disease and spermatoceles, the incidence is higher in males with this disease. Some studies are suggesting a link between mothers taking DES and son's risk in utero. Most spermatoceles are idiopathic with no clear etiology.

Physical Exam

Palpation of a smooth, firm lump, freely mobile, located on the caput of the epididymis may indicate a spermatocele. Transillumination of the mass will differentiate between a fluid-filled cyst and a solid mass. The mass is separate from and above the testis. Because of the possible differential diagnosis, the groin should be palpated for an inguinal hernia. Unexpected findings during the exam would include a mass that does not transilluminate, scrotal edema, inflammation, or significant pain. Such findings would warrant additional workup and referral to a urology provider.

Diagnostic Tests

Laboratory Evaluation
No lab workup is necessary to diagnose a spermatocele. A urinalysis and a urine culture may be recommended to rule out an infection.

Imaging Studies
Scrotal ultrasound with doppler: Highly sensitive in the diagnosis of a spermatocele. A scrotal ultrasound is indicated if the mass does not transilluminate or if other physical findings or patient history raise the concern for a more serious pathology. On ultrasound, a spermatocele should image as an anechoic cystic mass with posterior acoustic enhancement, usually 1–2 cm in size but can exceed 15 cm. It may appear as unilocular or oligolocular with thin-walled structure. These findings indicate a benign cystic mass.

Management

Most spermatoceles do not require treatment. Aspirin, acetaminophen, or anti-inflammatory drugs like ibuprofen may help if there is mild discomfort in the scrotum. Application of heat or ice packs may also provide symptomatic relief.

Surgical Options

If the size of the spermatocele is increasing and if the patient finds the associated pain burdensome, there are surgical options. Some infertile patients will undergo a spermatocelectomy in conjunction with a varicocelectomy to improve fertility. Patients should be counseled regarding the potential for infertility post-procedure due to injury to the epididymal tissue or vas deferens. Breach of the epididymis can also contribute to antisperm antibody formation, which can also contribute to lowered fertility.

Spermatocelectomy, an outpatient procedure, involves making a small incision in the scrotum and epididymis with removal of the spermatocele intact. This procedure is done either as an "open" procedure or with a microscopic approach.

Postoperative Management

Short Term A drain may be in place for 1 day. A scrotal support and/or scrotal elevation when supine is recommended for 1–2 weeks after surgery. Ice packs can be used for 2–3 days to help with swelling which is seen in 20–90 % of the patients. Heating pads may also be used. Postoperative pain is managed with narcotics short term. To help prevent infections, no baths are allowed until the incision is completely healed but showers are permitted after 48 h. No vigorous activity or contact sports for at least 2 weeks. Follow-up visit with the urologist is usually in 2 weeks. Other short-term complications include fever, infection (10 %), hematoma (17 %), and worsening pain (Kapoor 2008).

Long Term Long-term complications can include persistent scrotal pain, recurring spermatocele, hydroceles, and testicular atrophy. A more serious complication is possible injury to the epididymis or vas deferens which can lead to infertility.

Aspiration, with or without sclerotherapy, is also done as an outpatient. A needle is inserted into the spermatocele, and the fluid is aspirated. This procedure may be done in conjunction with a sclerotherapy procedure. Sclerotherapy involves injecting an irritating agent, sodium tetradactyl sulfate, into the spermatocele sac that will cause the sac to scar down.

Postoperative Management

Short-Term Complications A scrotal support and/or scrotal elevation when erect is recommended for 1–2 weeks after surgery, but no direct pressure should be used. Ice packs can be used for 2–3 days to help with swelling. Heating pads may also be used. Postoperative pain is managed with narcotics short term. To help prevent infections, no baths are allowed until the incision is completely healed but showers are permitted after 48 h. There are no restrictions on activity. Follow-up visit with the urologist is usually in 2 weeks. Other short-term complications include fever, hematoma, and worsening pain.

Long-Term Complications Long-term complications can include persistent scrotal pain or recurring spermatocele. A more serious complication is possible injury to the epididymis or vas deferens which can lead to testicular atrophy or infertility.

Hydrocele

Overview

A hydrocele is defined as an abnormal collection of peritoneal fluid located between the parietal and visceral layers of the tunica vaginalis that surround the testicles. Hydroceles are classified as communicating or noncommunicating. Communicating hydroceles with incomplete closure of the tunica vaginalis are present at birth and allow fluid movement between the scrotum and the peritoneal space. The size of these hydroceles, aided by gravity and increased abdominal pressure associated with crying and coughing, may be smaller in the morning and increase during the day as activity levels increase.

Acquired, noncommunicating hydroceles, also called simple hydroceles, have no opening between the peritoneum and the scrotum. Acquired hydroceles are further classified as primary or secondary. Primary hydroceles are idiopathic, usually slow growing, perhaps over years, and have no abnormal pathology. Secondary hydroceles are caused by trauma, infectious process, or inflammation. The fluid in the acquired hydroceles, produced by an inflammatory response, may accumulate at a rate faster than the body can reabsorb it.

Incidence

It is a common finding in children but only 1 % of adult males will develop a hydrocele. Worldwide, the most common cause for hydroceles in the adult males is related to a parasitic worm infection caused by the nematodes *Wuchereria bancrofti*. While rare in the United States, it is seen in over 70 countries, most predominantly Egypt and India. The incidence and prevalence in these endemic areas vary greatly by the country and the methods used to control the parasitic worm. In the endemic areas, filarial infection is acquired in early childhood but may not become clinically manifested until early adulthood. The adult worms are found in the intrascrotal lymphatic vessels causing lymphatic obstruction and formation of hydroceles as the most common manifestations. As the infection worsens, the hydroceles become very large and have significant morbidity including discomfort with walking and performance of other normal activities. As the disfigurement worsens, the patients experience social ostracism.

Differentiating filarial hydrocele from idiopathic hydrocele is difficult in many cases. A thorough history is necessary and often the key indicator is recent travel to the affected regions or exposure to recent travelers from those areas. The physical exam may demonstrate other symptoms of filariasis. The spermatic cord and epididymis may be thickened with multiple nodules. Excessive swelling of the scrotum and lymphedema in the pelvis and extremities may be seen. Precautions by the medical staff must be taken. Scrotal ultrasounds are used to diagnose and may demonstrate the filarial dance sign (FDS). The filial dance sign is the movement of the fluid in the hydrocele as the worms move. In this context, surgery is the treatment of choice. Filarial hydroceles are more difficult to excise surgically than idiopathic hydroceles, because of the effect of significant scarring and fibrosis associated with this disease.

Pertinent Anatomy and Physiology

In the last trimester of pregnancy, the testicles of the male fetus migrate from the abdomen through the inguinal canal and into the scrotum preceded by the processus vaginalis. In this early developmental stage, each testicle has a fluid-filled sac that encircles the testicles and allows fluid movement between the peritoneum and the sac. After passing through the inguinal ring, the processus vaginalis typically closes, and further fluid transfer between the peritoneum and the scrotum is impeded. A hydrocele may develop if this closure is not complete. Further, if the opening is significantly larger, a portion of the small intestine may also move into the scrotum causing an indirect inguinal hernia.

History

Information about the onset, location, size, and presence/absence of pain are the first components of the history. Medical history should include an updated list of any infections, trauma, and current medications. Surgical history should include any prior urologic procedure, any abdominal surgery, renal transplant, or AV shunt placement.

Signs and Symptoms

Frequently, hydroceles may be asymptomatic. They may change in size based on time of day or activity level, improving when lying down. Larger hydroceles may produce a feeling of "heaviness," "pulling," or "achiness" in the scrotum. This discomfort may radiate into the lower back and inguinal region. If GI symptoms of nausea, vomiting, constipation, or diarrhea are noted, the differential diagnosis includes an inguinal hernia.

Risk Factors

Prematurity and low birth weight are risk factors for hydrocele formation. Incomplete closure of the processus vaginalis is another risk factor. Exposure to the parasitic worm can predispose the individual to filarial hydrocele formation.

Physical Exam

In addition to the general scrotal exam recommended elsewhere in this chapter, there are some relevant findings specific to hydroceles. The hallmark presentation is a tense, smooth, usually non-tender scrotal mass that transilluminates when a small penlight is placed against the scrotal skin. The size and the consistency of hydroceles can vary at different times of the day based on activity. Hydroceles may become smaller when recumbent, and as the day progresses it may become larger and more tense.

It may also be difficult to feel the testicle if the hydrocele is large. The hydrocele is located superior and anterior to the testis. Palpation of the spermatic cord and inguinal ring above the hydrocele should be normal. Since there is an association between inguinal hernias and hydroceles, have the patient perform a Valsalva maneuver in a standing position and then palpate the inguinal canal area for palpable bowel. Patients with an incarcerated hernia may present with fever, chills, nausea, vomiting, diarrhea, or constipation. Approximately 10 % of testicular tumors may be accompanied by a hydrocele; therefore, assessment for lymphedema of the external genitalia and edema in the lower extremities may be indicated. See previous section for clinical findings related to filarial hydroceles.

Diagnostic Tests

Laboratory

Lab diagnostic testing is done to establish a differential diagnosis rather than for the definitive diagnosis of a hydrocele. Urinalysis and a urine culture would be done to rule out a urinary tract infection, epididymitis, or orchitis. Testing for sexually transmitted diseases (STD) could be ordered if the patient admitted to at-risk behaviors or recent STD infections, especially as the formation of a hydrocele may be reactive after epididymitis. Clinical findings concerning for a testicular tumor would suggest that AFP (alpha fetal protein), βHCG (human chorionic gonadotropin), and LDH (lactic acid dehydrogenase) should be added to the evaluation.

Imaging Studies

Imaging studies are not routinely needed and should only be ordered if the patient is symptomatic, if the scrotum did not transilluminate, if the diagnosis seems uncertain, or if abnormal findings during the exam raised concerns. A plain abdomen film would help to distinguish between a hydrocele and a hernia. If an incarcerated hernia were present, gas would be demonstrated over the groin area, but this is not ordered to definitively diagnose a hydrocele. A scrotal ultrasound with or without a Doppler study can help to diagnose a hydrocele and estimate the size. It can provide information about the testicular blood flow and differentiate between a hydrocele and a testicular torsion, a testicular tumor, a varicocele, or an incarcerated hernia.

Increased epididymal blood flow can assist the clinician in associating a hydrocele with epididymitis.

Management

Hydroceles in infants usually resolve by the second year and no treatment is needed. If a hydrocele develops after age 1, 75 % will resolve within 6 months (Hall et al. 2011). These patients require closer observation and follow-ups. In certain cases if there is concern about the viability of the individual testicle, an orchiectomy may be needed. Most hydroceles in adult men are benign and require no treatment.

Surgical repair, a hydroclelctomy, is considered the gold standard for symptomatic hydroceles. Indications for surgery include persistent pain, cosmetic concerns, disability due to the size of the hydrocele, or concern for an associated intratesticular mass. The approach may be inguinal or scrotal incision. Postoperative ultrasound imaging is recommended to assess structural integrity and testicular perfusion.

Another treatment option for hydroceles is the minimally invasive sclerotherapy. This procedure usually includes aspiration of the hydrocele fluid and then instillation of the sclerosants which may remain in the sac or may be aspirated out prior to the end of the procedure. This procedure is done in the clinic or outpatient surgery using local anesthetic, and the patient is discharged shortly after the procedure. Agents used for sclerosing are tetracycline derivatives, a 95 % alcohol-based solution, ethanolamine oleate, or other irritative agents. These agents may produce epididymal injury and obstruction, therefore, they are not recommended for males concerned about fertility.

Potential Complications The practitioner should present all options of care for treating hydroceles. Included in this discussion should be the short-term and potential long-term complications. These early complications of a hydrocelectomy could include fever, acute and chronic scrotal pain, infection, and formation of a hematocele, hematoma, and edema. A hematoma is the most common complication following a hydrocelectomy. Sclerotherapy is associated with a high risk of recurrence. So although the initial therapy is less costly than a hydrocelectomy, the need for repeat procedures lessens this benefit. Long-term complications include infertility related to injury to the epididymis or the vas deferens, the possibility of recurring hydroceles, and chronic pain.

Hematospermia

Overview

Hematospermia is defined as the macroscopic presence of blood in the semen. While usually a benign, self-limiting condition, it can be anxiety provoking for both the patient and the partner. Patients will present to their primary care provider with concerns about a malignancy or a sexually transmitted disease (STD). Hematospermia may present as a single incident or occur for weeks to months. The semen color can vary from bright red to coffee colored.

Incidence

The exact incidence and prevalence of hematospermia is unclear but it peaks in males between their 30s and 40s; it accounts for 1 in 5000 new patient visits in a urology clinic (Aslam et al. 2009). The cause of hematospermia was considered idiopathic in 70 % of the cases, but improved imaging techniques are helping to reduce these numbers to about 15 % (Ahmad and Krishna 2007; Kurkar 2007). In males under 40, it may be related to an infectious or inflammatory process. The list is quite extensive; the more common causes are epididymitis/orchitis, prostatic calculi, benign prostatic hyperplasia (BPH), or a sexually transmitted disease (STD). Common trauma-related causes include prostate biopsy, brachytherapy, and urethral instrumentation. There also has been an association with prolonged abstinence. In males older than 40, there is increased concern for a more serious pathology.

A new, emerging cause is linking hyperuricemia to hematospermia (Kukar et al. 2014). Uric acid crystals in the prostatic secretions and semen may produce an inflammatory response in the prostate or epididymis that results in mucosal inflammation, hyperemia, edema, and hematospermia.

Pertinent Anatomy and Physiology

Injury, inflammation, or obstruction at any point in the ejaculatory path can result in hematospermia.

History

A thorough detailed medical, surgical, and sexual history aids in the extent of the evaluation necessary. The sexual history should include the number of new partners, frequency of coitus (anal and vaginal), masturbation, and the prior history of and STD. Specifics about the ejaculate should include the character, color, timing, and frequency of the hematospermia. The examiner must rule out the female partner as a source of the blood in the semen. The blood could be related to micro-tears in the vaginal tissue, menstrual bleeding, or other gyne/anal pathology. This may include collecting an ejaculate specimen in a condom.

The medical history should include all comorbid conditions including hypertension, blood dyscrasias, liver disease, as well as the risk factors/symptoms for any inflammatory or infectious process. Travel to areas endemic for TB or schistosomiasis increases the risk for these infections. Urologic malignancy is not a common entity associated with hematospermia but it should be excluded. Medications such as aspirin and anticoagulants should also be recorded. The surgical history should include information about any recent prostate biopsy, brachytherapy, any invasive urologic procedure, and any at-risk sexual practices.

Signs and Symptoms

There are few symptoms associated with hematospermia but may include painful ejaculation, hematuria, dysuria, short-term urinary frequency, and scrotal discomfort. Symptoms associated with hyperuricemia associated with hematospermia also include foot arthralgia and chronic prostatitis.

Risk Factors

The risk factors listed are related to the pathologic conditions that may have hematospermia as a symptom. These include infections, inflammations, prostatic stones, and bleeding dyscrasias. Certain urologic procedures such as prostate biopsies, instrumentation, and brachytherapy can cause inflammation and infections that increase the risk for hematospermia

Physical Exam

The physical exam should begin with the assessment of the vital signs especially looking for hypertension, fever, and recent weight loss. A focused abdominal exam should be done assessing for any abdominal mass including hepatomegaly, splenomegaly, or pelvis swelling. The genital exam should be very detailed. The patient should be examined in an upright and prone position to better identify any abnormality. The penis should be examined for any unusual skin lesion that could represent an STD, torn frenulum, or skin cancer. Any lesion, rash, and skin eruption warrants a further review of the medical-sexual history. After completing a digital rectal exam (DRE), the meatus should be examined for any bloody discharge. The spermatic cord, epididymis, and testis should be palpated for tenderness, induration, or swelling. Based on the finding of the physical exam and the pertinent history, the evaluation will progress to rule out specific processes.

Diagnostic Tests

The diagnostic tests that are ordered vary based on the personal history and exam findings and are usually ordered to help reassure the patient. Persistent hematospermia, associated hematuria, and males older than 40 require a more in-depth evaluation. Basic initial testing for all patients should include a urinalysis and urine culture and PSA. A first voided urine sample for an STD is necessary only if risk factors are present. Additional testing could include a fresh semen sample, prostatic secretion sample, and an additional urine sample for cytology, TB, or schistosomiasis. Blood samples for a CBC, urea, electrolytes, liver function studies, and clotting studies may be ordered to R/O conditions associated with hematospermia.

Imaging Studies

Transrectal ultrasound (TRUS) is the most common imaging study used to diagnose hematospermia. The TRUS can locate prostatic stones, cysts in the seminal vesicle, dilated seminal vesicles, and blocked ejaculatory ducts. These conditions are associated with hematospermia. Malignancy is a rare cause of hematospermia, but TRUS can also identify prostate, bladder, and seminal vesicle tumors. MRI is rarely used now in the initial workup of hematospermia but may be ordered if more significant pathology is suspected. Ultrasound of the scrotum may be ordered if the scrotal examination was abnormal. CT urogram may also be ordered.

Procedures

A cystoscopy may be ordered if hematuria is also present. The cystoscopy will allow for direct visualization of the ejaculatory ducts, the prostate, and the bladder and may allow confirmation of a friable prostate.

Management

Since this is normally a benign condition, early management is usually observation and reassurance. If an infectious process is then identified, appropriate antibiotics or antiviral medications should be ordered. If the prostate is friable, a limited trial of finasteride or dutasteride may address the hematospermia. If hyperuricemia has been diagnosed, allopurinol 300 mg tablets twice daily for 8 weeks and then reduced to once daily has been effective in reducing the incidence of hematospermia and reducing the serum acid level. A low purine diet and increased fluid volume were also encouraged. Other treatment algorithms for hematospermia are based on treating the pathological condition.

Varicocele

Overview

A varicocele is a tortuous dilation of the pampiniform plexus and the internal spermatic veins. The pampiniform plexus is another term for the venous drainage system that consists of a deep and a superficial network. The deep network drains the testis, epididymis, and vas deferens. The superficial network drains the veins of the scrotum. These veins merge as they ascend the testicular cord forming a single testicular vein on each side. The right testicular vein drains into the right inferior vena cava and the left testicular vein drains into the left renal vein. The normal non-dilated diameter of the vein is between 0.5 and 2.0 mm. With a varicocele, it dilates to greater than 3.5 mm with a Valsalva maneuver.

Varicoceles are problematic because they can lead to damage to testicular tissue resulting in testicular atrophy, altered spermatogenesis, Leydig cell dysfunction, and infertility. Some varicoceles are problematic because of persistent/chronic pain.

The proposed pathogenesis of a varicocele is multifactorial, and left varicoceles are more common. Left varicoceles may also be the result of a spermatic vein that is 8–10 cm longer than the right side combined with the right angle insertion into the left renal vein which can also increase the pressure and turbulence in the vein. Compression of the left renal vein between the aorta and the superior mesenteric artery (the nutcracker phenomenon) can occur and results in hypertension in the left renal vein causing increased venous pressure, turbulence, and backflow, resulting in a left varicocele. The right side drains into the vena cava which allows more direct flow with less pressure and less dilation. Absence of valves in the internal, external, and cremasteric veins or incompetent valves are another potential cause for varicoceles. Any retrograde flow into the pampiniform plexus is less in the sitting or recumbent positions but increases significantly when standing.

Testicular hyperthermia may result from the increased stagnant venous blood circulating around the testis. The normal temperature of the testicles is approximately 1C to 2C lower than normal body temperature. This cooler temperature is necessary for optimal spermatogenesis. Hormonal changes associated with puberty may also play a role. Changes in the testosterone levels may increase the flow of blood into testis promoting dilation of the pampiniform plexus and subsequent varicocele formation. Early detection of a varicocele is key. The longer the palpable varicocele is present and the greater the size of the varicocele, the more likely it is to have significant alterations in testicular functioning.

Incidence

Varicoceles represent a common entity in urologic assessments and are seen in 15–20 % of the male general population but in 40 % of males who present for infertility evaluations (Crawford and Crop 2014). Varicoceles are most frequently diagnosed in males between the ages of 13 and 30. There is a lower incidence in obese males possibly related to the increased abdominal fat that limits compression between the superior mesenteric artery and the aorta.

Pertinent Anatomy and Physiology

Ninety percent of varicoceles occur on the left side (Wampler and Llanes 2010); absence of valves is seen more commonly on the left side. The prevalence of bilateral varicoceles varies significantly by studies but ranges from 30 to 80 % (Masson and Brannigan 2014). The normal diameter of the veins in the pampiniform plexus range from 0.5 to 1.5 mm, whereas the main testicular vein will have a diameter of 2 mm (Rubenstein et al. 2004). Palpable varicoceles (Grade I–III) can exceed 5–6 mm (Rubenstein et al. 2004).

The finding of a right-sided varicocele, especially in men under 40, raises concern for a pelvic/abdominal malignancy. This could include a renal cell cancer, a retroperitoneal fibrosis, a retroperitoneal mass, a sarcoma, or a lymphoma. Further evaluation is always indicated.

Risk Factors

Congenital absence of veins in the spermatic veins is a significant risk factor. There appears to be a familial link to varicoceles, that is not well understood. Having a first degree family member with a varicocele increases the risk for other members to develop a varicocele. Age is another common risk factor as mentioned above. The incidence of varicoceles increases in adolescents to 15 % where it stabilizes into adulthood (Masson and Brannigan 2014).

History

The pertinent history may vary, based on the reason the patient presents to the clinic. The visit could be a component of infertility evaluation, an evaluation for pain, or concern about the sudden occurrence of the varicocele. The age of the patient is another factor that can affect the history taking.

If the male of any age presents for infertility or is interested in fathering children at some future point, a reproductive and sexual history should be obtained and documented. Symptoms of androgen deficiency such as muscle loss ease of fatigability, low energy level, depressed mood, and low libido should be queried. Has there been a change in the position, the size, or consistency of the testicles, unilateral or bilateral? Has there been a change in erectile functioning? Obtain information about the onset, severity, and the outcomes of the different treatment choices. Is there a history of congenital anomalies, infections (mumps, orchitis, STDs), urologic surgery, or any known genital trauma? The patient should also be asked about past and current use/abuse of narcotics, alcohol, testosterone replacement therapy, or any other over-the-counter "hormonal" supplements.

If the patient presents primarily for pain, the onset, location, frequency, duration, and radiation of the pain should first be documented. Specifics about what makes the pain worse and what makes it better as well as previously tried comfort measures should be recorded. Based on the age of the patient, the questions about infertility may not be relevant but the provider should never make that assumption. The patient should always be asked if fertility is a concern. If the patient expresses concern, then the questions in the infertility section above should be reviewed.

Sometimes a patient will present with no symptoms other than a concern about the appearance of the "lump" or new abnormal finding. The full history should be collected.

Signs and Symptoms

Patients with varicoceles may present as asymptomatic or symptomatic. Some patients with varicoceles have been identified through incidental findings on a physical examination or an imaging study.

If a varicocele is symptomatic, the patient may present with a pain described as a dull, aching, persistent, heavy sensation in the ipsilateral scrotum. Some men note that these sensations may radiate up into the inguinal region. The discomfort may worsen with standing, straining, or increased activity. The discomfort may lessen when he becomes supine with the resolution of the varicocele in this position. The patient may describe a soft mass above the affected testis as a "bag of worms." The duration of these symptoms prior to seeking medical care ranges from 3 to 18 months.

Patients may present with concerns about recent changes in the testis or laboratory results showing a low testosterone level or abnormal semen analysis. While many patients with varicocele remain asymptomatic, varicoceles have been implicated in male-factor infertility, testicular pain, and impaired testosterone production. It is the most common and treatable cause of male infertility; there is a large body of evidence indicating that varicocele is associated with abnormal semen parameters and testicular atrophy. Development of these symptoms may be the result of elevated scrotal temperature, hypoxia secondary to venous stasis, and/or reflux of renal and adrenal metabolites.

Obese patients have a lower prevalence of varicoceles detected by ultrasound. The lower prevalence is independent of physical examination and more likely due to another factor.

Physical Exam

The physical exam is the cornerstone for varicocele investigation. The patient should be examined in a warm room to promote relaxation of the cremasteric and dartos muscles. A cold room, an anxious or embarrassed patient, or an inexperienced clinician can result in retraction or elevation of the scrotum, making the varicocele more difficult to palpate. The patient should be examined in both the supine and standing positions.

Inspection: Assess the symmetry of the scrotum. Assess for symmetry of each testis. Observe for any visible swelling in the scrotum. Look for any visible tortuous veins.

Auscultate: Place the stethoscope on some of the larger varicoceles and the pulsing blood may be heard.

Palpation: Palpate the spermatic cord with the patient supine and while standing with and without a Valsalva maneuver. The Valsalva maneuver will facilitate increased engorgement of the varicocele and assist the clinician in locating the varicocele. Feel for "a bag of worms" above the testis but in the testicular cord. With full engorgement, a pulse may be felt at the varicocele. Grade the varicocele using the scale proposed by Dubin and Amelar (Table 3.1). Document the change in size or resolution of the varicocele with the change in position. If no reduction in size is noted when supine, further evaluation with a CT scan or pelvic ultrasound is required to evaluate for a retroperitoneal mass such as a sarcoma, lymphoma, or a renal tumor.

In addition, a right-sided varicocele as a solo finding is rare and should also suggest a more in-depth physical exam looking for pelvic lymphadenopathy, abdominal lymphadenopathy, or a kidney mass.

Palpate the testis using the Prader orchidometer assessing for ipsilateral or bilateral testicular atrophy.

Diagnostic Tests

As discussed before, the associated medical history and the physical exam are the main diagnostic criteria for varicoceles. Laboratory evaluation could be considered and would include testing to assess for possible complications of a varicocele. Semen analysis is recommended as a baseline; for men seeking observation only, periodic semen analyses are recommended. Serum testosterone (T) and follicle-stimulating (FSH) hormone levels may also be drawn.

If imaging studies are needed, scrotal ultrasonography is the modality of choice. However, scrotal ultrasonography is not recommended for the routine evaluation of every male with varicoceles, especially in males with subclinical varicoceles.

The American Urological Association and the American Society for Reproductive Medicine (Appendix) suggest limiting the use of scrotal ultrasonography to only the cases that are inconclusive after the history and physical examination are completed.

Pilatz et al. (2011) noted that color Doppler ultrasound has a greater than 80 % sensitivity and specificity in linking the grade of the varicocele on exam with the findings on the Doppler study (Table 3.3). The use of the color Doppler may assist practitioners with determining the diagnostic grade of the varicocele and the optimal treatment choice. Posttreatment Doppler studies may be used to determine the success of the obliteration of the varicocele.

Although a retrograde spermatic venography study is highly sensitive for varicocele identification, it is rarely used unless coupled with the therapeutic occlusion procedure. In this procedure, a catheter is advanced into the testicular vein and a contrast dye is injected to identify the varicocele. A stainless steel coil is then placed which embolizes the varicocele. The venography in conjunction with the steel-coil

Table 3.3 Dubbin and Amelia varicocele grading system with the addition of color Doppler results

Grade of varicocele	Physical exam	US color Doppler results— median left gonadal vein diameter with Valsalva
Subclinical	Not palpable, found incidentally	
Grade I	Palpable only when standing and doing a Valsalva maneuver	3.65 mm
Grade II	Palpable when standing. Valsalva not necessary	3.75 mm
Grade III	Visible through scrotal tissue Palpable when standing "Bag of worms"	4.7 mm

embolization is indicated for persistent or recurrent varicoceles and has a success rate of 85 % (Punekar et al. 1996).

Management

Counseling: An adult male with a palpable varicocele, abnormal semen parameters, and a possible interest in future fertility should receive early counseling about the risks of infertility and the treatment options available (Chap. 2) and can be directed to the American Society of Reproductive Medicine for additional details. Similarly a male with a palpable varicocele and normal semen parameters should be counseled that untreated varicoceles can result in potential testicular dysfunction. These patients should undergo yearly evaluation of the varicocele and the testicular size and its consistency. Consideration for repeat semen analysis and testosterone and FSH levels should be discussed. A review of the risks and complications of untreated palpable varicoceles should be presented each year.

Treatment Options

Conservative measures: Conservative, nonsurgical treatments are usually the first recommendation offered to men with varicocele-related pain. Conservative measures consist of application of heat or ice, scrotal elevation, use of a scrotal support, nonsteroidal anti-inflammatory medications, analgesics, and physical activity limitations. Physical activity limitations include restrictions on heavy lifting, sports activities, and strenuous exercises. While conservative measures may lessen the discomfort of the varicocele, they may not negate the need for surgical repair. Patients may also benefit from a referral for pelvic floor physical therapy or consultation with a pain medicine specialist. When conservative measures prove inadequate, definitive treatment of the varicocele can be offered, although patients should be counseled that surgery may not completely relieve their discomfort.

Medical therapy: Currently there is no conclusive study that indicates there is any medical therapy recommended to improve the outcomes or lessen the complications of varicocele formation and repair. A study conducted by Pourmand et al. (2014) proposed the use of daily oral dose of 750 mg of L-carnitine, an antioxidant, for 6 months for patients having the standard inguinal varicocelectomy, but the results did not discover any improvement in semen analysis parameters or DNA damage.

Radiologic Interventional Percutaneous Embolization

Varicoceles can be ablated by embolization of the spermatic veins using coils, balloons, or sclerosants in a minimally invasive outpatient procedure using local anesthetic or sometimes with addition of light sedation. These procedures are performed by an interventional radiologist with or without the assistance of a urologist. A venography is always done first in all three procedures to help identify the size of the varicocele as well as the venous anatomy. It can identify possible collateral venous systems. Patients are discharged after stabilization from the procedure.

Retrograde sclerotherapy is the most common percutaneous embolization procedure done. In retrograde sclerotherapy, a small incision is made into the brachial, femoral, or internal jugular vein. Using fluoroscopy and a contrast dye, the catheter is advanced into the internal spermatic veins. When the site of the refluxing flow is identified, the sclerosing agent is injected. Sclerosing agents used include N-butyl cyanoacrylate (N2BCA), sodium tetradecyl sulfate (STS) (a foam preparation), and polidocanol. The agent chosen is physician preference.

An alternate procedure is the antegrade sclerotherapy. This procedure is also outpatient, using local anesthesia and takes only 20 min. In this procedure, a small incision is made directly into the scrotum, directly visualizing and isolating the spermatic vein. A small catheter is similarly advanced to the refluxing flow and the sclerosant is injected.

Complications of sclerotherapy include scrotal hematoma, scrotal swelling, allergic reaction to the contrast dye, retroperitoneal leaking of the dye, fever, or rupture of the gonadal vein. There is a potential for an unresolved varicocele or a recurrent varicoceles usually related to an alternate venous collateral system. Following the procedure, the scrotal pain noted preoperatively may be persistent. There may be a new pain associated with a recurrent varicocele.

Benefits of sclerotherapy include recurrence rates similar to surgical repair, less post-procedure pain, and earlier return to normal activities. Improvement in semen parameters are similar to outcomes noted with surgical repair.

Coil Embolization

During a coil embolization, a small incision is made in the groin and a catheter is advanced through the femoral vein and into the gonadal vein. A fluoroscopy with contrast dye is used to follow the path of the catheter to the site of the refluxing veins. The coil is deployed into the veins causing the varicocele, and the fluoroscopy is used to observe that occlusion of the appropriate vein is complete. The coils used today are MRI compatible. In addition, some radiologists will add a sclerosing agent to make sure that the collateral veins are also obstructed reducing the chances of recurrence.

Balloon Embolization

Balloon embolization is a similar procedure to coil embolization. This procedure is used mostly with large spermatic veins or in patients that have a bidirectional flow pattern. Again the fluoroscopy and administration of the contrast dye is used to tract the passage of the guide wire into the spermatic vein. Once the position has been confirmed, the balloon is used to occlude the retrograde blood flow. As with the coil procedure, some radiologists will add a sclerosing agent to improve success rates.

Complications of the coil and balloon embolization are similar to those seen with sclerotherapy. During the passage or adjustment of the coil or balloon, perforation of the vein may occur. An additional complication is migration of the coil or balloon. Hydrocele formation has not been seen with either procedure. Thrombophlebitis is another potential complication.

Advantages of the coil and balloon therapy include less discomfort, faster recovery, less infections, and comparable outcomes to surgery. An improvement in sperm count, motility, and normal forms is seen in 75 % of the infertile males (Hanno et al. 2014). Embolization procedures have a success rate of 83 % (Reynard et al. 2009). Cost analysis of the embolization procedure and surgical costs associated with a varicocelectomy show no significant difference.

Varicocelectomy

Criteria for Surgery

The American Urological Association Best Practice Policy "Report on Varicocele and Infertility" outlined the conditions in which a varicocele should be treated.

1. Infertility: Their recommendations suggested that all four of these criteria be met before the male partner should be considered for a surgical repair:
   (a) The varicocele should be palpable. Subclinical varicoceles are not recommended for surgical repair.
   (b) Infertility is present.
   (c) The female partner has no infertility or has only a potentially treatable cause of infertility.
   (d) The semen analysis is abnormal on one or more semen samples.

2. Other situations that meet the criteria for surgical repair:
   (a) An adult male with a palpable varicocele, abnormal semen parameters, and a possible interest in future fertility.
   (b) Adolescent males with a varicocele and documented ipsilateral testicular atrophy. Some studies suggest that a 20 % change in testicular size over a 1-year period constitutes adequate criteria. Semen analysis should be further evaluated in this population.
   (c) Males presenting with chronic scrotal pain longer than 3 months.
   (d) Males demonstrating abnormal testosterone levels on at least 2 occasions. Proposing a varicocelectomy for men with low testosterone levels is controversial, but multiple research studies indicate that progressive Leydig cell destruction and potential testicular atrophy result in impaired fertility and other complications of long-term hypogonadism.

Surgical

The goal of a surgical repair of a varicocele is to occlude the internal spermatic vein that is causing the varicocele, prevent any injury to the testicular artery, and minimize the risk of recurring varicoceles. There are multiple surgical approaches to the surgery. The scrotal approach for varicocele repair is outdated and has been replaced with procedures that cause less injury to the spermatic arteries and testicular tissues. The scrotal approach is associated with increased incidence of postoperative hydroceles.

Laparoscopic varicocelectomy is indicated for use in recurrent or bilateral varicoceles. It is used less frequently now since the advent of subinguinal microsurgical varicocelectomy, partly because of its association with a higher incidence of complications, increased operating room time, expensive equipment, and the need for general anesthesia. A laparoscopic Doppler probe is recommended during the surgery to identify the location of the spermatic artery. A port incision is made sub-umbilical for the working element and two smaller port incisions are made within inches of that site. Cautery, clips, or sutures are used to ligate the spermatic veins.

The open surgery techniques include retroperitoneal, inguinal (Ivanissevich), and subinguinal (Marmar) approach. In these procedures, the spermatic vein is accessed through a 2–3" incision on the abdomen. The inguinal and subinguinal techniques are the most common approaches used. The Ivanissevich approach makes the incision superior and medial to the external ring. Caution must be taken to not injure the ilioinguinal nerve or the testicular artery.

The Marmar approach makes the incision where the spermatic veins are most superficial, right over the superficial ring. This subinguinal microsurgical varicocelectomy has an improved ability to preserve the testicular and cremasteric arteries and lymphatics minimizing the risks for significant side effects and testicular atrophy. This microsurgical technique is also associated with less postoperative pain, lower recurrence rates, and lower incidence of hydrocele formation.

Preoperative Considerations

The most important preoperative consideration for all patients is their understanding of why they are having this procedure. Patients need to have realistic expectations of the outcomes whether this is done for pain control, infertility, testicular changes, or hypogonadism. The risks and benefits should be presented in verbal and written format. Further discussion on the impact of varicocelectomy on infertility will be found in the chapter on infertility.

Postoperative Management

External dressings covering the incisions may be removed in 2 days. If steri-strips are used to cover the incision, they should be allowed to fall off themselves. No baths until the incision is completely healed. Showers may be started after 48 h. Physical exertion is not recommended for 2 weeks. Sexual activity should be deferred for 1–2 weeks. If scrotal swelling or discomfort is noted, comfort measures of scrotal support, scrotal elevation, and application of ice should be employed. Most pain can be modulated with nonprescription medications. The patient should be instructed to call the physician if fever, unusual pain, bruising, swelling, or discharge is noted. An inability to urinate should prompt an immediate call. A postoperative visit should be scheduled from 2 to 8 weeks after the surgery and is likely to be surgeon and/or facility dependent. A second follow-up visit at 3–4 months is scheduled for evaluation of a recurrent varicocele and to collect a semen analysis. Additional visits are scheduled based on physician preference.

Complications of Surgery

Short-term complications can include scrotal swelling, bruising, postoperative pain, and infections. Long-term complications can include hydrocele formation which is one of the most frequent complications. A second long-term complication is the inadvertent ligation of the testicular artery that can result in testicular atrophy. Recurrence of a varicocele, a third complication, is related to type of procedure done. Subinguinal microscopic varicocelectomy has a less than 2 % recurrence rate (Gomel 2010)

With newer surgical approaches, the resolution of scrotal pain is seen in 94 % of the patients. New onset of scrotal pain after a varicocelectomy can be related to a recurrence of a varicocele in the collateral venous complex.

Resources for the Nurse Practitioner

American Urological Association: The Optimal Evaluation of the Infertile Male: AUA Best Practice Statement http://www.auanet.org/common/pdf/education/clinical-guidance/Male-Infertility-d.pdf

Men's Health Network (MHN): www.menshealthnetwork.org
Men's Health Month: www.menshealthmonth.org

Resources for the Patient
The Urology Care Foundation: www.urologyhealth.org
RESOLVE: The National Infertility Association: www.resolve.org
American Society for Reproductive Medicine: www.reproductivefacts.org
Men's Health Network (MHN): www.menshealthnetwork.org

Clinical Pearls
- If a patient's gait is normal, testicular torsion is unlikely.
- Torsion of the testicular appendage is rare in adults.
- The acute phase epididymo-orchitis can result in symptoms for up to 6 weeks, and males may need symptomatic support that is not antibiotics, e.g., NSAIDs.
- Retractile testes are a normal variant and can be unilateral or bilateral; they fully descended at puberty but may move out of the scrotum and return spontaneously.
- Acute idiopathic scrotal edema is typically seen in the prepubertal male <10 years old.
- Treatment for spermatoceles and hydroceles is almost always elective; unless an individual is not a surgical candidate, aspiration is rarely the treatment of choice due to rapid recurrence.
- A review of the risks and complications of untreated palpable varicoceles should be presented each year, especially in younger men with bilateral varicoceles.

Men's Health Month: www.menshealthmonth.org

References

Abaci A, Catli G, Anik A, Bober E (2013) Epidemiology, classification and management of undescended testes: does medication have value in its treatment? J Clin Res Pediatr Endocrinol 5(2):65–72

Ahmad I, & Krishna NS. (2007). Hemospermia. Journal of Urology, 177(5):1613–1618

Alzayyani NR, Wani AM, Al Miamini W, Al Harbi ZS (2011) Chronic epididymo-orchitis and scrotal ulcers. BMJ Case Rep 2011: doi:10.1136/bcr.03.2010.2825

Aslam MI, Cheetham P, Miller MA (2009) A management algorithm for hematospermia. Nat Rev Urol 6(7):398–402

Babu S, Nutman TB (2012) Immunopathogenesis of lymphatic filarial disease. Semin Immunooathol 34(6):847–861

Baldisserotto M, de Souza JC, Pertence AP, Dora MD (2005) Color Doppler sonography of normal and torsed testicular appendages in children. Am J Roentgenol 184(4):1287–1292

Beni-Israel T, Goldman M, Bar Chaim S, & Kozer E. (2010). Clinical predictors for testicular torsion as seen in the pediatric ED. American Journal of Emergency Medicine 28(7):786–789

Chanc Walters R, Marguet CG, Crain DS (2012) Lower prevalence of varicoceles in obese patients found on routine scrotal ultrasound. J Urol 187(2):599–601

Clin North America 31(1):237–260

Coutinho K, McLeod D, Stensland K, Stock JA (2014) Variations in the management of asymptomatic adolescent grade 2 or 3 left varicoceles: a survey of practitioners. J Pediatr Urol 10(3):430–434

Crawford P, Crop JA (2014) Evaluation of scrotal masses. Am Fam Physician 89(9):723–727

DaJusta DG, Granberg CF, Villanueva C, Baker LA (2013) Contemporary review of testicular torsion: new concepts, emerging technologies and potential therapeutics. J Pediatr Urol 9(6 Pt A):723–730

Docimo SG, Silver RI, Cromie W (2000) The undescended testicle: diagnosis and management. Am Fam Physician 62(9):2037–2044

Epididymo-orchitis 2010 Int J STD AIDS 22(7):361–365

Fantasia J, Aidlen J, Lathrop W, Ellsworth P (2015) Undescended testes: a clinical and surgical review. Urol Nurs 35(3):117–126

Geiger J, Epelman M, Darge K (2010) The fountain sign: a novel color Doppler sonographic finding for the diagnosis of acute idiopathic scrotal edema. J Ultrasound Med 29(8): 1233–1237

Gomella LG (2010) The 5-minute urology consult (2nd ed). Philadelphia: Wolters Kluwer/ Lippincott Williams & Wilkins

Haddad NG, Houk CP, Lee PA (2014) Varicocele: a dilemma in adolescent males. Pediatr Endocrinol Rev 11(Suppl 2):274–283

Hano P, Malkowicz SB and Wein AJ (2014). Penn clinical manual of urology.Philadelphia: Saunders Elsevier

Hall NJ, Ron O, Eaton S, & Pierro A (2011). Surgery for hydrocele in children-an avoidable excess? Journal of Pediatric Surgery 46(12):2401–2405

Hensle TW, & Deibert CM (2012). Adult male health risks associated with congenital abnormalities. Urologic Clinics of North America 39(1):109–114

Hunter SR, Lishnak TS, Powers AM, Lisle DK (2013) Male genital trauma in sports. Clin Sports Med 32(2):247–254

Hutson JM, Balic A, Nation T, Southwell B (2010) Cryptorchidism. Semin Pediatr Surg 19(3):215–224

Kapoor S (2008) Testicular torsion: a race against time. International journal of clinical practice 62(5):821–827.

Kauffman EC, Kim HH, Tanrikut C, Goldstein M (2011) Microsurgical spermatocelectomy: technique and outcomes of a novel surgical approach. J Urol 185(1):238–242

Keys C, Heloury Y (2012) Retractile testes: a review of the current literature. J Pediatr Urol 8(1):2–6

Kolon TF, Glassberg KI, Van Batavia JP (2014) Varicocele: early surgery versus observation. J Urol 192(3):645–647

Kolon TF, Herndon CD, Baker LA, Baskin LS, Baxter CG, Cheng EY, Diaz M, Lee PA, Seahore CJ, Tasian GE, Barthold J (2014) Evaluation and treatment of cryptorchidism: AUA guideline. American Urological association Education and Research, Inc. Downloaded www.guideline. gov

Kumar P, Kapoor S, Nargund V (2006) Haematospermia – a systematic review. Ann R Coll Surg Engl 88(4):339–342

Kurkar A, Elderwy AA, Awad SM, Abulsorour S, Aboul-Ella HA, & Altaher A (2014). Hyperuricemia: A possible cause of hemospermia. Urology 84(3):609–612

Kwak N, Siegel D (2014) Imaging and interventional therapy for varicoceles. Curr Urol Rep 15(4):399

Lao OB, Fitzgibbons RJ Jr, Cusick RA (2012) Pediatric inguinal hernias, hydroceles, and undescended testicles. Surg Clin N Am 92(3):487–504

Lee PA, Houk CP (2013). Cryptorchidism. Current Opinion in Endocrinology, Diabetes & Obesity 20(3):210–216

Lee YJ, Cho SY, Paick JS, Kim SW (2015) Usefulness of 2010 world health organization reference values for determining indications for varicocelectomy. Urology 85(4):831–835

Leocadio DE, Stein BS (2009) Hematospermia: etiological and management considerations. Int Urol Nephrol 41(1):77–83

Masson P, Brannigan RE (2014) The varicocele. Urol Clin N Am 41(1):129–144

Mestrovic J, Biocic M, Pogorelic Z, Furlan D, Druzijanic N, Todoric D, Capkun V (2013) Differentiation of inflammatory from non-inflammatory causes of acute scrotum using relatively simple laboratory tests: prospective study. J Pediatr Urol 9(3):313–317

Ng YH, Seeley JP, Smith G (2013) Haematospermia as a presenting symptom: outcomes of investigation in 300 men. Surgeon 11(1):35–38

Niederberger C (2015) Re: clinical outcome of microsurgical varicocelectomy in infertile men with severe oligozoospermia. J Urol 193(1):255

Palmer LS (2013) Hernias and hydroceles. Pediatr Rev 34(10):457–464

Pilatz A, Altinkilic B, Köhler E, Weidner W (2011) Color Doppler ultrasound imaging in varicoceles: is the venous diameter sufficient for predicting clinical and subclinical varicocele? World J Urol 29(5):645–650

Pogorelic Z, Mrklic I, Juric I (2013) Do not forget to include testicular torsion in differential diagnosis of lower acute abdominal pain in young males. J Pediatr Urol 9(6 Pt B):1161–1165

Pourmand G, Movahedin M, Dehghani S et al (2014) Does L-carnitine therapy add any extra benefit to standard inguinal varicocelectomy in terms of deoxyribonucleic acid damage or sperm quality factor indices: a randomized study. Urology 84(4):821–825

Practice Committee of the American Society for Reproductive Medicine, & Society for Male Reproduction and Urology (2014) Report on varicocele and infertility: a committee opinion. Fertil Steril 102(6):1556–1560

Puche-Sanz I, Flores-Martin JF, Vazquez-Alonso F, Pardo-Moreno PL, Cozar-Olmo JM (2014) Primary treatment of painful varicocele through percutaneous retrograde embolization with fibred coils. Andrology 2(5):716–720

Punekar SV, Prem AR, Ridhorker VR (1996) Post-surgical recurrent varicocele: efficacy of internal spermatic venography and steel-coil embolization. Br J Urol 77:124–128

Ramos-Fernandez MR, Medero-Colon R, Mendez-Carreno L (2013) Critical urologic skills and procedures in the emergency department. Emerg Med Clin North Am 31(1):237–260

Raviv G, Laufer M, Miki H (2013) Hematospermia--the added value of transrectal ultrasound to clinical evaluation: is transrectal ultrasound necessary for evaluation of hematospermia? Clin Imaging 37(5):913–916

Reynard J, Brewster S, & Biers S (2010). Oxford Handbook of Urology. England: Oxford University Press

Rioja J, Sanchez-Margallo FM, Uson J, Rioja LA (2011) Adult hydrocele and spermatocele. BJU Int 107(11):1852–1864

Rizvi SA, Ahmad I, Siddiqui MA, Zaheer S, Ahmad K (2011) Role of color doppler ultrasonography in evaluation of scrotal swellings: pattern of disease in 120 patients with review of literature. Urol J 8(1):60–65

Rubenstein RA, Dogra VS, Seftel AD, & Resnick MI (2004). Benign intrascrotal lesions. Journal of Urology 171(5):1765–1772

Sexual Health and HIV (2011) BASHH UK guideline for the management of

Shakiba B,Heidari K, Jamali A, Afshar K (2014) Aspiration and sclerotherapy versus hydrocoelectomy for treating hydroceles. Cochrane Database of Syst Rev (11):CD009735

Sharp VJ, Kieran K, Arlen AM (2013) Testicular torsion: diagnosis, evaluation, and management. Am Fam Physician 88(12):835–840

Shridharani A, Lockwood G, Sandlow J (2012) Varicocelectomy in the treatment of testicular pain: a review. Curr Opin Urol 22(6):499–506

Sigman M (2011) There is more than meets the eye with varicoceles: current and emerging concepts in pathophysiology, management, and study design. Fertil Steril 96(6):1281–1282

Sommers D, Winter T (2014) Ultrasonography evaluation of scrotal masses. Radiol Clin North Am 52(6):1265–1281

Sports. Clin Sports Med 32(2):247–254

Srinath H (2013) Acute scrotal pain. Aust Fam Physician 42(11):790–792

Stahl P, Schlegel PN (2011) Standardization and documentation of varicocele evaluation. Curr Opin Urol 21(6):500–505

Stewart A, Ubee SS, Davies H (2011) Epididymo-orchitis. BMJ 342:1543

Street E, Joyce A, Wilson J, Clinical Effectiveness Group, British Association for Sexual Health and HIV (2011) BASHH UK guideline for the management of epididymo-orchitis, 2010. Int J STD AIDS 22(7):361–365

Thomas RJ, Holland AJ (2014) Surgical approach to the palpable undescended testis. Pediatr Surg Int 30(7):707–713

Thorup J, McLachlan R, Cortes D, Nation TR, Balic A, Southwell BR, Hutson JM (2010) What is new in cryptorchidism and hypospadias – a critical review on the testicular dysgenesis hypothesis. J Pediatr Surg 45(10):2074–2086

Trojian TH, Lishnak TS & Heiman D (2009). Epididymitis and orchitis: An overview. Americani Family Physician 79(7):583–587

Urologic skills and procedures in the emergency department. Emerg Med

Van Langen AMM, Gal S, Hulsmann AR, De Nef JJEM (2001) Acute idiopathic scrotal oedema: four cases and a short review. Eur J Pediatr 160(7):455–456

Walker NA, Challacombe B (2013) Managing epididymo-orchitis in general practice. Practitioner 257(1760):21–25

Walsh TJ, Seeger KT, Turek PJ (2007) Spermatoceles in adults: when does size matter? Arch Androl 53(6):345–348

Wampler, S M, & Llanes, M. (2010). Common scrotal and testicular problems. Primary care, 37(3):613–26

Wilson C, Boyd K, Mohammed A, Little B (2010) A single episode of haematospermia can be safely managed in the community. Int J Clin Pract 64(10):1436–1439

Erectile Dysfunction: Identification, Assessment, Treatment, and Follow-Up

4

Penny Kaye Jensen and Jeffrey A. Albaugh

Contents

P.K. Jensen, DNP, APRN, FNP-C, FAAN, FAANP (✉)
Department of Veterans Affairs, Office of Nursing Services,
Washington, DC, USA
e-mail: penny.jensen@va.gov

J.A. Albaugh, PhD, APRN, CUCNS
Sexual Health, John & Carol Walter Center for Urological Health, North Shore University
Health System, Glenview, IL, USA

© Springer International Publishing Switzerland 2016   83
M. Lajiness, S. Quallich (eds.), *The Nurse Practitioner in Urology*,
DOI 10.1007/978-3-319-28743-0_4

Learning Objectives
1. Understand the incidence, prevalence, etiology, and risk factors associated with erectile dysfunction.
2. Identify the anatomy and physiology related to vascular, neurogenic, and hormonal components necessary for normal erectile function.
3. Identify the comorbidities associated with erectile dysfunction including cardiovascular disease, diabetes, obesity, metabolic syndrome, dyslipidemia, and hypertension.
4. Articulate the linkage of ED symptoms that are an early manifestation of endothelial dysfunction and should prompt further evaluation for cardiovascular risk.
5. Identify appropriate laboratory testing with interpretation of results.
6. Describe the role of both pharmacologic and non-pharmacologic treatment modalities.
7. Recognize that erectile dysfunction (ED) assessment can be a pathway for managing men's overall health.
8. Describe the use of guidelines to assist NPs in decision making, with integration into daily practice.

Introduction

Advances in the understanding of male sexuality have led to the development of a wide range of options for managing erectile dysfunction (ED). The availability of oral agents, particularly phosphodiesterase type-5 (PDE-5), inhibitors which are considered first-line treatment, has expanded the therapeutic choices for men with ED. The dynamic marketing of these agents has increased both public awareness and the number of men seeking treatment for ED. According to the National Ambulatory Medical Care Survey, for every 1000 men in the United States, 7.7 physician office visits were made for ED in 1985. By 1999 after the advent of the PDE-5 inhibitor, that rate had nearly tripled to 22.3 (Cherry and Woodwell 2002). Historically, ED was treated by urologists and mental health practitioners. Today ED is most often managed in the primary care setting initially with referrals to specialists as necessary when oral agents have failed. Primary care providers (PCPs) write approximately two-thirds of all PDE-5 inhibitors (Kuritzky and Miner 2004). Successful treatment with these agents requires attention to appropriate dosing and prescribing information. Furthermore, the association of ED with vascular disease risk factors, such as diabetes, hypertension, dyslipidemia, tobacco use, obesity, and coronary artery disease, may be initially identified by and treated by primary care providers. Thus, nurse practitioners (NPs) are in a unique position to identify men at risk for both vascular disease and ED.

Scope of the Problem

After decades as a problem considered off limits for discussion, erectile dysfunction is at the forefront of healthcare. The transformation from forbidden subject to well-publicized and accepted health problem began in 1993, when the National Institute of Health Consensus Development Panel on Impotence (1993) catapulted impotence into the limelight and labeled it an important public health problem. The panel proposed that the term "impotence" be replaced by the less disparaging and more acceptable term of "erectile dysfunction" (ED) to signify the inability to attain and/or maintain a penile erection sufficient for sexual performance (NIH Consensus Panel on Impotence 1993). Erectile dysfunction is a common problem; an estimated 30 million men in the United States have some degree of erectile dysfunction (Bacon et al. 2003). ED occurs in approximately 1 out of 5 men in their lifetime and is more common in men 40 and older (Selvin et al. 2007).

Prevalence of Erectile Dysfunction and Aging

The Massachusetts Male Aging Study (MMAS), the first large-scale, population-based study of ED, suggested that the prevalence of ED correlated highly with age. Feldman and colleagues (1994) found that as many as 52 % of men between the ages of 40 and 70 have some degree of ED. This frequency increases with age, so that 40-year-olds have a prevalence of approximately 40 %, and 70-year-olds have prevalence as high as 67 %. This high prevalence was later confirmed by the National Health and Social Life Survey, which revealed that sexual dysfunction affects over 30 % of men between 18 and 59 years of age (Laumann et al.1999a, b). Prevalence studies demonstrate that, when controlling for other factors, increasing age is a risk factor for the development of erectile dysfunction, especially after 50 years of age (Feldman et al. 1994). The patients in these age groups make up the majority of patients evaluated in the adult primary care setting; thus, up to half of all men seen in primary care clinics will have some degree of ED. According to the United Nations, by 2025, there will be more than 356 million worldwide over the age of 65, an increase of 197 million from the current number. In 1995, the global proportion of men older than age 65 was 4.2 %; this is expected to rise to 9.5 % by 2025 (Shabsigh 2006). Due to the correlation between ED and age, global aging will bring an increase in the number of men with ED in the future. Aging alone does not explain the high prevalence of ED in older men. Rather, the high prevalence of ED is explained by normal age-related changes in combination with the accumulation of risk factors and health conditions that accompany aging (Seftel et al. 2004). Since the penis is a vascular organ, it is true that a man is as old as his penis. Kinsey's classical work revealed that aging is crucial risk factor for the development of ED. In his early works, he found that the prevalence of ED increased with age from 0.1 % at 20 years of age to 75 % at 80 years of age (Kinsey et al. 1948). Almost

50 years later, the MMAS revealed the same trend (Feldman et al. 1994). The aging process causes longer latent periods between sexual stimulation and attaining an erection. There is also a decrease in erectile rigidity and tactile sensitivity, diminished ejaculation, decrease in ejaculatory volume, and a longer refractory period. Patients and partners may be advised that men in their 50s and 60s and those with diabetes may benefit from additional stimulation because of increased tactile sensory thresholds (Rowland et al. 2005).

Physiology of an Erection

An erection begins with physical and/or mental stimulation. This information is processed and integrated in the frontal lobe of the brain. The message then travels down the spinal cord to the sacral area (S2–4) and the parasympathetic impulses contribute to smooth muscle relaxation and the inflow of blood. Chemical mediators activate smooth muscle relaxation and blood vessel dilatation leading to filling of the erectile cylinders. Nitric oxide and cyclic guanosine monophosphate (cGMP) are the primary noncholinergic-nonadrenergic and cholinergic mediators for the relaxation of the cavernosal smooth muscle (Gratzke et al. 2010). There are three erectile cylinders within the penis including the paired corpus cavernosa and the corpora spongiosum, and when these cylinders fill to capacity, they press against the superficial veins locking blood in the penis causing penile engorgement. Testosterone is the primary male androgen and is regulated via the hypothalamus-pituitary-testis axis. Testosterone is involved in the maturation and the maintenance of penile tissue architecture (Carson et al. 2009). Although testosterone plays a major role in normal libido, it also plays a smaller role in erectile function and ability to achieve ejaculation. There can be many underlying etiological factors associated with ED, and it may be multifactorial. Blood flow into the penis and nervous system communication between the brain and penis are essential to erections. Any disease process that impacts blood or nerve conduction may impact erectile function.

Etiology of Erectile Dysfunction

A general classification of ED by etiology is useful in evaluating patients with ED when choosing treatment options. Erectile dysfunction may be classified as organic, psychogenic, or mixed in origin (Lue 2000). Until the early 1980s, 80 % of ED cases were attributed to psychogenic causes, and 20 % were attributed to organic etiologies (Boyle 1999). The primary cause of ED in the large proportion of patients is now attributed to arterial disorders such as hypertension, diabetes mellitus, dyslipidemia, and peripheral vascular disease. Clinical research suggests that the penile vascular bed may be a sensitive indicator of early systemic endothelial cell and smooth muscle dysfunction (Jones et al. 2002). Organic dysfunction is by far the most common form of ED and may be caused by multiple etiologies.

Psychogenic causes include performance anxiety, relationship problems, psychological stress, or depression, which causes a loss of libido, over inhibition, or impaired nitric oxide release. The most common psychogenic cause of ED is performance anxiety related to a man's fear that he will not be able to perform sexually. Anxiety may lead to an initial failure which further increases anxiety, resulting in a cycle that leads to future failures to achieve an erection. Stress, tension, worry, guilt, and anger can also inhibit sexual performance. Sexual performance is closely associated with a man's self-esteem; therefore, erectile dysfunction can be devastating not only to a man's sex life but also to his sense of self. Men with ED often develop feelings of inadequacy, embarrassment, or guilt. The psychological effects of ED can invade other areas of a man's life as well, such as social interactions and job performance. These psychological factors may occur secondary to and possibly as a result of the organic causes (Sachs 2003). Mixed etiologies can occur, and an organic etiology may become a secondary psychogenic problem.

Organic Etiologies of Erectile Dysfunction

Vasculogenic A common organic etiology of erectile dysfunction is vascular compromise, which can be either arterial or venous. Vasculogenic ED accounts for about two-thirds of patients with ED (Androshchuk et al. 2015). Vascular compromise may be related to hypertension, atherosclerosis, diabetes mellitus, pelvic irradiation, Peyronie's disease, and pelvic or perineal trauma, any of which can cause inadequate arterial flow or impaired venous occlusion. Traditionally, ED was viewed as an outcome of occlusive systemic vascular disease that occurred as a late consequence of atherosclerosis. Current and emerging clinical research investigators reveal that the penile vascular bed may be a sensitive indicator of early systemic endothelial cell and/or smooth muscle dysfunction. ED is likely among the initial signs of oxidative stress and subclinical cardiovascular disease (McCullough 2003). ED is becoming a barometer of overall cardiovascular risk factors and should be viewed in this context (McCullough 2003). In fact, the symptom of erectile difficulty, particularly the poor ability to maintain a firm erection, often occurs before the development of overt structural occlusive vascular problems that lead to adverse events such as myocardial infarction, stroke, or claudication (Kloner and Speakman 2002). The most important point of these findings is not that these comorbidities are related but that ED is an early end-organ manifestation of the disease process—one that manifests much earlier than a critical arterial stenosis of the coronary arteries, diabetic peripheral neuropathy, retinopathy, or hypertensive cardiomyopathy. ED is the body's "early warning system" (McCullough 2003). Because of its prevalence in CVD, diabetes, hypertension, and other systemic vascular illnesses, ED has traditionally been viewed as a secondary complication of these disorders. More recently, a growing body of clinical evidence has emerged to suggest that a paradigm shift is in order (McCullough 2003). Inman et al. (2009) have shown that when ED occurs in younger men, it is associated with a marked increase in the risk of future cardiac events and that overall ED may be associated with an approximately 80 % higher risk of subsequent CAD.

According to the Massachusetts Male Aging Study (MMAS), erectile dysfunction is strongly associated with significant health risks, such as diabetes, dyslipidemia, hypertension, and cardiac disease (Feldman et al. 1994). Billups and Friedrich (2005) found that 60 % of healthy men presenting ED had abnormal cholesterol levels, and over 90 % of these men had evidence of penile arterial disease when Doppler ultrasound was performed. The Minneapolis Heart Institute Foundation study initially reported that ED may be one of the first signs of cardiovascular disease, because the narrow vessels of the penis appear more sensitive to atherosclerotic blockage than the larger vessels in the heart (Pritzker 1999). Studies that suggested a link between coronary artery disease (CAD) and erectile dysfunction (ED) began to appear in the literature in the late 1980s. Men with cardiovascular disease, diabetes mellitus, and metabolic syndrome have a higher prevalence of ED than men who do not have these diseases (Grover et al. 2006).

Neurogenic A type of organic etiology, neurogenic etiologies include disorders such as Parkinson's disease, multiple sclerosis, Alzheimer's disease, stroke, spinal cord injury, and radical pelvic surgery, such as radical prostatectomy, diabetic neuropathy, or pelvic injury caused by failure to initiate nerve impulse or interruption of neural transmission. Injuries to the back, especially if they involve the vertebral column and the spinal cord, can cause erectile dysfunction. Diabetes mellitus, chronic renal failure, and coronary heart disease result in both neural and vascular dysfunction. A wide variety of operations performed for other conditions can cause incidental injury to the nerves of the penis resulting in ED.

Hormonal Approximately 10 % of erectile dysfunction is caused by hormonal imbalance. Testosterone declines with aging, with an average decrease in total serum testosterone levels of approximately 1.5 % per year (Feldman et al. 2002). The prevalence of low serum total testosterone levels is approximately 20 % by the age of 50 and 50 % by the age of 80 (Matsumoto 2002). Androgen deficiency decreases nocturnal erections and libido. Symptoms of low testosterone include decreased muscle mass and bone mineral density, increased fat mass, central obesity, insulin resistance, decreased libido, low energy levels, memory loss, irritability, and depression. Hypogonadism and hyperprolactinemia cause loss of libido and inadequate nitric oxide release. Kidney and liver disease also may lead to hormonal imbalances that can cause erectile dysfunction.

Diabetes The association between ED and diabetes is well established (Kolodny et al. 1974). The risk of ED in patients with diabetes approaches 50 %. Diabetics are not only at risk for developing macrovascular and microvascular disease, but these patients have an increased risk for neuropathies and hormonal abnormalities.

These conditions have been found at higher rates in diabetics than in the general population (Corona et al. 2004). Poor glycemic control as demonstrated by elevated glycosylated hemoglobin levels correlates with severe ED (Rhoden et al. 2005).

Lower Urinary Tract Symptoms   It is now recognized that men with lower urinary tract symptoms (LUTSs) have a high prevalence of ED (Rosen et al. 2003). LUTS is most often caused by benign prostatic hyperplasia (BPH), which is comprised of multiple voiding symptoms, including urinary frequency, urgency, nocturia, and slow stream. Although the etiology remains unclear, findings from several studies suggest that LUTS is a risk factor for ED, independent of age and other comorbidities (Braun et al. 2003). There is a strong epidemiological evidence for a link between ED and LUTS supported by theories for their shared pathogenesis. The quality of life of men with BPH is reduced by its effects on sexual function (Carson and McMahon 2008). Investigators suggest that LUTS associated with BPH may be improved with phosphodiesterase (PDE-5) inhibitors (Liu et al. 2011). These medications are commonly prescribed for ED. The inhibition of PDE isoenzymes relaxes the smooth muscle in the prostate or bladder and can improve LUTS in BPH patients (Kaplan and Gonzalez 2007).

Sleep Apnea   Several studies have suggested a link between sleep apnea and ED; the correlation between the severity of sleep apnea and the severity of ED is strong (Jankowski et al. 2008; Teloken et al. 2006; Zias et al. 2009). Sleep apnea disrupts rapid eye movement or REM sleep; this is the time when men routinely experience nocturnal erections. It is hypothesized that decreased REM sleep means fewer nocturnal erections. Nocturnal erections are a necessary process for men to maintain healthy sexual function. NPs should consider concomitant sleep disorders when evaluating patients with ED, especially in those refractory to routine therapy (Jankowski et al. 2008). Further studies are necessary to clearly define the causative link between sleep disorders and ED.

Depression   When depression is the primary illness, erectile dysfunction can be considered a symptom of the depressive illness. However, if ED is the primary diagnosis, men may develop depressive symptoms due to the loss of erectile function. Regardless of whether ED is a symptom of depression or depression is a consequence of ED, these conditions are frequently comorbid. Araujo and colleagues (1998) concluded that the relationship between depressive symptoms and ED in middle-aged men is robust and independent of important aging confounders such as demographics, lifestyle, health status, medication use, and hormones (Araujo et al. 1998).

Risk Factors for Erectile Dysfunction

Risk factors for ED are any underlying disease process that can impact blood flow, nerve conduction, or hormonal imbalance. In addition to sedentary lifestyle, obesity, and tobacco use, recreational drug use is also a risk factor for ED. Many commonly prescribed medications can diminish erectile function. Medications that can impact erectile function are antihypertensives (the most common are diuretics and beta-blockers), antidepressants (the most common are serotonin reuptake inhibitors (SSRIs) and tricyclic antidepressants), anti-anxiety medications, anti-psychotics, anticholinergics, antiarrhythmics, antiandrogens, antihistamines (the most common is pseudoephedrine), narcotics (opioids), and analgesics. It is important to obtain a history to assess the patient's potential underlying medical issues that may impact erectile function, current medications both prescribed and over the counter (OTC), and drugs of habituation (alcohol, marijuana, cocaine) for potential effects on erectile function and lifestyle choices in terms of exercise/activity, diet, and sexual activity.

Obesity nearly doubles the risk of ED (Bacon et al. 2003). A Danish community-based cross-sectional study reported that ED was more prevalent in men with a body mass index (BMI) of 30 or more (Andersen et al. 2008). Esposito et al. found that men with a BMI above 25 are at a higher risk of ED (Esposito et al. 2004). One-third of men who were obese improved their erectile function with moderate weight loss and an increase in the amount and duration of regular exercise (Esposito et al. 2004).

A healthy lifestyle prevents the occurrence of ED. Derby et al. (2000) conducted a study to prospectively examine whether changes in smoking, heavy alcohol consumption, sedentary lifestyle, and obesity were associated with the risk of erectile dysfunction. Data were collected as part of a cohort study of a random sample of men 40–70 years old. In-home interviews were completed by 1709 men at baseline in 1987–1989 and 1156 men at follow-up in 1995–1997 (average follow-up 8.8 years). Analyses included 593 men without erectile dysfunction at baseline were free of prostate cancer and had not been treated for heart disease or diabetes. Obesity status was associated with erectile dysfunction ($p = 0.006$), with baseline obesity predicting a higher risk regardless of follow-up weight loss. Physical activity status was associated with erectile dysfunction ($p = 0.01$), with the highest risk among men who remained sedentary and the lowest among those who remained active or initiated physical activity (Derby et al. 2000). Changes in smoking and alcohol consumption were not associated with the incidence of erectile dysfunction ($p > 0.3$). The authors concluded that midlife lifestyle changes may be too late to reverse the effects of smoking, obesity, and alcohol consumption on erectile dysfunction. In contrast, physical activity may reduce the risk of ED even if initiated in midlife; therefore, early adoption of healthy lifestyles may be the best approach to reduce the risk of developing erectile dysfunction (Derby et al. 2000).

Management of Erectile Dysfunction

A consensus guidelines model was developed for managing erectile dysfunction (ED) for healthcare clinicians. The model emphasizes a systematic approach in identification, assessment, intervention, and follow-up in patients with ED.

The guidelines are intended to provide a comprehensive care model for patients and their partners, which would be optimally cost effective and clinically relevant. This model allows quality sexual healthcare to be provided to increasing numbers of patients and their partners (Albaugh et al. 2002).

Identification of Erectile Dysfunction

Traditionally, sexual health has not been a high priority for primary care providers, including NPs. Men are often reluctant to bring up sexual issues (Eardley 2013) and often look to their nurse practitioner (NP) to initiate discussion about sexuality and intimacy. To provide holistic care to patients, NPs should ask patients about problems with sexuality and intimacy.

ED has been viewed as a quality-of-life issue rather than a relatively common medical condition that increases in prevalence as men age. Although ED is not perceived as a life-threatening condition, it is closely associated with many comorbidities and shared risk factors for those comorbidities. ED is a widespread and significant condition that warrants further investigation and is considered a marker for current or future cardiovascular and metabolic disease, as well as diabetes, dyslipidemia, depression, hypogonadism, and other disorders. Identifying ED represents an opportunity to screen for serious concomitant conditions.

While various cultures may approach sex and intimacy differently, cultural sensitivity may be helpful in approaching each individual patient and their partner. There is cultural variation regarding eye contact, thus, providers must be mindful of cultural issues. In some cultures or religions, it may be unacceptable to engage in sexual activity within a certain number of days before or after menstruation. Assessing for and understanding any individual or cultural inhibition are important in order to best advise a patient in moving forward with ED treatment.

Men who should be screened include those over age 40, those with predisposing comorbidities, or patients who may have difficulties with physical intimacy. Patients with sexual concerns often feel the most comfortable discussing these issues with an NP. More than 70 % of adult patients in a large sample considered sexual complaints an appropriate topic to discuss with their primary care clinician (Sadovsky and Curtis 2006). The rate of sexual dysfunction surveyed was 35 % for adult men and 42 % for adult women; evidence of discussion regarding these sexual complaints was documented in as few as 2 % of the clinician's notes (Sadovsky and Curtis 2006).

Sexual inquiry is most often conducted by face-to-face interview with the patient, although partner interviews, paper-and-pencil questionnaires, or computer-based methods may also be of value. Each of these methods has distinct advantages and limitations. Perhaps the most important aspect of the interview is the manner in which inquiry is conducted. A high level of sensitivity for each individual's unique ethnic, cultural, and person background should be taken into consideration. Administering self-evaluation questionnaires such as the Sexual Health Inventory for Men (SHIM) (Cappelleri and Rosen 2005) is a discrete way of screening patients while they are waiting in the office. The SHIM was developed and validated as a brief, easily administered, patient-reported diagnostic tool It is widely used for screening and diagnosis of ED as well as severity of ED in clinical practice and research (Cappelleri and Rosen 2005).

NPs can also approach patients using the PLISSIT model (Permission, Limited Information, Specific Suggestions, and Intensive Therapy) (Annon 1974). The approach begins with asking for and giving permission to discuss sexual concerns. Initiating discussion about sexual dysfunction opens the channels of communication and legitimizes the patient's concerns. The next step for the NP is to provide information about sexuality and sexual dysfunction. The information may include normal anatomy and physiology, dispelling myths about sexuality, and discussing common sexual problems. The next step is to provide specific recommendations on what may be helpful to improve the patient's sexual issue. These suggestions should be driven by the patient's sexual health goals. It is important to include the partner in the treatment plan and education process. The final step in the PLISSIT model is to guide the patient to intensive therapy (the IT of the model). The model should be instituted using a nonjudgmental and caring attitude while keeping in mind the patient's and partner's goals, feelings, and expectations. Including the partner in the visit can be very helpful and allow for sexual education of both the patient and their partner.

Sample Questions for Identifying ED
1. Do you have trouble achieving or maintaining an erection?
2. Do you have trouble all the time, some of the time, or infrequently?
3. Men with heart disease (or diabetes, high cholesterol, etc.) often have problems getting erections. Has this been a problem for you?
4. Did your erectile dysfunction begin suddenly or gradually?
5. Is erectile dysfunction (ED) global or dependent on circumstances, such as partner?
6. Are you having relationship conflicts with your partner not related to ED?
7. How often are intercourse attempts successful?
8. Is your interest still adequate?
9. Do you have early morning or nighttime erections?
10. Do you have any difficulties with ejaculation, too fast or too slow?
11. Are you able to achieve orgasm?
12. Have your tried any therapies to correct this problem?

Assessment of Erectile Dysfunction

A complete medical history should be obtained to evaluate for treatable organic and/or psychogenic etiologies. The successful treatment of erectile dysfunction begins with a detailed medical history, including both psychosocial and sexual components. Due to the close association between cardiovascular risk factors and ED, searching for potential cardiovascular disease in these patients is critical. ED may be a warning sign of latent cardiac disease before symptoms of heart disease are present. The NP should assume underlying cardiovascular disease until proven otherwise because of the link between ED and cardiovascular disease (Nehra et al. 2012).

The history should include a comprehensive targeted sexual, medical, and psychosocial history (Shamloul and Ghanem 2013). History taking should be aimed at characterizing the severity of the symptoms, triggers that exacerbate symptoms, onset of symptoms, duration of the problem, as well as any concomitant medical or psychosocial factors. Contributing factors including all medical conditions that may impact sex and intimacy, prescription or nonprescription drug use, relationship issues, depression, anxiety, or other psychiatric disorders should be carefully assessed. Screening for depression can also be integrated into the history-taking process (Jensen et al. 2004). Depression, post-traumatic stress syndrome (PTSD), anxiety, and other psychiatric conditions may be responsible for ED. It is imperative to obtain a social history since stress surrounding a relationship or problems with alcohol or substance abuse including tobacco can have a direct impact on erectile function (Jensen et al. 2004).

A complete physical examination with special emphasis placed on the review of genitourinary, endocrine, vascular, and neurologic systems should be performed. The physical examination of the genitalia provides an opportunity for patient education and reassurance regarding normal genital anatomy. During inspection, the NP should note the patient's secondary sex characteristics (facial/body hair, normal/abnormal breast tissue, deepness of voice), skin, scars from previous surgeries, and musculature development. Cardiovascular assessment should include blood pressure, heart sounds, and peripheral pulses in the lower extremities. The most useful physical finding is diminished femoral and/or popliteal pulses (LaRochelle and Levine 2006). This finding suggests that vascular disease, specifically arterial insufficiency, is the most likely cause or at least has a role in the patient's ED. If these large vessels have diminished pulsatility, it is likely that the cavernosal arteries, which are 0.5–1.0 mm in diameter, are also compromised (LaRochelle and Levine 2006). The neurologic evaluation may include muscle strength, muscle spasticity, assessment of gait, sensitivity to touch, and testing of the peripheral and genital reflexes. The genitourinary examination should involve assessment of the size of the penis, any indurations, nodules, fibrosis, lesions, or plaques along the penis or on the meatus. The scrotum and testicles should be evaluated for size and consistency. In addition, the NP should note any lesions, nodules, or abnormalities of the scrotum or testes. A digital rectal examination (DRE) should be performed to determine normal shape and consistency of the prostate and to determine the presence of any lesions, indurations, or abnormalities. The anal sphincter and the bulbocavernosus reflex may also be evaluated.

Laboratory Evaluation
Laboratory evaluation can range from simple to complex. Testing should be individualized to each patient and risk factors based on the patient history. Given the strong association between ED and vascular comorbidities, laboratory testing

should be conducted for all patients who have not been evaluated in the past 6 months. Selective laboratory testing should be considered to evaluate potential endocrine or other systemic causes of the patient's ED and identify likely comorbidities contributing to ED, such as diabetes or hyperlipidemia. Standard serum chemistries including fasting blood glucose or glycosylated hemoglobin, CBC, and lipid profile should be evaluated. Serum thyroid-stimulating hormone (TSH) determination may also be of some value. Plasma testosterone varies diurnally and may be decreased by anxiety, stress, or depression. Free testosterone levels may be more accurate of tissue hormone status but tend to be much more expensive. Low libido is associated with low testosterone levels; therefore, testosterone levels should be drawn on those patients complaining of a diminished sex drive. A prolactin level should be evaluated if the testosterone level is low, if there is a history of loss of libido, or if there are symptoms of prolactinoma, such as visual field loss or headache (Akpunona et al. 1994). Elevated prolactin levels can be indicative of a pituitary tumor, which should be further evaluated by MRI if no other etiology can be identified. A serum PSA may be indicated based upon the patient's age and relative risk status according to the American Urological Association (AUA) guidelines (American Urological Association 2005).

Specialized Diagnostic Assessment

Erectile dysfunction is diagnosed and treated through history and physical exam. Treatment does not vary greatly or hinge upon specialized diagnostic testing. Some patients may need referral for specialized testing when medically indicated for consideration of reconstructive surgery, failure of conventional therapy, or medicolegal reasons specialized diagnostic procedures may be indicated. These tests may include nocturnal penile tumescence and rigidity (NPTR) testing, color Doppler cavernosal studies (penile blood flow studies), or other specialized vascular or neurologic procedures, and they may play a role in further understanding selected cases. For example, these procedures may be of value in assessing young patients with pelvic or penile trauma who may be candidates for reconstructive vascular surgery. The tests may also be performed for medicolegal reasons (documenting organic erectile dysfunction in cases of litigation) or because the patient wishes to establish arterial insufficiency or venous leakage, but in general these tests do not change or impact the course of treatment and therefore may not be necessary. Patient referral to urology, endocrinology, cardiology, neurology, and/or psychiatry may be appropriate depending on diagnostic findings.

Intervention and Treatment of Erectile Dysfunction

A wide variety of medical treatments are now available for patients diagnosed with erectile dysfunction. These treatment options are classified according to efficacy, degree of invasiveness, safety, ease of use, and cost. Every treatment has pros and cons, and each patient and partner should understand these factors. Treatment plans should be goal oriented and ideally aimed at satisfying the needs of the patient and partner to maximize the chance of achieving partner satisfaction. By presenting all information, including advantages and disadvantages of each, patients can then make an informed decision about which treatment option is best for them.

First-Line Therapy

Counseling

Comprehensive sexuality education is an essential element of successful ED treatment. Patients need to not only understand each treatment option to make informed decisions about treatment choice but also information on how to integrate treatment into love play with their partner. Discussion should center on factual information and focus on resolving the patient's ED. Teaching strategies should include written, video, model reference, and verbal communication.

The key to patient success with the therapy lies in the NP's ability to effectively work one on one with the patient and/or their partner to understand and safely use the treatment. The NP should identify appropriate lifestyle changes that are recommended including smoking cessation, regular exercise, weight loss, limiting alcohol, and following a cardiovascular low fat, low cholesterol plant-based (Mediterranean) diet. These changes can help improve erectile function, reduce one's risk of heart disease or cancer, and improve overall general health (Gupta et al. 2011). Although the majority of ED has an underlying physiologic etiology, there is often a psychological component as well. It is important to encourage patients to seek counseling for themselves and their partner. Counseling may include individual counseling, couples' therapy, or sex therapy.

Oral Agents

NPs play an important role in prescribing treatments medications for their patients, including treat ED. Since its arrival, the class of agents known as type-5 phosphodiesterase (PDE$_5$) inhibitors has changed the management of ED. Type 5 phosphodiesterase (PDE$_5$) inhibitors are considered first-line therapy in the treatment of ED, as recommended by the American Urological Association (AUA) (Montague et al. 2005) and the European Association of Urology (EAU) (Wespes et al. 2006). Four PDE-5 inhibitors are now available by prescription: Viagra® (sildenafil), Levitra® & Staxyn® (vardenafil), Cialis® (tadalafil), and Stendra® (avanafil). The approval of sildenafil in 1998 revolutionized the treatment of ED worldwide. These agents are competitive and selective inhibitor of cyclic guanosine monophosphate (cGMP) type 5 phosphodiesterase (PDE). This inhibition increases the level of intracellular cGMP and results in the efflux of calcium ions from the cell, which causes smooth muscle relaxation. Increased levels of cGMP act to enhance the effect of nitric oxide in the penis. PDE type 5 inhibitors prevent the breakdown of cGMP, which is the intracellular second messenger of nitric oxide. Nitric oxide is released following sexual stimulation; therefore, these agents are only effective when a male is sexually stimulated. Libido is not affected by PDE-5 inhibitors (Porst et al. 2013).

The majority of patients prefer oral medications due to ease and convenience of use (Hatzichristou et al. 2000). There are no compelling data to support the superiority of one agent over another. Comparisons of efficacy among various agents in this class are limited. The main difference in these medications is their duration of action; tadalafil produces longer lasting effects offering a longer time period in which sexual activity may occur and increased spontaneity, while the shorter lasting avanafil reaches peak blood levels twice as fast as the other oral agents allowing for a shorter wait time before intercourse can occur. All PDE-5 inhibitors are contraindicated in patients using organic nitrates, in any form or frequency.

NPs should consider activity tolerance as a guide to the cardiovascular status of their patients, since there is a degree of cardiac risk associated with sexual activity. Treatment of ED, including PDE-5 inhibitors, should not be used in men for whom sexual activity is inadvisable. Guidelines for managing ED in patients with cardiovascular disease developed by the Princeton Consensus Panel recommend categorizing patients to one of three risk levels (high, intermediate, and low) based on their cardiovascular risk factors. The guideline recommends that patients at high risk should not receive treatment for sexual dysfunction until their cardiac condition has stabilized. Patients at low risk may be considered for oral agents (Jackson et al. 2006). Overall, controlled trials have revealed no increase in myocardial infarction, worsening CVD, or death rates among patients using PDE-5 inhibitors. Preliminary research indicates that these agents may be cardioprotective (Sesti et al. 2007).

PDE-5 inhibitors potentiate the hypotensive effects of nitrates, and administration to patients who are using organic nitrates, either regularly and/or intermittently, in any form is contraindicated. PDE-5 inhibitors are contraindicated in patients with a known hypersensitivity to any component of the tablet. They should be used cautiously in patients with cardiovascular conditions who are sensitive to the vasodilatory effects of PDE-5 inhibitors such as left ventricular outflow obstruction and severely impaired autonomic control of the blood pressure. They should not be used in patients who have had a myocardial infarction, stroke, or life-threatening arrhythmia in the last 6 months, unstable angina, BP <90/50 or >170/110, or retinitis pigmentosa. The concurrent use of a protease inhibitor can greatly increase PDE-5 inhibitor levels. Caution should be used in patients on multiple antihypertensive agents because PDE-5 inhibitors can lower the blood pressure further. When used in conjunction with alpha-blockers, PDE-5 inhibitors may decrease blood pressure and should be used cautiously. They should be used with caution in patients with penile curvature or deformities or in patients with sickle cell anemia, multiple myeloma, or leukemia. Common adverse reactions to these medications may include headache, flushing, nasal congestion or stuffiness, and nausea. Sildenafil may be associated with color change disturbances, often described as a "blue halo" effect. Tadalafil and avanafil may be associated with muscle or back pain. Full prescribing information should always be reviewed for more detailed information.

Patients should notify his or her NP of any changes in vision or hearing, stop the medication immediately, and seek immediate medical treatment. Vision changes may be a sign of non-arteritic anterior ischemic optic neuropathy (NAION). NAION, a cause of decreased vision including permanent loss of vision, has been reported rarely postmarketing in temporal association with the use of PDE-5 inhibitors, including Viagra (Federal Drug Administration 2007). Most, but not all, of these patients had underlying anatomic or vascular risk factors for developing NAION, including but not necessarily limited to low cup to disk ratio ("crowded disk"), age over 50, diabetes, hypertension, coronary artery disease, hyperlipidemia, and smoking. It is not possible to determine whether these events are related directly to the use of PDE-5 inhibitors, to the patient's underlying vascular risk factors or anatomical defects, to a combination of these factors, or to other factors (VIAGRA® (sildenafil) New York, NY: Pfizer Inc. 2005).

A case report in the published literature of sudden hearing loss in a male patient using Viagra® prompted Federal Drug Administration (FDA) to search the Adverse Event Reporting System (AERS) for postmarketing reports of hearing loss for all PDE-5 inhibitors. The FDA identified a total of 29 reports of sudden hearing loss, both with and without tinnitus, vertigo or dizziness, in strong temporal relationship to dosing with Viagra® (sildenafil), Cialis® (tadalafil), or Levitra® (vardenadil). There have also been cases of hearing loss reported in patients using Revatio® (sildenafil) for the treatment of pulmonary arterial hypertension (PAH). Even though no causal relationship has been demonstrated, the FDA believed that the strong temporal relationship between the use of PDE-5 inhibitors and sudden hearing loss in these cases warranted revisions to the product labeling for the drug class (Federal Drug Administration 2007).

Patients should also avoid a high-fat diet for 2 h before administration, and be advised of onset of the particular medication prescribed. PDE-5 inhibitors do not affect ejaculation, orgasm, or libido. Guay et al. (2001) found that as testosterone levels fell, the response to sildenafil decreased and eventually became ineffective; therefore, it is important to evaluate testosterone levels if oral therapy is not effective.

A management strategy, in which patients take tadalafil on a consistently scheduled basis, rather than on demand, is now being implemented. In 2008, the FDA-approved once-daily use of tadalafil in a dose of 5 mg or a 2.5-mg dose for the treatment of ED. Theoretically, chronic dosing would result in continuous inhibition of PDE-5, therefore increasing a higher concentration of cyclic guanosine monophosphate, which may benefit men who have not responded to on-demand treatment. Once-daily tadalafil may be appropriate for men with ED who anticipate sexual activity more than twice per week and allow greater spontaneity in the patients' sexual encounters while improving tolerability, patient satisfaction, and adherence (Hatzimouratidis and Hatzichristou 2007; McMahon 2004; Porst et al. 2006). The majority of treatment failures with oral PDE-5 inhibitors can be salvaged with re-education. Men who are not responsive may have issues with intimacy or establishing relationships, are not able to tolerate side effects, or have advanced endothelial dysfunction. Patients with advanced vascular disease or multiple comorbidities may have a poor response to PDE-5 inhibitors.

Vacuum Constriction Devices

Vacuum constriction devices (VCDs) are the least invasive and least expensive of all treatment options and can be used regardless of etiology. The efficacy and safety of vacuum constriction devices are well documented (Kohler et al. 2007; Pahlajani et al. 2012; Raina et al. 2006). VCDs are often used by individuals who wish to avoid taking medications or in combination with medications when the PDE-5 inhibitor is not completely or consistently effective. A VCD consists of a cylinder attached to a vacuum pump and tension rings. VCDs are noninvasive and may be a less least expensive treatment option. Medical grade devices have a pressure release valve on the pump or cylinder and may be either manual or battery operated. The devices produce an erection by creating negative pressure around the penis to pull blood into the penis. The erection is maintained by applying the tension band or ring around the base of the penis off the edge of cylinder. The band/ring does not completely constrict penile arterial blood flow but should be removed and should never be worn for greater than 30 min at a time maximum.

There are no major adverse effects reported when the vacuum device is used carefully and according to instructions. Adverse effects may include hematoma, ecchymosis, petechiae, numbness of the penis, pain, pulling of scrotal tissue, and blocked or painful ejaculation. The use of vacuum devices requires thorough one-on-one training for treatment success. The advantages of VCDs are that they are noninvasive and with proper instruction and practice have a high success rate. The disadvantages of VCDs are that they are cumbersome, awkward, and the resulting erection is often not viewed as natural. The erection must be maintained with a tension ring during intercourse.

A venous flow constriction loop/or ring alone can also be used to maintain erections. They consist of bands or rings of various designs and materials that are placed around the base of the penis to diminish venous return holding the blood within the penis. The device is placed on the penis after achieving an erection to assist in maintaining the erection. VCDs have been used successfully in combination with intracavernosal injection, intraurethral therapy, and PDE-5 inhibitors. A VCD can also be alternatively recommended for the initiation of programmed cavernosal oxygenation to accelerate penile erection recovery after prostatectomy (Kendirici et al. 2006).

Second-Line Therapy

Intracavernosal Injection Therapy

The introduction of intracavernosal injections (ICIs) revolutionized the diagnosis and treatment of erectile dysfunction in the mid-1980s. Before oral agents became available, intracavernosal self-injection was the most common medical therapy for ED. This therapy is effective in approximately 89 % in most cases of ED, regardless of etiology (Coombs et al. 2012). These are vasoactive drugs that are injected directly into the corpora, causing erection as the smooth muscles of the arterioles and the cavernous trabeculae relax. Intracavernosal injections may be effective in those patients who have failed intraurethral or oral therapies.

Medications most commonly used in injection therapy are papaverine hydrochloride, phentolamine, prostaglandin (PGE1), and/or atropine. These agents are injected in bimix, trimix, or quadmix solutions and are available through compounding pharmacies and various urology clinics. Even though these agents have been available since the 1980s and documentation of efficacy is well established, they are not approved by the FDA and commonly injected mixtures are only available through an accredited compounding pharmacy. The injectable form of alprostadil (Edex® or Caverject®) is the only FDA-approved injectable agent for ED. All of these medications are used in parenteral form and require the patient to self-administer intracavernosal injections. Patient education is the key to penile injections. The patient must understand the need to rotate injection sites to prevent fibrosis or plaque. Adverse effects include penile pain, priapism, fibrosis, facial flushing, dizziness, hematoma, and ecchymosis. Injections are contraindicated in those patients with penile implants, have a hypersensitivity to prostaglandins, or have a condition that would predispose them to priapism (sickle cell anemia or trait, multiple myeloma, leukemia, hypervaricosity, thrombocytopenia, polycythemia, and those prone to venous thrombus) (Auxillium Pharmaceuticals Inc. 2011). The patient should press over the injection site for 5 min after removing the needle (especially if using any type of anticoagulant therapy or aspirin).

Penile injections may be used up to 3 times/week and never more than once in a 24 h period (even if the injection is not effective, the patient should be instructed not to re-inject related to the risk of priapism). In some older patients, the effect of intracavernous agents seems to decline with time. The erection occurs with or without sexual stimulation. To decrease pain or burning associated with alprostadil, the patient may take acetaminophen 30–45 min before injection. It is important to teach patients what to do in case of priapism and to provide an information card to carry them in case of emergency (American Urological Association's Guidelines for treating priapism). One-on-one teaching and in-office trial of the first self-injection for the patient and/or partner is essential to success with penile injections. The NP should encourage partners to be involved in the learning process. Take-home educational materials should be utilized during face-to-face visits, as well as return demonstration of self-injection technique after instruction. Written and video instruction are available for both FDA-approved injectables via the website for each medication and can be accessed and studied before the self-injection visit to help the patient prepare for the process.

Intraurethral Therapy

Alprostadil may also be introduced intrauretrally in the form of a semisolid pellet that is partially absorbed into the surrounding corpora cavernosa. MUSE® is an intraurethral suppository containing alprostadil, which is a form of prostaglandin E1. It is inserted from within a special plastic applicator into the distal urethra. MUSE® is less invasive with a lower risk of priapism as compared to injection therapy. MUSE® is contraindicated in patients with a hypersensitivity to alprostadil or prostaglandins, and anyone who has a condition that would predispose them to priapism (sickle cell anemia, leukemia or multiple myeloma); patient with anatomical deformity of the penis (curvature, fibrosis, severe hypospadias).

MUSE® should not be used for sexual activity with pregnant women. Almost 10 % of female partners report symptoms of vaginitis following exposure to intraurethral alprostadil. Adverse effects include urethral irritation, bleeding, or pain in pelvis or upper thighs (Meda Pharmaceuticals Inc 2014).

Initial dosing should take place in the office setting. Patients should be monitored for syncope and hypotension secondary to orthostatis. The use of a Venoseal® band (constriction device) may increase absorption and help maintain the erection. Stress, anxiety, or the consumption of alcohol may reduce the efficacy of MUSE®. The patient should be given written, verbal, and video instructions prior to dosing. The NP should encourage partners to be involved in the patient education process.

Third-Line Therapy

Penile Implant

Penile prostheses were first introduced in the 1970s and are considered the final treatment for ED after less invasive treatments have failed. Penile prostheses are available in two forms: malleable or inflatable devices. The malleable implant is always semirigid, while the inflatable implant can be inflated or deflated. The inflatable implant is the most popular device and most consist of two cylinders that are implanted into the corpora cavernosa area, a reservoir for the fluid, and a pump mechanism which dwells within the scrotum. The pump is used to move the fluid into the chambers in the penis for intercourse and the release mechanism on the pump is used to deflate the chambers and return fluid to the reservoir after sex. This option is highly invasive, irreversible, and should be reserved for select cases failing other treatment modalities. Following surgery, other medical therapies will no longer be effective in producing erection due to the damage of the corporal bodies by the prosthesis. These devices produce a natural erection with a high degree of patient and partner satisfaction but are only available in specialized medical centers and costly. A 4- to 8-week postoperative recovery period is necessary before the prosthesis can be used for sexual intercourse (American Urological Association 2005). Outcomes are not guaranteed, and surgical risk is associated with this procedure. The patient and his partner should be informed that penile prosthesis implantation may preclude subsequent use of a vacuum device or vasoactive injection therapy. Complications include erosion, infection, and mechanical failure. When these occur, the prosthesis must be surgically removed. After erosion or infection has resolved, a new prosthesis may be placed; however, a second surgery is technically more difficult and results may be less satisfactory.

Vascular Surgery

Young men with vascular insufficiency may benefit from surgical revascularization. Microvascular arterial bypass and venous ligation may increase arterial inflow and decrease venous outflow. Surgical revascularization is an expensive option and available only in large medical centers. Patients must be evaluated with specialized testing by an experienced surgeon.

Penile Rehabilitation

Men who undergo radiation therapy or surgical intervention such as radical prostatectomy for prostate cancer treatment will experience changes in erectile function. These changes can be attributed to a cascade of events that affect normal erectile function. The overall effect is a loss of smooth muscle tissue, increase in corporal collagen formation, and an increase in fibrosis leading to erectile dysfunction. Vascular changes caused by arterial injury result in ischemic and hypoxic insult which may cause penile shortening up to 2 cm. Neuropraxia or damage to the cavernosal nerve is triggered by mechanical stretch during the procedure, thermal injury from cautery, and inflammation attributed to surgical trauma or ischemia from the vascular injury (Rabbani et al. 2010). Men post radical prostatectomy should understand that the erectile recovery may take up to 2 or more years (Rabbani et al. 2010).

Some men with prostate cancer undergo external beam radiation therapy (EBRT) or brachytherapy as opposed to surgical intervention. Both treatments are associated with delayed and progressive onset of ED (Stember and Mulhall 2012). Similar to radical prostatectomy, the most common long-term adverse effect of radiation therapy is ED. The mechanism of injury is due to damage done postradiation exposure leading to vascular changes, neurogenic injury and structural changes resulting in fibrosis, increased collagen formation, damage to the smooth muscle tissue, and ultimately an inability to obtain or maintain a rigid erection (Stember and Mulhall 2012).

Treatment options for penile rehabilitation are similar for men undergoing radical prostatectomy or radiation therapy. Multiple factors should be taken into consideration when determining the likelihood of restoring erectile function after prostate cancer treatment. Most importantly, the NP must consider the patient's preoperative erectile function as previous erectile dysfunction is a factor in erectile recovery post treatment. In addition, other important factors are age and the presence of comorbid conditions, such as diabetes, hypertension, hyperlipidemia, cardiovascular disease, and neurological disorders. Pretreatment assessment of erectile function should be initially assessed through the use of the Sexual Health Inventory for Men (SHIM/

IIEF5) or the international Index of Erectile Functioning (IIEF) (Rosen et al. 1999; Shamloul and Ghanem 2013). Men with comorbid conditions or those who have utilized medications for erectile dysfunction prior to prostate cancer therapy, such as an oral agent are at greater risk for worsened erectile dysfunction post prostate cancer treatment (McCullough 2001).

Penile rehabilitation involves early intervention with the PDE-5 inhibitors, vacuum constriction devices (VCDs), intraurethral suppositories, and penile injections to improve erectile function; however, further research is needed to validate long-term outcomes (Tal et al. 2011). The ultimate goal of penile rehabilitation is to preserve preoperative erectile function by establishing regular blood flow to the penis to enhance erectile response. During the period of neuropraxia following radical prostatectomy, the lack of blood flow and smooth muscle activity during erections and subsequent tumescence, can lead to atrophic structural changes. Penile rehabilitation is accomplished by trying to reduce the complications of prostate cancer therapies through preserving endothelial cell function, reducing the development of fibrosis, venous leakage, and penile shortening by encouraging regular erectile activity using medical treatments (McCullough 2008; Mulhall 2008; Padma-Nathan et al. 2008). The International Consensus of Sexual Medicine (ICSM) 2001 concluded that early intervention after prostate cancer treatment improves long-term penile tissue recovery (Mulhall et al. 2010).

PDE-5 inhibitors are considered first-line therapy and work at the cellular level to preserve endothelial cell function, improve cavernosal oxygenation, decrease apoptotic cell death, and decrease corporal fibrosis and collagen production (Tal et al. 2011). Many protocols recommend nightly use, while others suggest 2–3 times/week which is expensive and not often covered by insurance plans. The failure rate of PDE-5 inhibitors early after radical prostatectomy has been reported to be 69–80 % (Blander et al. 2000; Mydlo et al. 2005). The use of oral agents for penile rehabilitation has produced mixed research results. Padma-Nathan et al. (2008) demonstrated in a study of 76 men after nerve-sparring radical prostatectomy that 4 % of the men taking placebo reported an erection sufficient for sexual activity versus 27 % of men taking sildenafil 50 or 100 mg. Another research demonstrated improvement in nocturnal penile tumescence with nightly sildenafil (Montorsi et al. 2000). Subsequent large, multicenter, placebo-controlled studies have failed to demonstrate benefit from regular use of PDE-5 inhibitors for penile rehabilitation (Montorsi et al. 2000, 2008; Pavlovich et al. 2013).

Vacuum constriction devices (VCDs) can be used for penile rehabilitation, the vacuum pulls venous and arterial blood into the corpora bringing the PO_2 levels to 80 mmHg, thus providing improved oxygenation of penile tissue and reducing the risk of collagen formation and fibrosis (Mazzola and Mulhall 2011). Regular VCD use post prostatectomy may prevent penile shrinkage in both length and girth (Pahlajani et al. 2012). Post-prostatectomy patients reported improved erectile function and less penile shrinkage after using the vacuum device (Raina et al. 2006). An additional study by Kohler et al. revealed that early intervention with the vacuum constriction device was associated with a higher IIEF score and reduced penile shrinkage (Kohler et al. 2007). A study suggests improved results are achieved with a combination of sildenafil and a VCD; this combination resulted in almost a third of the men reporting return of spontaneous erections and improved satisfaction compared to therapy with oral medications or the vacuum device alone (Raina et al. 2005).

Alprostadil (MUSE) increases arterial flow to the corpora suppressing collagen synthesis and most likely preventing fibrosis. Rehabilitation protocols vary from nightly use to 3×/week with dose ranges of 125–250 mcg. McCullough (2008) found that 125–250 mcg of alprostadil improved cavernosal oxygen saturation, although these men often did not experience penile rigidity.

Intracavernosal injections increase blood flow to penile tissues resulting in increased oxygenation, preservation of endothelial cells, and reduction of permanent erectile damage. Intracavernosal injections produce an erection sufficient for sexual intercourse in men post prostatectomy, and also improve return of spontaneous erections. Montorsi et al. (1997) conducted a study in men who had undergone bilateral nerve-sparing radical prostatectomy. Fifteen men received intracavernosal alprostadil 3 times/week for a 12-week period and 15 men received no injections. The results revealed that men performing injection therapy experienced a 67 % return of spontaneous erections which were sufficient for intercourse versus a 20 % return of spontaneous erections of those receiving no treatment (Montorsi et al. 1997). Raina et al. (2008) reported that 56 % (10 of 18 patients) who had used a combination of either oral agents or injections of alprostadil experienced a return of partial erection at approximately 6 months, but required additional treatment in order to engage in sexual intercourse (Raina et al. 2008). Mulhall et al. (2005) conducted a study with a penile rehabilitation regimen that began with regular use of oral PDE-5 inhibitors. If oral agents were not working, the participants advanced to using penile injections regularly. If patients failed to respond to oral agents, they were treated with intracavernosal injections. The rehabilitation group was compared to a similar group of men who choose to not do penile rehabilitation. After 18 months, the men receiving rehabilitation treatment ($n = 58$) had a greater percentage of men able to engage in intercourse without medication compared to the men who did not do rehabilitation [$n = 74$, 52 % versus 19 %, $p < 0.001$] (Mulhall et al. 2005). There are no published reports of controlled trials using injection therapy.

A challenge when using penile injections for penile rehabilitation is convincing patients to self-inject 3 times/week, since injections are perceived as invasive and associated with pain early after radical prostatectomy. Although patients were told to do injections 3 times/week, Albaugh and Ferrans (2010) found that most men in their study did not follow the recommended protocol and only injected an average of once per week. Oral agents, intraurethral suppositories, VCDs, and penile injections all have pros and cons and may not be appealing to all patients. In addition, there is a high dropout rate related to various factors even when optimal results were achieved. The International

Consensus of Sexual Medicine (ICSM) 2001 committee failed to recognize a specific regimen that is preferred for penile rehabilitation (Mulhall et al. 2010). Although current research shows that working closely with each individual man to encourage regular blood flow to the penis early after prostate treatment for erectile function preservation, further research is needed to evaluate each treatment option and the role it plays in penile rehabilitation.

Erectile dysfunction is a common adverse effect of radical prostatectomy or radiation therapy, the effects of which can be severe for both the patient and their partner. Penile rehabilitation can be initiated as an attempt to preserve pre-prostate cancer treatment erectile function. Several medical treatments can be used for penile rehabilitation to encourage improved erectile response and increased blood flow into the penis including oral agents (PDE-5 inhibitors), the vacuum constriction device, intraurethral alprostadil, and/or penile injections. The ideal strategy, personalized to the individual patient, would involve using various treatment modalities in both the peri- and postoperative periods to maximally enhance erectile recovery. When counseling patients about treatment options, realistic expectations should be provided by the NP. Further research is needed to determine the best strategies to individualize rehabilitation regimens for patients.

Follow-Up of Erectile Dysfunction

As with any treatment plan, regular follow-up visits are necessary to evaluate the treatment and progress of therapy. Modifying risk factors may facilitate erection directly or improve response to ED treatments. Patients should be evaluated 1 month after initiation of treatment; during the visit, a brief history along with administration of standardized scales such as the SHIM may be used to evaluate erectile function. Although PDE-5 inhibitors are effective, safe, and well tolerated, they are often used suboptimally, and patient discontinuation rates are substantial. Patients may need additional assistance and information or wish to try another treatment option. Switching to a different PDE-5 inhibitor is another option for nonresponders. For example, a study revealed that one-third of patients who failed sildenafil therapy achieved normal erectile function after switching to vardenafil (Carson et al. 2004). Regular follow-up promotes long-term adherence and optimizes treatment outcomes (including patient and partner satisfaction) by assessing effectiveness and tolerability and making any needed "mid-course adjustments" in treatment expectations (Jensen and Burnett 2002). At follow-up visits, NPs should ask their patients (and/or partners) "Were you satisfied with your erection (or the sexual experience)?" Early success may increase the likelihood that a patient will continue treatment (Table 4.1).

Table 4.1 Erectile Dysfunction Treatment

Drug/onset/duration	Dosage	Contraindications	More common side effects	Teaching/instruction
Sildenafil (Viagra)®	25, 50, 100 mg PO	Absolutely contraindicated with nitrates including amyl nitrates (poppers) Contraindicated in patients with retinitis pigmentosa Known hypersensitivity to medication See full list of precautions and drug interactions in prescribing information	Headache, dyspepsia, visual changes (bright, blurred or blue), often described as a "blue halo," flushing, nasal congestion, dizziness	Take on empty stomach or 2 h after eating Works only in presence of sexual stimulation Not approved for females Does not protect against STIs Use no more than once in a 24 h period Take at least 60 min or more prior to sexual activity May need multiple attempts for optimal results Excessive alcohol intake can cause orthostatic hypotension and tachycardia
Vardenafil (Levitra)® (Staxyn)®	5, 10, 20 mg PO 10 mg only (orally disintegrating tablet)	Absolutely contraindicated with nitrates including amyl nitrates (poppers) Use with caution in men with unstable angina and ischemic CV disease, QT interval- slight prolongation – precaution in labeling Contraindicated in patients with retinitis pigmentosa Known hypersensitivity to medication See full list of precautions and drug interactions in prescribing information	Headache, dyspepsia, flushing, nasal congestion, dizziness	Although it can be taken with food, food and fat may delay absorption Not approved for females Does not protect against STIs Use no more than once in a 24 h period Take 60 min or more prior to sexual activity May need multiple attempts for optimal results Works only in presence of sexual stimulation Excessive alcohol intake can cause orthostatic hypotension and tachycardia

(continued)

Table 4.1 (continued)

Drug/onset/duration	Dosage	Contraindications	More common side effects	Teaching/instruction
Tadalafil (Cialis)® Long half-life	5, 10, 20 mg PO	Cannot be taken with nitrates or nitric oxide donor, patients with MI in last 90 days, unstable angina, class 2 heart failure, uncontrolled arrhythmias, hypotension, HTN, or stroke within 6 months. Known hypersensitivity to drug See full list of precautions and drug interactions in prescribing information	Headache, dyspepsia, flushing, nasal congestion, dizziness, myalgias, back pain	Although it can be taken with food, food and fat may delay absorption Improved spontaneity Does not protect against STIs Do not use more than 20 mg in a 24 h period Take 60 min or more prior to sexual activity May need multiple attempts for optimal results No effect on libido, ejaculation, or orgasm Works only in presence of sexual stimulation Excessive alcohol intake can cause orthostatic hypotension and tachycardia
Daily dosing with steady state within 5 days	2.5–5 mg PO			
Avanafil (Stendra)®	50–200 mg PO	Absolutely contraindicated with nitrates including amyl nitrates (poppers) Patients taking CY3A4 inhibitors (ketoconazole, clarithromycin, ritonavir, nefazodone, etc.) Safety is unknown in patients with bleeding disorders and those with active peptic ulceration Known hypersensitivity to drug See full list of precautions and drug interactions in prescribing information	Headache, flushing, nasal stuffiness/congestion, back pain	No food restriction, large meals may decrease absorption, improved results if taken on empty stomach. Not approved for use in females Provides no protection from STIs. Use no more than once in a 24 hours Take 20–40 min prior to sexual activity May need multiple attempts for optimal results No effect on libido, ejaculation, or orgasm Works only in presence of sexual stimulation Excessive alcohol intake can cause orthostatic hypotension with hypotension and tachycardia

Venoseal® 30 min duration maximum	NA	Latex or rubber hypersensitivity Precautions: abnormally formed penis, sickle cell anemia, leukemia, tumor of bone marrow or conditions that increase or decrease blood clotting	Ecchymosis, petechiae, numbness of the penis, pain, pulling of scrotal tissue, blocked or painful ejaculation	Remove after 30 min Allow 60 min period before reapplying
Vacuum therapy	NA	No contraindications Precautions: history of priapism, sickle cell, bleeding disorders	Hematoma, ecchymosis, petechiae, numbness of the penis, pain, pulling of scrotal tissue, blocked or painful ejaculation	Requires thorough initial instruction, good dexterity, water-soluble gel and reconditioning for up to 2 weeks Do not use the tension ring for more than 30 minutes maximum
MUSE® Onset 5–10 min Duration 30–60 min	125, 250, 500, 1000 mcg	Hypersensitivity to drug Abnormally formed penis Conditions causing prolonged erections like sickle cell, leukemia, tumor of bone marrow Not for intercourse with pregnant women without a barrier	Penile and urethral pain Warmth or burning in the urethra Erythema of the penis Hypotension Lightheadedness/dizziness Vaginal burning	First dose must be administered in clinic in accordance with prescribing information related to dizziness, lightheadedness, and hypotension Check HR and BP before and after trail dose. Physical activity is necessary to improve blood flow after dose is administered (i.e., walking) Refrigerate unopened package Can be kept at room temp for up to 14 days at < 86 degrees

(continued)

Table 4.1 (continued)

Drug/onset/duration	Dosage	Contraindications	More common side effects	Teaching/instruction
Intracavernosal injection FDA-approved Alprostadil Off label Compounded Trimix: papaverine/ phentolamine/ prostaglandin E1 or Bimix: papaverine/ phentolamine	2.5–40 mcg Or as prescribed with compounds in units	Hypersensivity to drug Conditions that may lead to priapism like sickle cell, multiple myeloma, leukemia, deformed penis Penile implants Inability to visualize the penis for injections related to central obesity	Pain Injection site bleeding or bruising Priapism (prolonged erection) Peyronie's disease (curvature) due to fibrosis	Comprehensive one-on-one teaching In office titration of first dose; start low and titrate slow to avoid priapism Store at or below 77° Single use item Rotate sites, avoid visible veins Press over injection site for 5 min after injection with alcohol wipe Once in 24 h, 3 times/week maximum use Provide very specific instruction in case priapism occurs
Penile implant	NA	Poor surgical risk	Infection Erosion Mechanical failure Following surgery, other medical therapies will no long be effective due to damage of corporal bodies	Invasive Expensive Provide pre- and postoperative teaching 4–8 weeks postoperative recovery period Provide specific instructions for operating the device

Conclusion

ED is a common disorder that is frequently underreported and under treated in clinical practice. It is important for NPs to screen for ED in at-risk patients to identify individuals who may benefit from treatment and/or have other serious conditions. NPs can play an integral role in the identification, assessment, treatment and follow up of erectile dysfunction. Diagnosis may lead to early recognition of other comorbidities, such as diabetes, vascular disease, and hormone deficiency. Most medical treatment can be initiated in the primary care setting, those patients requiring more complex treatment should be referred. The mounting body of clinical and basic science research strongly suggests that ED is a harbinger and very early warning sign of incipient endothelial dysfunction and associated vascular damage (Billups et al. 2005, 2008). The recognition of ED as a precursor of systemic CVD represents a significant opportunity for prevention. Future large-scale, longitudinal studies that prospectively monitor cardiovascular risk and emergent disease in young men with ED will ultimately support aggressive diagnostic and treatment recommendations.

There are multiple treatment options for men with ED, as with all therapies there are specific advantages and disadvantages inherent to the method of treatment. The NP can play a critical role in affecting treatment outcomes through patient education and facilitation of therapy.

Sexual Health Inventory for Men (SHIM)

Patient Instructions

Sexual health is an important part of an individual's overall physical and emotional well-being. Erectile dysfunction, also known as impotence, is one type of a very common medical condition affecting sexual health. Fortunately, there are many different treatment options for erectile dysfunction. This questionnaire is designed to help you and your provider identify if you may be experiencing erectile dysfunction.

Each question has several possible responses. Circle the number of the response that best describes your own situation. Please be sure that you select one and only one response for each question.

Over the Past 6 Months

1. How do you rate your confidence that you could get and keep an erection?

1	2	3	4	5
Very low	Low	Moderate	High	Very high

2. When you had erections with sexual stimulation, how often were they hard enough for penetration?

0	1	2	3	4	5
No sexual activity	Almost never/never	A few times	Sometimes	Most times	Almost always/always

3. During sexual intercourse, how often were you able to maintain an erection after penetration?

0	1	2	3	4	5
Did not attempt	Almost never/never	A few times	Sometimes	Most times	Almost always/always

4. How difficult was it to maintain your erection to the completion of intercourse?

0	1	2	3	4	5
Did not attempt	Extremely difficult	Very difficult	Difficult	Slightly difficult	Not difficult

5. How often was sexual intercourse satisfactory to you?

0	1	2	3	4	5
Did not attempt	Almost never/never	A few times	Sometimes	Most times	Almost always/always

Total Score: _____

Scoring Key:

22–25: No ED	**12–16**: Mild-to-moderate ED	**1–7**: Severe ED
17–21: Mild ED	**8–11**: Moderate ED	

Used with permission from Rosen et al. (1999).

References

Akpunona AZ, Mutgi AB, Federman DJ (1994) Routine prolactin measurement is not necessary in the initial evaluation of male impotence. J Gen Intern Med 9:336–338

Albaugh JA, Ferrans CE (2010) Impact of penile injections on men with erectile dysfunction after prostatectomy. Urol Nurs 30(1):64–77

Albaugh J, Amargo I, Capelson R, Flaherty E, Forest C, Goldstein I, Jensen PK, Jones K, Kloner R, Lewis J, Mullin S, Payton T, Rines B, Rosen R, Sadovsky R, Snow K, Vetrosky D, University of Medicine and Dentistry of New Jersey (2002) Health care clinicians in sexual health medicine: focus on erectile dysfunction. Urol Nurs 22(4):217–231; quiz 232

American Urological Association (2005) Management of erectile dysfunction, 3rd edn. Retrieved 15 Oct 2015, from http://www.auanet.org/content/guidelines-and-quality-care/clinical-guidelines.cfm?sub=ed

Andersen I, Heitmann BL, Wagner G (2008) Obesity and sexual dysfunction in younger Danish men. J Sex Med 5(9):2053–2060. doi:10.1111/j.1743-6109.2008.00920.x

Androshchuk V, Pugh N, Wood A, Ossei-Gerning N (2015) Erectile dysfunction: a window to the heart. BMJ Case Rep. doi:10.1136/bcr-2015-210124

Annon JS (1974) The behavioral treatment of sexual problems, 1st edn. Kapiolani Health Services, Honolulu

Araujo AB, Durante R, Feldman HA, Goldstein I, McKinlay JB (1998) The relationship between depressive symptoms and male erectile dysfunction: cross-sectional results from the Massachusetts Male Aging Study. Psychosom Med 60(4):458–465

Auxillium Pharmaceuticals Inc. (2011) Edex. Retrieved 2015, from http://www.edex.com/_assets/pdf/prescribing_information.pdf

Bacon CG, Mittleman MA, Kawachi I, Giovannucci E, Glasser DB, Rimm EB (2003) Sexual function in men older than 50 years of age: results from the health professionals follow-up study. Ann Intern Med 139(3):161–168

Billups K, Friedrich S (2005) Assessment of fasting lipid panels and Doppler ultrasound testing in men presenting with erectile dysfunction and no other medical problem. Am J Cardiol 96(Suppl):57M–61M

Billups KL, Bank AJ, Padma-Nathan H, Katz S, Williams R (2005) Erectile dysfunction is a marker for cardiovascular disease: results of the minority health institute expert advisory panel. J Sex Med 2(1):40–50. doi:10.1111/j.1743-6109.2005.20104_1.x; discussion 50–52

Billups KL, Bank AJ, Padma-Nathan H, Katz SD, Williams RA (2008) Erectile dysfunction as a harbinger for increased cardiometabolic risk. Int J Impot Res 20(3):236–242. doi:10.1038/sj.ijir.3901634

Blander DS, Sanchez-Ortiz RF, Wein AJ, Broderick GA (2000) Efficacy of sildenafil in erectile dysfunction after radical prostatectomy. Int J Impot Res 12(3):165–168

Boyle P (1999) Epidemiology of erectile dysfunction. In: Carson C, Kirby RS, Goldstein I (eds) Textbook of erectile dysfunction. ISIS Medical Media, Oxford, pp 15–29

Braun MH, Sommer F, Haupt G, Mathers MJ, Reifenrath B, Engelmann UH (2003) Lower urinary tract symptoms and erectile dysfunction: co-morbidity or typical "Aging Male" symptoms? Results of the "Cologne Male Survey". Eur Urol 44(5):588–594

Cappelleri JC, Rosen RC (2005) The Sexual Health Inventory for Men (SHIM): a 5-year review of research and clinical experience. Int J Impot Res 17(4):307–319. doi:10.1038/sj.ijir.3901327

Carson C, McMahon C (2008) Fast facts: erectile dysfunction, 4th edn. Health Press, Ocford

Carson CC, Hatzichristou DG, Carrier S, Lording D, Lyngdorf P, Aliotta P, Auerbach S, Murdock M, Wilkins HJ, McBride TA, Colopy MW, Patient Response with Vardenafil in Slidenafil Non-Responders Study Group (2004) Erectile response with vardenafil in sildenafil nonresponders: a multicentre, double-blind, 12-week, flexible-dose, placebo-controlled erectile dysfunction clinical trial. BJU Int 94(9):1301–1309. doi:10.1111/j.1464-410X.2004.05161.x

Carson CC, Kirby RS, Goldstein I, Wyllie MG (eds) (2009) Textbook of erectile dysfunction, 2nd edn. Informa Healthcare, New York

Cherry DK, Woodwell DA (2002) National ambulatory medical care survey: 2000 summary. Adv Data (328):1–32

Coombs PG, Heck M, Guhring P, Narus J, Mulhall JP (2012) A review of outcomes of an intracavernosal injection therapy programme. BJU Int 110(11):1787–1791. doi:10.1111/j.1464-410X.2012.11080.x

Corona G, Mannucci E, Mansani R, Petrone L, Bartolini M, Giommi R, Forti G, Maggi M (2004) Organic, relational and psychological factors in erectile dysfunction in men with diabetes mellitus. Eur Urol 46(2):222–228. doi:10.1016/j.eururo.2004.03.010

Derby CA, Mohr BA, Goldstein I, Feldman HA, Johannes CB, McKinlay JB (2000) Modifiable risk factors and erectile dysfunction: can lifestyle changes modify risk? Urology 56(2):302–306

Eardley I (2013) The incidence, prevalence, and natural history of erectile dysfunction. Sex Med Rev 1(1):3–16. doi:10.1002/smrj.2

Esposito K, Giugliano F, Di Palo C, Giugliano G, Marfella R, D'Andrea F, D'Armiento M, Giugliano D (2004) Effect of lifestyle changes on erectile dysfunction in obese men: a randomized controlled trial. JAMA 291(24):2978–2984. doi:10.1001/jama.291.24.2978

Federal Drug Administration (2007) FDA announces revisions to labels for Cialis, Levitra, and Viagra: potential risk of sudden hearing loss with ED drugs to be displayed more prominently. Retrieved 1 July 2015, from www.fda.gov/NewsEvents/Newsroom/PressAnnouncements/2007/ucm109012.htm

Feldman HA, Goldstein I, Hatzichristou DG, Krane RJ, McKinlay JB (1994) Impotence and its medical and psychosocial correlates: results of the Massachusetts Male Aging Study. J Urol 151(1):54–61

Feldman HA, Longcope C, Derby CA, Johannes CB, Araujo AB, Coviello AD, Bremner WJ, McKinlay JB (2002) Age trends in the level of serum testosterone and other hormones in middle-aged men: longitudinal results from the Massachusetts male aging study. J Clin Endocrinol Metabol 87(2):589–598. doi:10.1210/jcem.87.2.8201

Gratzke C, Angulo J, Chitaley K, Dai YT, Kim NN, Paick JS, Simonsen U, Uckert S, Wespes E, Andersson KE, Lue TF, Stief CG (2010) Anatomy, physiology, and pathophysiology of erectile dysfunction. J Sex Med 7(1 Pt 2):445–475. doi:10.1111/j.1743-6109.2009.01624.x

Grover SA, Lowensteyn I, Kaouache M, Marchand S, Coupal L, DeCarolis E, Zoccoli J, Defoy I (2006) The prevalence of erectile dysfunction in the primary care setting: importance of risk factors for diabetes and vascular disease. Arch Intern Med 166(2):213–219. doi:10.1001/archinte.166.2.213

Guay AT, Perez JB, Jacobson J, Newton RA (2001) Efficacy and safety of sildenafil citrate for treatment of erectile dysfunction in a population with associated organic risk factors. J Androl 22(5):793–797

Gupta BP, Murad MH, Clifton MM, Prokop L, Nehra A, Kopecky SL (2011) The effect of lifestyle modification and cardiovascular risk factor reduction on erectile dysfunction: a systematic review and meta-analysis. Arch Intern Med 171(20):1797–1803. doi:10.1001/archinternmed.2011.440

Hatzichristou DG, Apostolidis A, Tzortzis V, Ioannides E, Yannakoyorgos K, Kalinderis A (2000) Sildenafil versus intracavernous injection therapy: efficacy and preference in patients on intracavernous injection for more than 1 year. J Urol 164(4):1197–1200

Hatzimouratidis K, Hatzichristou D (2007) Phosphodiesterase type 5 inhibitors: the day after. Eur Urol 51(1):75–88. doi:10.1016/j.eururo.2006.07.020; discussion 89

Inman BA, Sauver JL, Jacobson DJ, McGree ME, Nehra A, Lieber MM, Roger VL, Jacobsen
SJ (2009) A population-based, longitudinal study of erectile dysfunction and future coronary
artery disease. Mayo Clin Proc 84(2):108–113. doi:10.4065/84.2.108

Jackson G, Rosen RC, Kloner RA, Kostis JB (2006) The second Princeton consensus on sexual
dysfunction and cardiac risk: new guidelines for sexual medicine. J Sex Med 3(1):28–36.
doi:10.1111/j.1743-6109.2005.00196.x; discussion 36

Jankowski JT, Seftel AD, Strohl KP (2008) Erectile dysfunction and sleep related disorders. J Urol
179(3):837–841. doi:10.1016/j.juro.2007.10.024

Jensen PK, Burnett JK (2002) Erectile dysfunction. Primary care treatment is appropriate and
essential. Adv Nurse Pract 10(4):45–47, 51–52

Jensen PK, Lewis J, Jones KB (2004) Improving erectile function: incorporating new guidelines
into clinical practice. Adv Nurse Pract 12(4):40–50

Jones RW, Rees RW, Minhas S, Ralph D, Persad RA, Jeremy JY (2002) Oxygen free radicals and
the penis. Expert Opin Pharmacother 3(7):889–897

Kaplan SA, Gonzalez RR (2007) Phosphodiesterase type 5 inhibitors for the treatment of male
lower urinary tract symptoms. Rev Urol 9(2):73–77

Kendirici M, Bejma J, Hellstrom WJG (2006) Radical prostatectomy and other pelvic surgeries:
effects on erectile function. In: Mulcahy JJ (ed) Male sexual function: a guide to clinical management, 2nd edn. Humana Press, Totowa, pp 135–154

Kinsey AC, Pomeroy WB, Martin CE (1948) Sexual behavior in the human male. W. B. Saunders,
Philadelphia

Kloner RA, Speakman M (2002) Erectile dysfunction and atherosclerosis. Curr Atheroscler Rep
4(5):397–401

Kohler TS, Pedro R, Hendlin K, Utz W, Ugarte R, Reddy P, Makhlouf A, Ryndin I, Canales BK,
Weiland D, Nakib N, Ramani A, Anderson JK, Monga M (2007) A pilot study on the early use
of the vacuum erection device after radical retropubic prostatectomy. BJU Int 100(4):858–862.
doi:10.1111/j.1464-410X.2007.07161.x

Kolodny RC, Kahn CB, Goldstein HH, Barnett DM (1974) Sexual dysfunction in diabetic men.
Diabetes 23(4):306–309

Kuritzky L, Miner M (2004) Erectile dysfunction assessment and management in primary care
practice. In: Broderick G (ed) Oral pharmacotherapy for male sexual dysfunction. Humana
Press, Totowa, pp 149–183

LaRochelle JC, Levine L (2006) Evaluation of the patient with erectile dysfunction. In: Mulcahy
JJ (ed) Male sexual function: a guide to clinical management, 2nd edn. Humana Press, Totowa,
pp 253–270

Laumann EO, Paik A, Rosen RC (1999a) The epidemiology of erectile dysfunction: results from
the National Health and Social Life Survey. Int J Impot Res 11(Suppl 1):S60–S64

Laumann EO, Paik A, Rosen RC (1999b) Sexual dysfunction in the United States: prevalence and
predictors. JAMA 281(6):537–544

Liu L, Zheng S, Han P, Wei Q (2011) Phosphodiesterase-5 inhibitors for lower urinary tract
symptoms secondary to benign prostatic hyperplasia: a systematic review and meta-analysis.
Urology 77(1):123–129. doi:10.1016/j.urology.2010.07.508

Lue TF (2000) Erectile dysfunction. N Engl J Med 342(24):1802–1813. doi:10.1056/
NEJM200006153422407

Matsumoto AM (2002) Andropause: clinical implications of the decline in serum testosterone
levels with aging in men. J Gerontol A Biol Sci Med Sci 57:M76–M99

Mazzola C, Mulhall JP (2011) Penile rehabilitation after prostate cancer treatment: outcomes and
practical algorithm. Urol Clin N Am 38(2):105–118. doi:10.1016/j.ucl.2011.03.002

McCullough AR (2001) Prevention and management of erectile dysfunction following radical
prostatectomy. Urol Clin North Am 28(3):613–627

McCullough AR (2003) The penis as a barometer of endothelial health. Rev Urol 5(Suppl 7):S3–S8

McCullough AR (2008) Rehabilitation of erectile function following radical prostatectomy. Asian
J Androl 10(1):61–74. doi:10.1111/j.1745-7262.2008.00366.x

McMahon CG (2004) Efficacy and safety of daily tadalafil in men with erectile dysfunction previously unresponsive to on-demand tadalafil. J Sex Med 1:292–300

Meda Pharmaceuticals Inc. (2014) MUSE full prescribing information. Retrieved 23 Oct 2016, from http://www.muserx.com/hcp/global/full-prescribing-information.aspx

Montague DK, Jarrow JP, Broderick GA, Dmochoski RR, Heaton JP, Lue TF, Milbank AJ, Nehra A, Sharlip ID (2005) Erectile dysfunction guideline update panel: the management of erectile dysfunction. J Urol 174(1):230–239

Montorsi F, Guazzoni G, Strambi LF, Da Pozzo LF, Nava L, Barbieri L, Rigatti P, Pizzini G, Miani A (1997) Recovery of spontaneous erectile function after nerve-sparing radical retropubic prostatectomy with and without early intracavernous injections of alprostadil: results of a prospective, randomized trial. J Urol 158(4):1408–1410

Montorsi F, Maga T, Strambi LF, Salonia A, Barbieri L, Scattoni V, Guazzoni G, Losa A, Rigatti P, Pizzini G (2000) Sildenafil taken at bedtime significantly increases nocturnal erections: results of a placebo-controlled study. Urology 56(6):906–911

Montorsi F, Brock G, Lee J, Shapiro J, Van Poppel H, Graefen M, Stief C (2008) Effect of nightly versus on-demand vardenafil on recovery of erectile function in men following bilateral nerve-sparing radical prostatectomy. Eur Urol 54(4):924–931. doi:10.1016/j.eururo.2008.06.083

Mulhall JP (2008) Penile rehabilitation following radical prostatectomy. Curr Opin Urol 18(6):613–620. doi:10.1097/MOU.0b013e3283136462

Mulhall J, Land S, Parker M, Waters WB, Flanigan RC (2005) The use of an erectogenic pharmacotherapy regimen following radical prostatectomy improves recovery of spontaneous erectile function. J Sex Med 2(4):532–540. doi:10.1111/j.1743-6109.2005.00081_1.x; discussion 540–542

Mulhall JP, Bella AJ, Briganti A, McCullough A, Brock G (2010) Erectile function rehabilitation in the radical prostatectomy patient. J Sex Med 7(4 Pt 2):1687–1698. doi:10.1111/j.1743-6109.2010.01804.x

Mydlo JH, Viterbo R, Crispen P (2005) Use of combined intracorporal injection and a phosphodiesterase-5 inhibitor therapy for men with a suboptimal response to sildenafil and/or vardenafil monotherapy after radical retropubic prostatectomy. BJU Int 95(6):843–846. doi:10.1111/j.1464-410X.2005.05413.x

Nehra A, Jackson G, Miner M, Billups KL, Burnett AL, Buvat J, Carson CC, Cunningham GR, Ganz P, Goldstein I, Guay AT, Hackett G, Kloner RA, Kostis J, Montorsi P, Ramsey M, Rosen R, Sadovsky R, Seftel AD, Shabsigh R, Vlachopoulos C, Wu FC (2012) The Princeton III Consensus recommendations for the management of erectile dysfunction and cardiovascular disease. Mayo Clin Proc 87(8):766–778. doi:10.1016/j.mayocp.2012.06.015

NIH Consensus Panel on Impotence (1993) Impotence. NIH Consensus Development Panel on Impotence. JAMA 270(1):83–90

Padma-Nathan H, McCullough AR, Levine LA, Lipshultz LI, Siegel R, Montorsi F, Giuliano F, Brock G, Study Group (2008) Randomized, double-blind, placebo-controlled study of postoperative nightly sildenafil citrate for the prevention of erectile dysfunction after bilateral nerve-sparing radical prostatectomy. Int J Impot Res 20(5):479–486. doi:10.1038/ijir.2008.33

Pahlajani G, Raina R, Jones S, Ali M, Zippe C (2012) Vacuum erection devices revisited: its emerging role in the treatment of erectile dysfunction and early penile rehabilitation following prostate cancer therapy. J Sex Med 9(4):1182–1189. doi:10.1111/j.1743-6109.2010.01881.x

Pavlovich CP, Levinson AW, Su LM, Mettee LZ, Feng Z, Bivalacqua TJ, Trock BJ (2013) Nightly vs on-demand sildenafil for penile rehabilitation after minimally invasive nerve-sparing radical prostatectomy: results of a randomized double-blind trial with placebo. BJU Int 112(6):844–851. doi:10.1111/bju.12253

Porst H, Giuliano F, Glina S, Ralph D, Casabe AR, Elion-Mboussa A, Shen W, Whitaker JS (2006) Evaluation of the efficacy and safety of once-a-day dosing of tadalafil 5mg and 10mg in the treatment of erectile dysfunction: results of a multicenter, randomized, double-blind, placebo-controlled trial. Eur Urol 50(2):351–359. doi:10.1016/j.eururo.2006.02.052

Porst H, Burnett A, Brock G, Ghanem H, Giuliano F, Glina S, Hellstrom W, Martin-Morales A, Salonia A, Sharlip I, ISSM Standards Committee for Sexual Medicine (2013) SOP conservative (medical and mechanical) treatment of erectile dysfunction. J Sex Med 10(1):130–171. doi:10.1111/jsm.12023

Pritzker MR (1999) The penile stress test: a window to the hearts of man? Circ J 100(Suppl 1):3751

Rabbani F, Schiff J, Piecuch M, Yunis LH, Eastham JA, Scardino PT, Mulhall JP (2010) Time course of recovery of erectile function after radical retropubic prostatectomy: does anyone recover after 2 years? J Sex Med 7(12):3984–3990. doi:10.1111/j.1743-6109.2010.01969.x

Raina R, Agarwal A, Allamaneni SS, Lakin MM, Zippe CD (2005) Sildenafil citrate and vacuum constriction device combination enhances sexual satisfaction in erectile dysfunction after radical prostatectomy. Urology 65(2):360–364. doi:10.1016/j.urology.2004.09.013

Raina R, Agarwal A, Ausmundson S, Lakin M, Nandipati KC, Montague DK, Mansour D, Zippe CD (2006) Early use of vacuum constriction device following radical prostatectomy facilitates early sexual activity and potentially earlier return of erectile function. Int J Impot Res 18(1):77–81. doi:10.1038/sj.ijir.3901380

Raina R, Pahlajani G, Agarwal A, Zippe CD (2008) Early penile rehabilitation following radical prostatectomy: Cleveland clinic experience. Int J Impot Res 20(2):121–126. doi:10.1038/sj.ijir.3901573

Rhoden EL, Ribeiro EP, Teloken C, Souto CA (2005) Diabetes mellitus is associated with subnormal serum levels of free testosterone in men. BJU Int 96(6):867–870. doi:10.1111/j.1464-410X.2005.05728.x

Rosen RC, Cappelleri JC, Smith MD, Lipsky J, Pena BM (1999) Development and evaluation of an abridged, 5-item version of the International Index of Erectile Function (IIEF-5) as a diagnostic tool for erectile dysfunction. Int J Impot Res 11(6):319–326

Rosen R, Altwein J, Boyle P, Kirby RS, Lukacs B, Meuleman E, O'Leary MP, Puppo P, Robertson C, Giuliano F (2003) Lower urinary tract symptoms and male sexual dysfunction: the multinational survey of the aging male (MSAM-7). Eur Urol 44(6):637–649

Rowland DL, Incrocci L, Slob AK (2005) Aging and sexual response in the laboratory in patients with erectile dysfunction. J Sex Marital Ther 31(5):399–407. doi:10.1080/00926230591006520

Sachs BD (2003) The false organic-psychogenic distinction and related problems in the classification of erectile dysfunction. Int J Impot Res 15(1):72–78. doi:10.1038/sj.ijir.3900952

Sadovsky R, Curtis K (2006) How a primary care clinician approaches erectile dysfunction. In: Mulcahy JJ (ed) Male sexual function: a guide to clinical management, 2nd edn. Humana Press, Totowa, pp 77–104

Seftel AD, Sundi P, Swindle R (2004) The prevalence of hypertension, hyperlipidemia, diabetes mellitus and depression in men with erectile dysfunction. J Urol 171:2341–2345

Selvin E, Burnett AL, Platz EA (2007) Prevalence and risk factors for erectile dysfunction in the US. Am J Med 120(2):151–157. doi:10.1016/j.amjmed.2006.06.010

Sesti C, Florio V, Johnson EG, Kloner RA (2007) The phosphodiesterase-5 inhibitor tadalafil reduces myocardial infarct size. Int J Impot Res 19:55–61

Shabsigh R (2006) Epidemiology of erectile dysfunction. In: Mulcahy JJ (ed) Male sexual function: a guide to clinical management, 2nd edn. Humana Press, Totowa, pp 47–59

Shamloul R, Ghanem H (2013) Erectile dysfunction. Lancet 381(9861):153–165. doi:10.1016/S0140-6736(12)60520-0

Stember DS, Mulhall JP (2012) The concept of erectile function preservation (penile rehabilitation) in the patient after brachytherapy for prostate cancer. Brachytherapy 11(2):87–96. doi:10.1016/j.brachy.2012.01.002

Tal R, Teloken P, Mulhall JP (2011) Erectile function rehabilitation after radical prostatectomy: practice patterns among AUA members. J Sex Med 8(8):2370–2376. doi:10.1111/j.1743-6109.2011.02355.x

Teloken PE, Smith EB, Lodowsky C, Freedom T, Mulhall JP (2006) Defining association between sleep apnea syndrome and erectile dysfunction. Urology 67(5):1033–1037. doi:10.1016/j.urology.2005.11.040

Wespes E, Amar E, Hatzichristou D, Hatzimouratidis K, Montorsi F, Pryor J, Vardi Y, EAU (2006) EAU Guidelines on erectile dysfunction: an update. Eur Urol 49(5):806–815. doi:10.1016/j.eururo.2006.01.028

Zias N, Bezwada V, Gilman S, Chroneou A (2009) Obstructive sleep apnea and erectile dysfunction: still a neglected risk factor? Sleep Breath 13(1):3–10. doi:10.1007/s11325-008-0212-8

Benign Prostatic Hyperplasia

5

Gail M. Briolat

Contents

Objectives
1. Define the pathophysiology, incidence, presenting symptoms, and risk factors of BPH.
2. Discuss assessment techniques associated with BPH.
3. Explain treatment options including pharmacologic, watchful waiting, and surgical.
4. Discuss complications and side effects of treatments options.

Incidence and Epidemiology

Benign prostatic hyperplasia (BPH) is a histologic diagnosis that refers to the proliferation of smooth muscle and epithelial cells within the prostatic transition zone (Djavan and Kazzazi 2012). On autopsy studies BPH was not found in men

G.M. Briolat, ANCP-BC
Michigan Institute of Urology, Michigan Institute of Urology, St Clair Shores, MI, USA
e-mail: gamawo@hotmail.com

© Springer International Publishing Switzerland 2016
M. Lajiness, S. Quallich (eds.), *The Nurse Practitioner in Urology*,
DOI 10.1007/978-3-319-28743-0_5

117

less than 30 years old (Paolone 2010) but is the fourth most common condition in men over 50 years old (Russo and La Croce 2014). It is estimated that greater than 70 % of men between the ages of 60 and 69 suffer from BPH (Parsons 2014), and the incidence in men over 70 years of age is over 80 % (Russo and La Croce 2014). In the United States, greater than 15 million men are affected leading to health-care cost of greater than three billion dollars annually (Sandeep Bagla 2014).

BPH is not life threatening but causes a significant impact on quality of life. Symptoms of BPH lead to loss of sleep, anxiety, depression, decreased mobility, increased falls, and impairment of activities of daily living as well as leisure activities and sexual activity (Gacci and Carini 2014; Parsons 2014). In the last decade, hospitalizations in the United States for acute renal failure secondary to acute urinary retention from BPH have increased (Parsons 2014).

Risk factors for the development of BPH have not been well understood. Studies have suggested a genetic component, racial differences, and possibly half the men under age 60 undergoing surgery for BPH may have an inherited form of the condition. It is thought to be an autosomal dominant trait and first-degree male relatives carry a fourfold increased risk (Presti 2004). Recent studies suggest correlations with obesity, increased animal protein in diets, and decreased exercise as risk factors for developing symptomatic BPH. Increased BMI, body weight, and waist circumference have been associated with increased prostate volume in ultrasound and MRI studies evaluating prostate volume (Parsons 2014). Moderate to vigorous physical activity has been associated with up to 25 % decreased risk of BPH (Parsons 2014). Consuming at least four servings of vegetables daily, lycopene and green tea added to diets have shown a significantly lower risk of BPH (Espinosa 2013).

Pathophysiology

The prostate is composed of three zones of glandular tissue made of stromal and epithelial cells. The three zones are known as the transition, central, and peripheral zones. The prostate is attached superiorly to the bladder neck and inferiorly bound by the urogenital diaphragm, and posteriorly it is next to the rectum and the anterior surface lies against the pubis (Resnick 2003). BPH is an increase in epithelial and stromal cells in the periurethral area leading to the use of the current term "hyperplasia" versus "hypertrophy" in previous literature (Roehrborn 2012). The exact mechanism of the hyperplastic development is not certain but may be caused by epithelial and stromal proliferation or caused by impairment in programmed cell death leading to the cellular hyperplasia (Roehrborn 2012). Testicular androgens are necessary for the development of BPH. Patients castrated prior to puberty or with impaired androgen production do not develop BPH (Roehrborn 2012). At the end of puberty, the prostate gland is approximately 26 g and maintains that weight unless BPH develops (McConnell 1998). More recent studies are suggesting a role of inflammatory cells in the development of BPH. Activated T cells which are capable of producing and secreting growth factors have been found in BPH in humans (Roehrborn 2012). These factors may be contributing to stromal and glandular prostatic growth (Roehrborn 2012).

Table 5.1 LUTS in BPH

Obstructive symptoms – secondary to the obstruction of the bladder outlet from the growing prostate	Irritative symptoms – caused by the effects on the bladder due to prolonged bladder outlet obstruction
Decreased force of urinary stream	Urgency
Hesitancy – trouble starting stream/straining to pass urine	Urge incontinence
Double voiding/post-void dribbling	Frequency
Acute or chronic urinary retention	Nocturia
Feeling of incomplete bladder emptying	
Prolonged micturition	
Overflow incontinence	

Presentation

Symptoms and presentation of patients suffering from BPH include various lower urinary tract symptoms (LUTS). Among the most common symptoms are decreased force of stream, hesitancy, intermittent stream, post-void dribbling, hematuria, and nocturia. As BPH advances and bladder outlet obstruction (BOO) progresses, symptoms of overactive bladder (OAB) such as urgency and frequency may also develop (Wieder 2010). There is little correlation between the overall size of the prostate and the degree of symptoms. Frequency and urgency of symptoms vary from patient to patient. BPH is characterized by a spectrum of obstructive and irritative symptoms, referred to as lower urinary tract symptoms or "LUTS" (See Table 5.1)

History and Physical Examination

In making the diagnosis of BPH, care must be taken to rule out other pathologies of the urinary tract which can exhibit similar symptoms. The first step is obtaining a detailed medical history from the patient. Determine if the patient has any preexisting neurologic disorders such as multiple sclerosis and Parkinson's disease or has had a stroke in the past. Determine if the patient ever experienced any urinary tract trauma or urethral stricture disease. Obtain a history of current prescriptions and over-the-counter medications which may impact bladder emptying such as anticholinergics or regular use of muscle relaxants or narcotics. Determine if the patient has chronic constipation (Thomas Anthony McNicholas MBBS 2012)

When assessing patients for BPH, it is important to ask very specific questions in history taking. BPH symptoms develop very slowly, and patients tend to adapt to the abnormal voiding pattern and lifestyle and do not consider their voiding pattern abnormal. Older patient tend to blame it on "getting older" and accept it as normal. Consider asking patients about details such as: frequency of nocturia; evening fluid restrictions, fluid restrictions during the day to prevent interference with activities; strength of urinary stream; a need to push or strain to start the urinary stream; and quality of sleep.

Physical examination focuses on digital rectal exam (DRE), neurologic exam, and examination of the external genitalia. When performing DRE, note should be made of the anal sphincter tone; decreased tone may suggest neurologic etiology, while increased tone may suggest pelvic floor dysfunction. Physical exam of the prostate determines approximate size of the gland, and particular attention is directed to examining for any indurated areas which could be concerning for malignancy. Exam of the external genitalia evaluates for meatal stenosis or palpable masses of the urethra which could contribute to abnormal voiding symptoms.

The international prostate symptom score (IPPS) is a seven-question tool used to quantitate the subjective symptoms of BPH. The tool asks patients to evaluate their sensation of incomplete bladder emptying, frequency, intermittency, urgency, stream strength, and nocturia on a scale of 0–5. The higher the number, the greater the urinary symptoms. The tool is very useful in monitoring improvement and deterioration in symptoms (Resnick 2003).

Abnormal Findings

Abnormal digital rectal exam (DRE) findings include a specific firm area or nodule which is of different texture from the rest of the gland or extreme tenderness on palpation of the gland. When doing the DRE, it is important to note and correlate lax or spastic anal sphincter tone which may suggest neurologic etiology contributing to symptoms (Thomas Anthony McNicholas MBBS 2012). External genitalia abnormalities include meatal stenosis, palpable ureteral mass, or phimosis. Other abnormal physical findings are a palpable bladder (Thomas Anthony McNicholas MBBS 2012).

Diagnostic Tests

A urinalysis must be done to rule out hematuria or a urinary tract infection both of which could suggest a non-BPH pathology for the symptoms. Serum creatinine should be obtained to exclude renal insufficiency in the presence of obstructive uropathy. If the serum creatinine is elevated, imaging studies such as ultrasound should be obtained.

Prostate-specific antigen (PSA) should also be obtained in BPH evaluation and is directly proportional to prostate volume. Men with higher prostate volume will tend to have higher PSA. Many conditions other than BPH can elevate PSA and must be considered. Other causes for increased PSA include prostate cancer, infections, manipulation or trauma, and ejaculation within few days of obtaining sample. It is also important to note conditions which can lower PSA as well. Medications such as 5-α reductase inhibitors, androgen deprivation, or castration will reduce the PSA (Wieder 2010).

Much discussion has and continues to take place among the experts regarding PSA screening. In May of 2013, the American Urological Association (AUA) released a new guideline regarding PSA screening. The changes which are specific to BPH and PSA measurement include offering PSA testing to patients who have at least a 10-year life expectancy and for those in which the detection for prostate cancer would change the management plan or the plan for management of their voiding symptoms and shared decision-making (American Urological Association 2013). The AUA has developed a tool to guide practitioners in this process (see appendix). Other useful diagnostic studies include uroflowmetry and post-void residual. Uroflowmetry is a noninvasive electronic recording of the urinary flow rate during voiding. Post-void residual is obtained immediately after the patient has voided and can be done noninvasively by transabdominal ultrasound or invasively by catheterization (Silva and Silva 2014). Both studies have limitations and variability but decreased flow rates and increased post void residuals can be consistent with BPH. Another useful tool in determining the level of bother in a patient is the the *international prostate symptom score* (*IPSS*), an eight-question (seven *symptom* questions + one quality-of-life question) written screening tool used to screen for, rapidly diagnose, track the symptoms of, and suggest management of the symptoms of the disease BPH (see resources).

Management

The first treatment option for patient with BPH is watchful waiting. Patients with mild symptoms of LUTS (IPSS score of <8) or those with moderate to severe symptoms who are not bothered by the symptoms and are not experiencing medical complications (see Table 5.2) can opt for no intervention and be followed by active surveillance or watchful waiting. Often behavior modifications such as decreasing evening fluid intake and reducing alcohol or caffeine intake can improve mild symptom relief (Paolone 2010). These patients should be evaluated annually with repeat of the initial exam. Symptom score via IPSS to determine subjective changes in voiding pattern should be repeated. Patients are usually aware of a four-point change on the scale (Paolone 2010). Increase in post-void residual and decrease in flow rate are some objective changes noted in progressive BPH and possibly increased PSA or increase in gland volume (Paolone 2010) Some patients never require further treatment and approximately 65 % of patients continue to be satisfied at 5 years (Silva and Silva 2014).

Many patients will seek nonprescription therapy for mild-to-moderate symptoms of BPH. The herbal product saw palmetto has been popular in the treatment of

Table 5.2 Long-term complications of bladder outlet obstruction	Formation of bladder diverticula(e)
	Bladder wall trabeculation
	Detrusor decompensation
	Hydroureteronephrosis
	Renal insufficiency
	Recurrent urinary tract infections

BPH. After review of several randomized trials involving over 3000 patients, no benefits of saw palmetto over placebo were noted (Espinosa 2013; Parsons 2014).

Medical therapies for moderate-to-severe BPH symptoms include α-blockers and 5-α reductase inhibitors (5ARIs) or a combination of the two classes of medication. Recent studies have investigated three other drug classes, antimuscarinics, β3-adrenoceptor agonists, and 5-phosphodiesterase inhibitors (PDE5i) in the treatment of LUTS in BPH when urine storage problems exist (Silva and Silva 2014). Currently five α-blockers, doxazosin, terazosin, tamsulosin, alfuzosin, and silodosin, are available to treat BPH. Alpha-blockers inhibit α-1 adrenergic receptors relaxing smooth muscle tone in the prostate and bladder neck and improve voiding symptoms (Wieder 2010; Silva and Silva 2014). Alpha-1 adrenergic receptors have three subtypes: α-1A, α-1B, and α-1D. Alpha-1A relaxes smooth muscle in the prostate, bladder neck, seminal vesicles, and vas deferens. These are the primary subtype of α-1 receptors in the prostate. Alpha-1B is mainly located in the vasculature; hypotension can be caused by blockage of this receptor. Alpha-1D is located in the nasal passages, bladder, and spinal cord; blocking this receptor often results in nasal congestion (Wieder 2010). The most common side effects of α-blockers are dizziness, headache, asthenia, postural hypotension, rhinitis, sexual dysfunction, and retrograde ejaculation. Studies have suggested all five of these drugs are statistically significant and better than placebo in improving flow and decreasing BPH symptoms. Silodosin is the only drug in the class to be selective to the α-1A receptor subtype. Due to being α-1A selective, silodosin has less incidence of cardiovascular side effects but increased incidence of ejaculatory dysfunction (Silva and Silva 2014).

A significant side effect of α-blockers to be aware of is intraoperative floppy iris syndrome. This syndrome was described in 2005 by Chang and Campbell as miosis intraoperatively during cataract surgery, despite dilation preoperatively. The condition does not seem to occur with the older agents doxazosin and terazosin. If a patient is planning a cataract surgery, it is recommended to avoid initiation of alpha-blockers until the surgery is completed; 5α-reductase inhibitors work to decrease BPH-related symptoms by preventing the conversion of testosterone to dihydrotestosterone. The two drugs currently available in this class are finasteride and dutasteride. Unlike the α-blockers the benefits of these drugs can take up to 6 months but reduce the prostate gland volume up to 25 % (Wieder 2010). When taking either of these medications for 9–12 months, a 50 % decrease in PSA is expected. Common side effects with these drugs include erectile dysfunction, decreased libido, and decreased volume of ejaculate (Silva and Silva 2014).

Two large long-term studies (the Medical Therapy of Prostatic Symptoms study (MTOPS) and Combination of Avodart® and Tamsulosin study (ComBat)) were conducted comparing α-blockers, 5α-reductase inhibitors, and a combination of using both together. Conclusions of these studies suggested combination therapy works better on larger prostates. Combination therapy of an α-blocker and a 5α-reductase inhibitor should be considered for patients with prostate gland volumes >40 ccs, PSA > 4.0 ng/ml, moderate-to-severe voiding symptoms and advanced age. Combination therapy does increase the cost of medication for the patient and increases the side effects of the medications (Silva and Silva 2014) (Wieder 2010).

Neither the MTOPS nor ComBat studies indicate when combination therapy should be initiated or how long the patient should remain on a single agent before adding combination mediations. Most clinicians begin with combination therapy in patients with severe symptoms and high risk for progression of BPH (Silva and Silva 2014). The AUA guidelines support the use of combination therapy for patients with LUTS and demonstrated prostate enlargement (American Urological Association 2013).

Up to half the men suffering from BPH report detrusor overactivity, the more severe the obstruction, the greater the overactivity (Silva and Silva 2014). The overactive bladder symptoms associated with detrusor overactivity may include nocturia, urgency, or frequency. Antimuscarinic therapy can be safe and helpful to these patients. Tolterodine 4 mg has been studied against placebo and found to reduce the associated symptoms. The incidence of increased post-void residual and acute urinary retention was similar to the placebo groups. Benefits of adding an antimuscarinic to patients already on α-blockers or 5α-reductase inhibitors with detrusor overactivity symptoms were also found to be effective and well tolerated (Silva and Silva 2014).

Another drug class having success with bladder capacity is the β3-adrenoceptor agonists. Mirabegron dosed at 50–100 mg showed a significant decrease in voiding frequency, and patients studied taking the 50 mg dose had a statistically significant decrease in urgency as well (Silva and Silva 2014). The most common reported side effects of mirabegron were hypertension, nasopharyngitis, and urinary tract infections (Russo and La Croce 2014).

Several studies have suggested a strong correlation between BPH/LUTS and erectile dysfunction (ED) (Gacci and Carini 2014). 5-Phosphodiesterase inhibitors (PDE-5) have been used for the treatment of ED and more recently studied in daily use for the treatment of BPH. The mechanism of action of the PDE-5 receptor is thought to relax prostatic smooth muscle, have antiproliferative effects, improve blood flow to the pelvis, and act on the afferent sensory nerves or the prostate and bladder (Paolone 2010). Of the PDE-5 products, only tadalafil 5 mg daily is approved for the treatment of BPH. At this time the efficacy of combining use of an α-blocker and tadalafil for BPH treatment is not recommended due to the risk of hypotension from combining these drugs. The most common side effects of tadalafil include headache dyspepsia, back pain, nasopharyngitis, diarrhea, pain in the extremity, myalgia, and dizziness (Russo and La Croce 2014).

Surgical Management

When medication therapy fails or is unable to relieve symptoms adequately, the historical gold standard treatment of BPH has been transurethral resection of the prostate (TURP) (Turini 2009). However, there are also varieties of minimally invasive options for the treatment of symptomatic enlarged prostate. Indications for further treatment include urinary retention, recurrent urinary tract infections, bladder stones, renal insufficiency from BPH, increase of symptoms, low flow rates, and increased post-void residual along with a IPPS score of eight or greater (Wieder

2010). Many patients experiencing significant symptoms of BPH are not candidates for surgical procedures or are not willing to accept the risks of having a TURP. Over the last decade, several laser techniques which use energy to ablate tissue to relieve symptoms associated with BPH have emerged (Georg Muller 2014).

Currently four lasers are used for BPH interventions: the holmium, thulium, diode lasers, and the potassium-titanyl-phosphate and lithium triborate lasers. The major differences in the lasers are their wavelength, fiber type, and surgical technique used (Gilling 2013). The major advantages to laser procedures when compared with TURP are less risk of bleeding, less erectile dysfunction and retrograde ejaculation, shorter hospital stays, and less risk of TUR syndrome (Paolone 2010). TUR syndrome is defined as clinical cardiovascular and neurologic symptoms associated with a sodium less than or equal to 125 mmol/l (Junichi Ishii 2015). The syndrome can develop as a result of dilutional hyponatremia secondary to the necessary use of a nonconductive irrigation fluid during a TURP. A nonconductive fluid must be used due to the use of monopolar electrodes as cautery for the excision. Since the nonconductive fluid contains no electrolytes, it can be absorbed into the blood stream leading to hyponatremia and therefore cardiac and or neurologic symptoms of hyponatremia (Junichi Ishii 2015). These endoscopic laser procedures are well accepted by patients and have replaced open prostatectomy and TURP approaches in many facilities. Whether the laser is used and which laser is used depends on the patients overall presentation and the surgeon's preference, experience, and availability of the equipment (Gilling 2013).

Over the last 15 years, minimally invasive treatments such as transurethral microwave thermotherapy (TUMT) have emerged (Djavan and Kazzazi 2012). Advantages of the TUMT include being an outpatient procedure often office based, is usually performed with local or oral pain medications avoiding spinal or general anesthesia, and is associated with less risk of bleeding, TUR syndrome, retrograde ejaculation and the development of strictures (Turini 2009). The treatment systems have evolved since the first system was developed and currently operate by the placement of a special urethral catheter by which microwave energy is delivered to the prostate. The heat delivered destroys the hyperplastic prostatic tissue through coagulation necrosis. The body reabsorbs the destroyed tissue and returns the prostate to a more normal size. Patients must be aware that the maximum effects of the TUMT are likely to occur 3–6 months after the procedure. In the immediate post-procedure period, increased incidence of urinary retention requiring catheterization or the need for α-blockers may be necessary until maximum recovery has occurred (Turini 2009; Djavan and Kazzazi 2012).

Another minimally invasive technique is the transurethral radiofrequency needle ablation (TUNA). This procedure is accomplished by placing several needles directly in the urethra which deliver low-frequency energy to the area which then result in coagulation and necrosis of the prostatic tissue. This procedure usually requires a pelvic block, spinal or general anesthesia therefore somewhat more invasive than TUMT (Turini 2009). Some other minimally invasive therapies include water-induced thermotherapy (WIT) in which hot water is used to induce coagulation necrosis of the prostatic overgrowth, transurethral ethanol ablation (TEAP) in which hemorrhagic coagulation necrosis is the process in which the tissue is ablated. Both WIT and TEAP can be performed with minimal anesthesia or topical anesthetic (Turini 2009). High intensity focused ultrasound (HIFU) is yet another emerging therapy (Wieder 2010).

These newer minimally invasive options do have favorable characteristics such as fewer side effects, less anesthesia, and being done outpatient but have not proven to be better for long-term results as the transurethral resection procedures (Turini 2009).

One surgical procedure effective for men with smaller prostates (<30 g) is the transurethral incision of the prostate (TUIP). This procedure is achieved by incising the urethra with one or two incisions in the urethra. This procedure has similar effects as the TURP but less incidence of retrograde ejaculation (Wieder 2010).

TURP involves inserting a sheath in the urethra in which the electrified resecting loop is placed to resect prostate tissue often referred to as "chips" from the bladder neck to the verumontanum (Wieder 2010). TURP requires the use of spinal or general anesthesia and usually requires a 1–2 days hospital stay (Presti 2004; Turini 2009). Immediate complications of TURP include hemorrhage potentially requiring transfusion and TUR syndrome, in which absorption of the irrigation fluid can lead to significant hyponatremia. Long-term complications seen after a TURP include development of urethral strictures, bladder neck contracture, incontinence, reoccurrence of lower urinary tract symptoms, retrograde ejaculation, and impotence (Paolone 2010; Resnick 2003).

When prostates are very large (over 100 g), an open simple prostatectomy can be considered. The choice to use in this approach is dependent on the surgeon's experience and coupled with a potential need to perform other procedures, such as treat a bladder diverticulum or bladder stone. Two approaches can be taken to perform open prostatectomies. The suprapubic approach is typically used if a secondary bladder procedure is intended, while the retrobubic approach does not involve entry into the bladder (Presti 2004).

Clinical Pearls

I find it helpful after reviewing the IPPS score to review the questions with the patient. Often I find they do not clearly understand the question and therefore do not answer accurately. They may have adapted to the changed in their stream and do not perceive their stream to be weak. After asking more specific questions such as "How is your stream today compared to 5 years ago?" pt's will go into more detail and give you a better picture of their true voiding pattern. I have found some patient's to be embarrassed to ask for clarification if they do not understand the question.

When discussing treatment plans with the patient, it is important to individualize the plan. Many patients cannot afford mediations and are embarrassed to tell the provider and therefore do not take the medications and symptoms progress. The medications are considered long term and if the patient will not be able to obtain them, an invasive procedure may be indicated sooner.

Resources for the Nurse Practitioner

http://www.auanet.org/education/guidelines/benign-prostatic-hyperplasia.cfm

https://www.youtube.com/playlist?list=PLF38D35BBEFD7740F&feature=plcp

Resources for the Patient
http://www.uptodate.com/contents/benign-prostatic-hyperplasia-bph-beyond-the-basics

References

American Urological Association (2013) Retrieved 21 Sept 2014. From http://www.auanet.org/education/guidelines/benign-porstatic-hyperplasia.cfm

Bagla S, Martin CP, van Breda A, Sheridan MJ, Sterling KM, Papadouris D, Rholl KS, Smirniotopoulos JB, van Breda A (2014) Early results from a United States trial of prostatic artery embolization in the treatment of benign prostatic hyperplasia. J Vasc Interv Radiol 25(1):47–52.

Djavan B, Kazzazi A, Bostanci Y (2012) Revival of thermotherapy for benign prostatic hyperplasia. Curr Opin Urol 22(1):16–21

Espinosa G (2013) Nutrition and benign prostatic hyperplasia. Curr Opin Urol 23(1):38–41

Gacci M, Carini M, Salvi M, Sebastianelli A et al. (2014) Management of benign prostatic hyperplasia: role of phosphodiesterase-5 inhibitors. Drugs Aging 31:425–439

Georg Muller AB (2014) Vaporization techniques for benign prostatic obstruction: Green Light all the way? Curr Opin Urol 24(1):42–48

Gilling AA (2013) Which laser works best for benign prostatic hyperplasia? Curr Urol Rep 141:614–619

Ishio J, Nakahira J, Sawai T, Inamoto T, Fujiwara A, Minami T (2015) Change in serum sodium level predicts clinical manifestations of transurethral resection syndrome: a retrospective review. BMC Anesthesiol. doi:10.1186/s12871-015-0030-z

McConnell JD (1997) Epidemiology, etiology, pathophysiology, and diagnosis of benign prostatic hyperplasia. In: Campbell's urology, 7th edn, vol. 2. W. B. Saunders

McConnell JD (1998) Epidemiology, etiology, pathophysiology, and diagnosis of benign prostatic hyperplasia. In: John D. McConnell M, Patrick C. Walsh MA (ed) Campbell's urology, 7th edn, vol. 2. W.B. Saunders Company, Philadelphia, pp 1429–1452

McNicholas TA, Kirby RS, Lepor H (2012) Evaluation and nonsurgical management of benign prostatic hyperplasia. Campbell-Walsh Urology. Elsevier Saunders, Philadelphia, pp 2611–2654

Paolone DR (2010) Benign prostatic hyperplasia. Clin Geriatr Med 26:223–239

Parsons OA (2014) Associations of obesity, physical activity and diet with benign prostatic hyperplasia and lower urinary tract symptoms. Curr Opin Urol 24(1):10–14

Prescribing information (copyright 2003–2014) Eli Lilly and Company pp 1–29. Marketed by Lilly USA LLC Indianapolis in 46285, USA. http://www.cialis.com

Presti JC (2004) Neoplasms of the prostate gland. In: McAninch EA, editor. Smith's general urology. 16th ed. Lange Medical Books/McGraw-Hill, New York, pp 367–385

Resnick MI (2003) Benign prostatic hyperplasia. In: Resnick MI (ed) Urology secrets, 3rd edn. Hanley & Belfus, Inc, Philadelphia, pp 98–101

Russo A, La Croce G, Capogross P, Ventimislia E et al. (2014) Latest pharmacotherapy options for benign prostatic hyperplasia. Expert Opin Pharmacother 1–10

Silva J, Silva CM, Cruz F (2014) Current medical treatment of lower urinary tract symptoms/BPH: do we have a standard? Curr Opin Urol 24(1):21–28

Turini GA III (2009) Update on minimally invasive therapies for benign prostatic hyperplasia. Med Health/Rhode Island 92(10):336–338

Wein AJ, Kavoussi LR, Campbell ME (2012) Benign prostatic hyperplasia. In: Roehrborn G. Claus, Campbell-Walsh Urology. Elsevier Saunders, Philadelphia, pp 2570–2610

Wieder JA (2010) Benign prostatic hyperplasia, prostate specific antigen (PSA). In: Wieder JA, Pocket guide to urology, 4th edn. J. Wieder Medical in association with Griffith Publishing, Caldwell. pp 172–183, 160–163

Hematuria

6

Michelle J. Lajiness and Susanne A. Quallich

Contents

Objectives
1. Distinguish between the clinical presentation of microscopic hematuria and gross hematuria.
2. Differentiate among potential causes for both conditions.
3. Determine the appropriate evaluation and management for the hematuria patient.

M.J. Lajiness, FNP-BC (✉)
Department of Urology and Department of Infectious Disease,
Beaumont Health System, Royal Oak, MI, USA
e-mail: Michelle.Lajiness@beaumont.org

S.A. Quallich, ANP-BC, NP-C, CUNP, FAANP
Division of Andrology and Urologic Health, Department of Urology,
University of Michigan Health System, Ann Arbor, MI, USA
e-mail: quallich@umich.edu

© Springer International Publishing Switzerland 2016
M. Lajiness, S. Quallich (eds.), *The Nurse Practitioner in Urology*,
DOI 10.1007/978-3-319-28743-0_6

Overview

Hematuria is the presence of blood in the urine; greater than three red blood cells per high-power microscopic field (HPF) are significant. Hematuria is a common problem seen in the urology office, one that cannot be ignored. Patients with gross hematuria (visible) are usually frightened by the sudden onset of blood in the urine and frequently present to the emergency department for evaluation. Hematuria of any degree should never be ignored and, in adults, should be regarded as a symptom of urologic malignancy until proven otherwise. Hematuria is classified by its site of origin: nephrologic, urologic, or pseudo-hematuria (origin from outside the urinary system, such as menstruation).

Studies have shown that the incidence of hematuria, both gross and microscopic, ranges from 2 to 30 % (Lee et al. 2013; Harmanil and Yuksel 2013). Hematuria can be caused from urologic and nephrologic causes, and the nurse practitioner must have a thorough understanding of the causes, history, physical exam, and diagnostic studies to properly evaluate these patients. Any patient that presents with gross hematuria not related to recent surgery, trauma, or UTI in a female should complete a hematuria work-up. Patients with gross hematuria usually have an underlying pathology, whereas it is quite common for patients with microscopic hematuria to have a negative work-up (evaluation).

Microscopic hematuria is defined as one properly collected, non-contaminated urinalysis, with greater than 3 RBCs per 10 HPF (AUA Guideline 2012), that has no other attributable cause. Microscopic hematuria can result from both urologic and nephrologic causes; it can be the result of either anatomic issues or physiologic issues with the kidney (glomerular bleeding, Box 6.1). It is rarely the result of a patient complaint and is usually found incidentally during the evaluation for another condition. Long-term use of anti-inflammatory medications and other over-the-counter medications can result in medical renal disease that produces microscopic hematuria.

Box 6.1. Examples of Conditions Contributing to Medical/Renal Hematuria
- Berger's disease (IgA nephropathy)
- Bleeding disorder
- Bleeding dyscrasias/sickle cell disease
- Diabetes mellitus
- Drug-induced interstitial disease
- End-stage renal disease
- Exercise (marathon running)
- History of analgesic abuse
- HIV
- Infections (e.g., hepatitis)
- Postinfectious glomerulonephritis
- Systemic lupus erythematosus

Hematuria can be caused by menstruation, vigorous exercise, sexual activity, viral illness, trauma, or infection, such as a urinary tract infection (UTI). More serious causes of hematuria include malignancy (kidney or bladder); inflammation of the kidney, urethra, bladder, or prostate; polycystic kidney disease; blood clotting disorders, such as hemophilia; and sickle cell disease. Gross hematuria can be the only indication of urologic malignancy and is usually an indicator of an anatomic issue within the genitourinary tract or non-glomerular bleeding (Boxes 6.2 and 6.3).

Box 6.2. Examples of Conditions Contributing to Gross Hematuria
- Autosomal dominant polycystic kidney disease (ADPCKD)
- Benign prostatic hypertrophy (BPH)
- BPH regrowth post-transurethral resection
- Contamination from menstruation
- Hemorrhagic cystitis
- Interstitial cystitis
- Posterior urethritis
- Poststreptococcal glomerulonephritis
- Renal/ureteral/bladder stone
- Renal/ureteral/bladder tumor
- Sickle cell disease
- Trauma
- Tuberculosis
- Urethritis
- Urethral cancer
- Urethral stricture
- Vigorous exercise

Box 6.3. Medications that May Cause Red Urine
- Chloroquine
- Ibuprofen
- Levodopa
- Methyldopa
- Nitrofurantoin
- Phenacetin
- Phenazopyridine
- Phenytoin
- Quinine
- Rifampin
- Sulfamethoxazole

In evaluating hematuria, several questions should always be asked, and the answers will guide the work-up:

Is the hematuria gross or microscopic?
At what time during urination does the hematuria occur (beginning or end of stream or during entire stream)?
Is the hematuria associated with pain?
Is the patient passing clots?
If the patient is passing clots, do the clots have a specific shape?

Although inflammatory conditions may result in hematuria, all patients with hematuria, except perhaps young women with acute bacterial hemorrhagic cystitis, should undergo urologic evaluation. Older women and men who present with hematuria and irritative voiding symptoms may have cystitis secondary to infection arising in a necrotic bladder tumor or, more commonly, flat carcinoma in situ of the bladder. The most common cause of gross hematuria in a patient older than age 50 years is bladder cancer.

History

When obtaining the history from the patient it is very important to clarify the timing of the hematuria. The patient may note that the hematuria is at the beginning of the stream (initial) throughout the whole stream (total) or at the end of the stream (terminal). It is very helpful to establish the timing of blood in the urinary stream, which can help predict the source of bleeding and narrow the diagnostic evaluation (Table 6.1). Other items to consider are whether this is the first occurrence and were there any precipitating events and if duration of the hematuria has lasted (weeks, months).

Is there any associated pain? Hematuria is usually not painful unless it is associated with inflammation or obstruction. Thus patients with cystitis and secondary hematuria may experience painful urinary irritative symptoms, but the pain is usually not worsened with passage of clots. More commonly, pain in association with hematuria usually results from upper urinary tract hematuria with obstruction of the ureters with clots. Passage of these clots may be associated with severe, colicky flank pain similar to that produced by a ureteral calculus, and this helps identify the source of the hematuria.

The presence of clots usually indicates a significant urologic pathology. Usually, if the patient is passing clots, they are solid and of bladder or prostatic urethral origin. However, the presence of vermiform (wormlike) clots, particularly if associated with flank pain, identifies the hematuria as coming from the upper urinary tract.

There are certain distinct points that should be elicited from history, because they can indicate a higher risk factor for malignancy in the presence of microhematuria. This includes a history of smoking, chronic urinary tract infections, pelvic irradiation, irritative voiding symptoms, past episodes of gross hematuria, and male gender.

Table 6.1 Timing of blood in the urinary stream

Description of hematuria	Possible cause
Microscopic hematuria *Any site within the upper or lower urinary tract*	UTI, prostatitis, urethritis, medical renal disease, bladder/ureteral/renal malignancy, stone disease
Initial gross hematuria *Anterior urethra*	Stricture, meatal stenosis, urethral cancer
Total gross hematuria *Source above bladder neck: bladder, kidney, ureter*	Renal/ureteral/bladder stone or tumor; trauma, including vigorous exercise; hemorrhagic cystitis; interstitial cystitis; sickle cell disease; nephritis; ADPCKD; poststreptococcal glomerulonephritis
Terminal gross hematuria *Bladder neck, prostate, posterior urethra*	BPH or regrowth BPH post-transurethral resection, bladder neck polyps,

ADPCKD autosomal dominant polycystic kidney disease, *BPH* benign prostatic hyperplasia, *UTI* urinary tract infection

Physical Examination

There is no specific physical examination for the patient with hematuria, unless associated with trauma or kidney stones (Chap. 8, appendix). Physical examination should always include blood pressure. A routine genitourinary examination accompanied by a pelvic exam for female patients and a digital rectal exam for male patients is mandatory. Unfortunately, the physical exam tends to be unrevealing but can increase suspicion for other conditions, such as kidney stones, with a positive finding of costovertebral angle tenderness.

Other noted findings in the physical exam such as edema or cardiac arrhythmia may suggest nephrotic syndrome. Costovertebral angle tenderness suggests ureteral obstruction, such as due to stone disease. A careful history and physical examination will help stratify an individual patient's risk for underlying urologic disease.

Diagnostic Tests

Laboratory Evaluation

The urinalysis dipstick and microscopic assessment are key to deciding how to proceed in a patient with hematuria; this should be obtained via a midstream voided clean-catch specimen, unless the patient is unable to void. Unless there is concern about compromise to renal function, or hematuria is present in a patient with known compromise renal function, the value of additional laboratory work is debatable but should include an estimation of renal function. Additional tests could include CBC, serum electrolytes, serum creatinine and blood urea nitrogen, PT/PTT, or PSA testing. Choice of studies will be guided by the patient's presentation and risk factors.

Urine cytology is a necessary part of the microscopic or gross hematuria evaluation and will help eliminate low-risk patients from additional evaluation. A positive cytology may indicate that malignancy is present at any point in the genitourinary tract. Ideally the urine cytology should be obtained on a patient's first voided morning urine on three separate days, if possible, for the greatest degree of accuracy. It can also be obtained at the time of cystoscopy. Depending on individual's risk factors, the provider may consider tumor markers as well.

Imaging Studies

The patient should also have the appropriate imaging study based on the suspected cause of the hematuria and will help establish an anatomic cause for hematuria. The appropriate imaging study will be selected based on patient's comorbidities and suspected causes for the hematuria. Other considerations will be influential as well, such as the speed with which the work-up is intended to be completed, coupled with available resources, as well as potential insurance coverage and preauthorization issues. CT urogram is the preferred initial imaging study because of its higher sensitivity and specificity for upper tract pathology. If this test is not available, an IVU and renal ultrasound is a suitable alternative.

Procedures

In a patient who presents with gross hematuria, cystoscopy should be performed as soon as possible, because frequently the source of bleeding can be readily identified. Cystoscopy will determine whether the hematuria is coming from the urethra, bladder, or upper urinary tract. In patients with gross hematuria secondary to an upper tract source, it may be possible to see red urine pulsing from the involved ureteral orifice. Ideally, the patient will also undergo a CT urogram, especially when there is a concern for malignancy.

In patients under age 35 without significant risk factors for malignancy of cystoscopy is considered at the discretion of the provider. Patients greater than age 35 and any patient with significant risk factors for malignancy will have a cystoscopy.

Management

The potential causes for both microscopic and gross hematuria are numerous and include such variable conditions as renal stones, interstitial cystitis, urothelial malignancy, radiation cystitis and an enlarged prostate. Management depends on determining and treating the underlying cause of the hematuria and can include medical or surgical management. Conservative methods for managing these conditions includes recommending that patients increase their fluid intake to help dilute their urine and stop taking analgesics that could potentially contribute to hematuria.

In the presence of renal insufficiency, hypertension, significant proteinuria, dysmorphic red blood cells, or red blood cell casts, the patient should be referred to the nephrologist for additional renal disease evaluation.

Initial management of gross hematuria will be determined by the suspected cause of the gross hematuria, such as reversing excessive anticoagulation. Frequently this involves placement of a three-way hematuria catheter for irrigation and may involve additional surgical procedures and possible inpatient stay. Placing the catheter on light traction may tamponade bleeding. Gross hematuria that is refractory to management can be managed in some instances with medication (5α reductase inhibitors for prostate bleeding) or surgical remedies (embolization of specific arteries or veins).

Long-Term Management

There is no specific long-term management for hematuria; rather its management is determined by cause. If after evaluation, no significant urologic or nephrologic disease is established, patients can be followed yearly with a routine urinalysis. If they have two consecutive negative annual urinalyses, no further evaluation is necessary. If a clear source of hematuria is established, the urinalysis should be repeated once treatment has been completed.

The exception to this is persistent microscopic hematuria, such as can be seen with diabetic patients and other patients with comorbidities the compromise their renal function. In this population, yearly urinalyses should continue to monitor for changes in the degree of microhematuria. The urinalysis is a low-cost test with little patient burden but may provide insight into patients who may be at risk for nonmalignant urologic disease. Serial urinalysis can be followed through an individual's primary care provider or through yearly visits with a urology provider.

Clinical Pearls
- Patients are often frightened and require reassurance. One drop of blood can color the urine and patients often believe they are hemorrhaging.
- Always include recent history of exercise with patients (male or female) who present with microscopic hematuria, especially those of a younger age.
- Gross hematuria must be evaluated urgently with accompanying studies arranged and, if possible, completed before the appointment.
- Therapeutic anticoagulation should not result in gross hematuria or microscopic hematuria. The anticoagulated patient presenting with either gross hematuria or microscopic hematuria needs to complete a urologic and nephrologic evaluation, beginning with coagulation studies.
- A patient is unlikely to lose enough blood through GU bleeding to compromise their hemodynamics, with a possible exception for gross hematuria that the patient has ignored.

- Helpful mnemonic: Pee Pee ON TTTTHIS – Prostate, obstructive uropathy, nephritis, trauma, tumor, tuberculosis, thrombus, hematologic, infection/inflammation, stones

Resources for the Nurse Practitioner

Diagnosis, Evaluation and Follow-up of Asymptomatic Microhematuria(AMH) in Adults: AUA Guidelines http://www.auanet.org/education/asymptomatic-microhematuria.cfm

Resources for the Patient

Urology Care Foundation Blood in the Urine http://www.urologyhealth.org/urology/index.cfm?article=113

National Kidney and Urologic Diseases Information Clearinghouse (NKUDIC) http://kidney.niddk.nih.gov/kudiseases/pubs/hematuria

References

American Urological Association (2012) Diagnosis, evaluation and follow-up of Asymptomatic microhematuria (AMH). Retrieved 14 Sept 2015 from http://www.auanet.org/education/asymptomatic-microhematuria.cfm

Harmanil O, Yuksel B (2013) Asymptomatic microscopic hematuria in women requires separate guidelines. Int Urogynecol J 24:203–206

Lee Y, Chang J, Koo C, Lee S, Choi Y, Cho K (2013) Hematuria grading scale: a new tool for gross hematuria. J Urology 82(2):284–289

Prostatitis and Chronic Male Pelvic Pain

7

Kaye K. Gaines

Contents

K.K. Gaines, FNP-BC, CUNP
Department of Medicine, C.W. Bill Young V.A. Medical Center, Bay Pines, FL, USA
e-mail: kaye.gaines@outlook.com

© Springer International Publishing Switzerland 2016
M. Lajiness, S. Quallich (eds.), *The Nurse Practitioner in Urology*,
DOI 10.1007/978-3-319-28743-0_7

Overview

Prostatitis (inflammation of the prostate gland) and chronic male pelvic pain represent a complex problem ranging from an acute and possibly life-threatening bacterial infection to a challenging set of chronic and debilitating symptoms that can defy effective treatment. Prostatitis is a common genitourinary infection affecting 10–15 % of all men. It is more common in younger and middle-aged men and is responsible for up to 25 % of all urology office visits (Nguyen 2014; Wagenlehner et al. 2013a).

Prostatitis was classified into four categories by the National Institutes of Health (NIH) in 1999:

I. Acute prostatitis [<5 % of all cases]—acute symptoms, +bacterial infection
II. Chronic bacterial prostatitis—recurrent symptoms, +bacterial infection with the same organism
III. Chronic prostatitis/chronic pelvic pain syndrome (CP/CPPS) [90–95 % of all cases]:
    A. Inflammatory (IIIA)—semen/prostatic secretion leukocytes—inflammation, NO infection
    B. Noninflammatory (IIIB)—NO semen/prostatic secretion leukocytes, NO inflammation or infection
IV. Asymptomatic inflammatory prostatitis—no symptoms, incidental finding, requires no treatment (Krieger et al. 1999)

Symptoms and Risk Factors: Acute and Chronic Bacterial Prostatitis

Most common symptoms	Risk factors
Perineal, rectal, or testicular pain	Trauma
Abdominal, pelvic, or groin pain	Recent prostate biopsy
Back pain	Recent urethral instrumentation

Most common symptoms	Risk factors
Dysuria	Dehydration
Urinary urgency or frequency	Intermittent catheterization
Urinary hesitancy or dribbling	Indwelling catheter
Urge incontinence	Urethral stricture
Hematospermia or hematuria	Benign prostate hypertrophy (BPH)
Nausea and vomiting	Recurrent urinary tract infection
Fever, chills	Chronic constipation
Prostate tenderness on DRE	Sexually transmitted diseases (chlamydia/gonorrhea)
Elevated PSA	Chronic pain syndromes (IBS, CFS, fibromyalgia, etc.)
Painful ejaculation	HIV
Erectile dysfunction	
Malaise, flu-like symptoms	

Brede and Shoskes (2011), Meyrier and Fekete (2015a, b), Sharp et al. (2010)

Acute Prostatitis

Clinical Presentation

Acute prostatitis affects all age groups, tends to occur more frequently in young and middle-aged men, and typically has a rapid and severe onset. It is the most easily recognized and is less common than chronic bacterial prostatitis or CP/CPPS. Etiology includes ascending urethral infection or intraprostatic reflux, and it was historically more common prior to advent of antibiotics, especially those used to treat sexually transmitted infections. Patients will be acutely ill—most commonly with fever and chills, UTI symptoms (dysuria, urinary frequency, urgency), perineal and/or low back pain, possible generalized arthralgia/myalgia, and exquisitely tender prostate on DRE. Prompt diagnosis and treatment are critical to prevent complications of sepsis; clues in this context include high fever and chills, cardiovascular instability, and mental status changes. Prostate abscess is rare, but should be suspected if there is no improvement or if symptoms worsen on initial antibiotic therapy.

Risk factors for acute prostatitis are multifactorial, influenced by the overall health of the patient, any dysfunctional voiding, chronic constipation, inflammation from urine substrates, potential psychological factors, and pelvic floor dysfunction. It is more common in diabetics or HIV-related immunosuppression, and there is approximately an 8 % increase in a man's risk for acute prostatitis for every 5-year increase in his age. Coexisting conditions such as phimosis or urethral stricture disease will also increase an individual's risk (Meyrier and Fekete 2015b; Sharp et al. 2010; Wagenlehner et al. 2013a).

Diagnosis/Evaluation

Obtain urinalysis, gram stain, and culture; complete blood count, basic metabolic panel, and ESR, C-reactive protein. PSA is likely to be elevated. Blood cultures are needed only if sepsis is suspected. Imaging is not usually needed except in the case of possible abscess. If abscess is suspected, obtain transrectal ultrasound (TRUS) or CT. Perform abdominal, genitalia, and rectal exams. On DRE, the prostate may be firm, edematous, and exquisitely tender; avoid vigorous DRE to reduce the risk of urosepsis. Men may also be at risk for acute urinary retention due to swelling of the prostate; an ultrasound post-void residual can aid in treatment decisions.

Expected findings include elevated WBCs, pyuria/bacteriuria, and positive urine culture. Causative organisms are primarily gram-negative and are often the same as for UTI or urethritis (*Escherichia coli* (~80 %), *Klebsiella* (3–11 %), *Proteus* (3–6 %), *Pseudomonas* (3–7 %)). Less frequent pathogens include *Staphylococcus aureus*, *Streptococcus faecalis*, *Chlamydia*, or anaerobes like *Bacteroides* species. Rare findings would include granulomatous prostatitis, TB, or systemic mycosis. Instrumentation (prostate biopsy or resection) may be a factor in acute prostatitis with resistant pathogens, possibly secondary to peri-procedure antibiotics (Meyrier and Fekete 2015b; Nguyen 2014; Sharp et al. 2010).

Treatment

See Table 7.1—fluoroquinolones are usually the first-line therapy unless contraindicated (optimal prostate concentration levels). Some patients may require hospitalization for hydration and IV antibiotics, while others will improve with outpatient antibiotics. Monitor culture/sensitivity results to be certain the patient is on appropriate antibiotic regimen. Treat for 2–4 weeks, emphasizing increased fluid intake and avoidance of pressure to the prostate. Men may benefit from a probiotic such as Align® which can help prevent GI distress, due to the lengthy course of antibiotics. Avoid urethral catheterization—if catheter is needed, use suprapubic catheter. Treat fever and pain with NSAIDs and constipation with stool softeners. Alpha-blockers may help with obstructive symptoms. Reassess voiding function and bladder emptying and repeat UA/culture posttreatment (Brede and Shoskes 2011; Meyrier and Fekete 2015b; Nguyen 2014).

It may be necessary to perform an ultrasound-guided perineal puncture in the case of an abscess to better tailor antibiotic regimens. Surgical debridement may also be necessary in cases of sepsis (Brede and Shoskes 2011).

Follow-Up

Once treatment is completed, some men may benefit from assessment of voiding function and evaluation for stricture disease or pelvic floor dysfunction, and emphasis should be placed on safe sex practices. Emphasis should also be placed on avoiding constipation and maintaining hydration.

Table 7.1 Antibiotic treatment for acute and chronic bacterial prostatitis

Type of prostatitis	Medication regimen	Treatment time/considerations
	(First choice listed first)	
Acute bacterial (uncomplicated)	Ciprofloxacin 500 mg q12h, Levofloxacin 500–750 mg q24h, or TMP-SMX DS q12h	Duration: 14–28 days, decrease dosage for renal impairment. Repeat urine culture 2 and 4 weeks posttreatment
Acute bacterial with possible STD	Ceftriaxone 250 mg IM, or cefixime 400 mg × 1 dose plus doxycycline 100 mg q12h × 14 days, or azithromycin 500 mg q24h × 14 days	Fluoroquinolones not used for gonorrhea. Urine test for *N. gonorrhoeae* and *C. trachomatis*
Acute bacterial with sepsis or prostate abscess	Ciprofloxacin 400 mg IV q12h or levofloxacin 500 mg IV q24h. Alternative: ceftriaxone 1–2 g IV q24h plus levofloxacin 500–750 mg po q24h, or ertapenem 1 g IV q24h, or piperacillin-tazobactam 3.375 g IV q6h Gentamicin 1.7 mg/kg q8h IV may be added	Duration: 4 weeks. Ultrasound/CT scan to confirm abscess. Switch IV to oral when blood culture neg. or abscess drained
Chronic bacterial	Ciprofloxacin 500 mg q12h or levofloxacin 500–750 mg q24h TMP-SMX DS q12h Possible macrolide, doxycycline, and cephalexin use in cases of allergy and resistance	Duration: 4–12 weeks

Sources: Brede and Shoskes (2011), Nguyen (2014), Sharp et al. (2010)

Men should also be advised that they may experience lingering symptoms of prostate irritation for several weeks after completion of antibiotics, and this should be managed symptomatically.

Chronic Bacterial Prostatitis (CBP)

Clinical Presentation

Chronic bacterial prostatitis (CBP) tends to occur more often in middle-aged to older men, with a more gradual and less severe onset of symptoms. CBP almost always involves recurrent documented bacterial infections with the same pathogens as previous episode of acute prostatitis. CBP is accompanied by urogenital symptoms similar to those in acute prostatitis. It may be a complication of inadequate treatment of acute prostatitis. Some men may have persistent bacteriuria without the urogenital symptoms. Risk factors are the same as for acute prostatitis, but possible additional risk factors for CBP are prostate or bladder calculi, diabetes, tobacco abuse, and a shorter treatment course for acute prostatitis. Presentation is similar to that for acute prostatitis, but men may give a history of symptoms waxing and waning.

Men are at risk for CBP because glands in the periphery of the prostate have a poor drainage system, offering a possible explanation for the peripheral zone of the prostate being the most common area of CBP. Bacteria may colonize deep into these prostatic ducts, affecting the success of short-term antibiotic treatments that may be reflexively prescribed. Men may also be labeled with "chronic epididymitis" when in fact the issue is recurrent migration from the prostate to the epididymis after inadequate treatment for acute prostatitis or CBP (Meyrier and Fekete 2015a; Schiller and Parikh 2011; Wagenlehner et al. 2013a).

Diagnosis/Evaluation

The gold standard of bacterial localization for CBP is the Meares and Stamey 4-glass test: first-voided urine, midstream urine, expressed prostatic secretions, and post-prostatic massage urine are sampled. The simpler 2-glass pre- and post-massage test uses a midstream urine before massage and first-stream urine after as an alternative. Both tests, while classic for diagnosis purposes, are labor intensive and infrequently used in clinical practice.

Semen culture is also used, but is not as accurate and may identify pathogens in only about 50 % of specimens. Gram-negative rods (primarily *E. coli)* are the most prevalent organisms causing CBP. Gram-positive pathogens and chlamydia also may be isolated. As noted, the same pathogens causing acute prostatitis are responsible for CBP. If CBP is suspected and cultures are all negative, test for chlamydia. DRE may reveal hypertrophy, tenderness, irregularity, or edema, but the exam is often normal.

Imaging studies might include TRUS, bladder scan after voiding to check PVR, and bladder ultrasound, but imaging studies are often not necessary. Laboratory values (CBC/diff, inflammatory markers, PSA) may all be normal. Most often, CBP is diagnosed on the basis of recurrent or chronic urogenital symptoms and/or bacteriuria. However, in the absence of proven bacterial infection, it is difficult to distinguish CBP from chronic prostatitis/chronic pelvic pain syndrome (CP/CPPS), which requires further evaluation (CP/CPPS should not be treated routinely with long-term antibiotics) (Meyrier and Fekete 2015b; Sharp et al. 2010; Wagenlehner et al. 2013a).

Treatment

See Table 7.1—fluoroquinolones are usually the first-line therapy in CPB also, again because higher drug concentrations can be achieved in the prostate. The length of treatment should be at least 4 weeks, but can range between 4 and 12 weeks. Fluoroquinolone resistance is a growing concern, so in cases of allergy or resistance, use TMP-SMX DS. Alpha-blockers may also be useful for obstructive symptoms or if BPH is suspected. NSAIDS may be used to treat inflammation. Recurrence of chronic bacterial prostatitis is common and requires retreatment and longer duration. Consider antibiotic resistance, impaired absorption, and failure to complete prior treatment. Some men may be candidates for suppressive antibiotic regimens with medications such as low-dose TMP-sulfa, nitrofurantoin, or tetracycline.

Transurethral resection of the prostate (TURP) is a consideration when CBP is refractory and well documented (Meyrier and Fekete 2015b; Nguyen 2014; Wagenlehner et al. 2013a), but this is a treatment of last resort.

Follow-Up

Similar to men with acute prostatitis, some men may benefit from assessment of voiding function and evaluation for stricture disease or pelvic floor dysfunction, and emphasis should be placed on safe sex practices. Emphasis should also be placed on avoiding constipation and maintaining hydration, especially when on suppressive antibiotics.

Men should also be advised that they may experience lingering symptoms of prostate irritation for several weeks after completion of antibiotics, and this should be managed symptomatically.

Chronic Prostatitis/Chronic Pelvic Pain Syndrome (CP/CPPS)

Chronic prostatitis/chronic pelvic pain syndrome (CP/CPPS) is a clinical syndrome defined as pelvic pain associated with urinary symptoms and/or sexual dysfunction, lasting for at least 3 of the past 6 months in the absence of other identified causes (NIH standardized definition). CP/CPPS (previously called abacterial/nonbacterial prostatitis or prostatodynia) is the most common type of prostatitis and occurs in 2–10 % of all adult men, but there is no precise incidence for this condition. The symptoms and clinical presentation are similar to prostate infection, yet with no evident source of infection. Since the exact cause of pain is unknown, the diagnosis is one of exclusion.

In CP/CPPS, the term "prostatitis" may not be indicative that the source of symptoms is really the prostate. Recent research indicates an association between nonurological somatic syndromes and symptom severity of CP/CPPS. Breaking research by the MAPP network has identified overrepresentation of *Burkholderia cenocepacia* (gram-negative bacteria) in the initial urine stream of men with chronic pelvic pain syndrome (Krieger et al. 2015; Nickel et al. 2015) and suggests there may be two types of patients: those with pelvic and urinary symptoms and those with both urological symptoms and nonurological syndromes, suggesting a more systemic condition (Table 7.2) that may be influenced by other chronic pain conditions (Pontari 2015; Pontari and Giusto 2013; Schiller and Parikh 2011).

Inflammatory and noninflammatory delineations are used primarily for research purposes. Both subgroups have similar symptoms and treatment responses.

Table 7.2 Discussion of chronic prostatitis/chronic pelvic pain syndrome

Chronic prostatitis/chronic pelvic pain syndrome (CP/CPPS)	
Possible causes (speculative)	Associated nonurological somatic syndromes
Persistent infection	Chronic fatigue syndrome
Inflammation due to trauma	Irritable bowel syndrome
Pelvic muscle spasms	Fibromyalgia
Neurogenic inflammation/pain	TMJ disorder
Increased prostate tissue pressure	Anxiety disorder
Autoimmune factors	Widespread chronic pain
Somatic, psychological factors (stress, anxiety, fear)	Interstitial cystitis/painful bladder syndrome (IC/PBS)
Depression	

Krieger et al. (2015), Pontari (2015), Wagenlehner et al. (2013b)

Inflammatory (IIIA) CP/CPPS includes patients with positive inflammatory cells in expressed prostatic secretions, post-prostate massage urine, or seminal fluid. Noninflammatory (IIIB) CP/CPPS includes all other patients with chronic prostatitis symptoms or pelvic pain (Krieger et al. 1999; Sharp et al. 2010).

Clinical Presentation

CP/CPPS is characterized by frequent, relapsing, and often debilitating symptoms including, but not limited to, pelvic pain (perineal, abdominal, penile, scrotal, prostate, and/or rectal pain), low back pain, painful intercourse or ejaculation, dysuria, urinary urgency or hesitancy, obstructive voiding symptoms, hematuria or hematospermia, malaise, and fatigue. CP/CPPS usually does not involve fever or chills. Sexual dysfunction may also be a complaint, but the primary issues for these men are pelvic floor tenderness, depression, and catastrophizing. The precise etiology is often unclear and may be influenced by autoimmune disorders, inflammation, or urine reflux into prostatic ducts (Krieger et al. 2015; Pontari 2015; Pontari and Giusto 2013; Wagenlehner et al. 2013b).

Diagnosis/Evaluation

It is important to exclude other possible causes of pelvic pain. Differential diagnoses include urethritis/UTI, cancer, stricture, and neurological bladder dysfunction. A detailed history is essential and should include urinary symptoms; pain; sexual history and current sexual activity; mental health history; any history of physical, emotional, or sexual trauma; PTSD; and quality of life. Review history of any other nonurological somatic disorders (Table 7.2).

The physical exam should include an assessment of the abdomen, groin, spermatic cord, epididymis, and testes. A digital rectal exam assesses for tenderness, irregular prostate, rectal mass, hemorrhoids, muscle spasms, or myofascial tenderness. Labs should include urinalysis and culture, urine cytology if hematuria is noted, PSA, and inflammatory markers. Cystoscopy and/or prostate ultrasound or biopsy, bladder ultrasound, and/or catheterization for post-void residual may be indicated. Imaging studies could include renal/abdominal/pelvic ultrasound, KUB, CT, and/or MRI (Pontari 2015; Sharp et al. 2010; Stein et al. 2014).

CP/PPS diagnostic and assessment tools:

- NIH Chronic Prostatitis Symptom Index (NIH-CPSI)
- AUA/IPSS Symptom Questionnaire
- UPOINT (phenotypic classification system) six domains: urinary (U), psychosocial (P), organ specific (O), infection (I), neurologic/systemic (N), and tenderness of pelvic floor skeletal muscles (T) (Nickel and Shoskes 2010; Shoskes and Nickel 2013)

The UPOINT website suggests:

Urinary: A post-void residual measured by ultrasound.
Psychosocial: Ask about clinical depression and catastrophizing (feeling helpless and hopeless about the condition).
Organ specific: Pain improvement with bladder emptying and prostate tenderness.
Infection: Culture for mycoplasma and ureaplasma, urine culture and (in men) expressed prostatic secretions, or a post-prostate massage urine.
Neurologic/systemic: Ask about pain outside the pelvis and a diagnosis of other pain syndromes.
Tenderness: Palpate the abdominal and pelvic skeletal muscles (via the rectum or vagina) and check for spasm and trigger points (http://www.upointmd.com/index.php) (Kartha et al. 2013; Nickel and Shoskes 2010).

For CP/CPPS, there is no universally accepted treatment regimen, and there is no therapy that will be effective in all cases, but the UPOINT screening tool helps direct individualized, multimodal therapeutic approaches to CP/CPPS. Treating CP/CPPS must be a joint venture between patient and clinician, and the relationship must be based on mutual trust and respect. The goals of management are to improve functional status, quality of life, and sexual function. Cognitive-based therapy may assist with psychosocial aspect and stress reduction, and men may benefit from involvement of the spouse and/or family. Successful management involves managing expectations and introducing the concept that condition has to be managed, like other chronic pain conditions. Surgical treatment is rarely indicated (Nickel et al. 2013; Pontari and Giusto 2013; Riegel et al. 2014; Stein et al. 2014).

Chronic prostatitis/chronic pelvic pain syndrome (CP/CPPS)
Multimodal therapies should be considered and offered on a patient-specific basis

Lifestyle measures	Alternative therapy	Psychological/medical interventions
Meditation	Acupuncture	Biofeedback
Yoga	Phytotherapy	Psychological counseling
Aerobic Exercise	Herbal medications	Prostate massage
		Pelvic muscle rehabilitation
		Myofascial trigger point release
Frequent ejaculation	Homeopathy	Transurethral resection of the prostate (TURP)
Sitz baths		Transurethral microwave thermotherapy (TUMT)
Emotional support group		Prostatectomy

Herati and Moldwin (2013), Ismail et al. (2013), Pontari and Giusto (2013), Stein et al. (2014)

Chronic Prostatitis/Chronic Pelvic Pain Syndrome—Medications to Consider

- Antibiotics (consider resistance issues) (see Table 7.1) (not indicated for chronic use)
- Alpha-blockers
- Five-alpha reductase inhibitors
- Anticholinergics
- Antispasmodics
- Anti-inflammatories
- Glucocorticoids
- Gabapentin (Neurontin)
- Pregabalin (Lyrica)
- Pentosan (Elmiron)
- Tricyclic antidepressants (amitriptyline, nortriptyline)
- Antidepressants—SSRI/SRNI (particularly duloxetine)
- Ismail et al. (2013), Nguyen (2014), Pontari (2015), Sharp et al. (2010).

Asymptomatic Inflammatory Prostatitis

Clinical Presentation/Diagnosis

Asymptomatic inflammatory prostatitis is an incidental finding in men who undergo urological procedures—usually prostate biopsy, infertility, or cancer workup. There are no definitive symptoms. Chronic inflammation may be noted on prostate biopsy or in pathology post-prostate resection. Leukocytospermia (elevated WBCs) without infection may be noted in semen on fertility evaluation. Elevated PSA and/or male infertility may be associated (not proven).

Treatment

No treatment is required unless symptoms develop. Antibiotics are often prescribed in men with chronically elevated PSA and negative biopsies or for leukocytospermia in male infertility. There is insufficient research to document either the natural history or evidence-based treatment for asymptomatic inflammatory prostatitis at this time (Krieger et al. 1999; Schiller and Parikh 2011; Sharp et al. 2010).

Clinical Pearls
- If acute prostatitis is suspected, avoid vigorous DRE—painful and may cause bacteremia.
- Imaging studies are not usually needed to diagnose acute prostatitis unless prostate abscess is suspected (then get TRUS or CT).
- Fluoroquinolones are effective for 2/3 of patients and are usually the first-line therapy for acute or chronic bacterial prostatitis unless contraindicated (optimal prostate concentration levels).
- A possible severe adverse effect of fluoroquinolones is tendonitis/tendon rupture.
- Recurrence of chronic bacterial prostatitis is common and requires retreatment for longer duration. Consider antibiotic resistance, impaired absorption, and failure to complete prior treatment.
- More than 90 % of prostatitis is chronic prostatitis/chronic pelvic pain syndrome (CP/CPPS), and it is a diagnosis of exclusion.
- CP/CPPS is a male pelvic pain associated with urinary symptoms and/or sexual dysfunction, lasting for at least 3 of the past 6 months in the absence of other identified causes.
- There is NO universally accepted treatment regimen for CP/CPPS.

Resources for the Nurse Practitioner
1. The National Institutes of Health Chronic Prostatitis Symptom Index (NIH-CPSI). http://www.proqolid.org/instruments/national_institute_of_health_chronic_prostatitis_symptom_index_nih_cpsi?private=yes&fromSearch
2. AUA/IPSS Symptom Questionnaire (attach PDF unless already in BPH chapter).
3. UPOINT clinical phenotyping system for CP/CPPS to guide multimodal treatment. http://www.upointmd.com/index.php
4. National Guideline Clearinghouse: Chronic Pelvic Pain. http://www.guideline.gov/content.aspx?id=38626#Section424
5. The Multidisciplinary Approach to the Study of Chronic Pelvic Pain (MAPP) is a research network conducting collaborative research on urological chronic pelvic pain disorders—specifically, interstitial cystitis/painful bladder syndrome

(IC/PBS) and chronic prostatitis/chronic pelvic pain syndrome (CP/CPPS). http://mappnetwork.org/
6. Up to Date—Acute, Chronic Bacterial and CP/CPPS. http://www.uptodate.com
7. SUNA's "Core Curriculum."

Resources for the Patient

1. SUNA: "Prostatitis—Patient Fact Sheet" (English and Spanish). https://www.suna.org/download/members/prostatitis.pdf
2. NIH: "What I need to know about Prostate Problems" (English and Spanish). http://www.niddk.nih.gov/health-information/health-topics/urologic-disease/prostatitis-disorders-of-the-prostate/Pages/ez.aspx
3. Up to Date—"Patient Information: Prostatitis (The Basics)." http://www.uptodate.com
4. AUA: Urology Care Foundation (2015). "Prostatitis (Infection of the Prostate)." http://www.urologyhealth.org/urologic-conditions/prostatitis-(infection-of-the-prostate)/symptoms
5. *British Medical Journal* (BMJ) "Prostatitis" (patient handout—note that some of the information refers to European medication names, but overall topic coverage is solid). http://bestpractice.bmj.com/best-practice/pdf/patient-summaries/532707.pdf

---

References

American Urological Association (AUA): Urology Care Foundation (2015) Prostatitis (Infection of the Prostate). http://www.urologyhealth.org/urologic-conditions/prostatitis-(infection-of-the-prostate)/symptoms

Brede C, Shoskes D (2011) The etiology and management of acute prostatitis. Nat Rev Urol 8:207–212. doi:10.1038/nrurol.2011.22

Herati A, Moldwin R (2013) Alternative therapies in the management of chronic prostatitis/chronic pelvic pain syndrome. World J Urol 31:761–766. doi:10.007/s00345-011097-0

Ismail M, Mackenzie K, Hashim H (2013) Contemporary treatment options for chronic prostatitis/chronic pelvic pain syndrome. Drugs Today 49(7):457–462. doi:10.1358/dot.2013.49.7.1990152

Kartha GK, Kerr H, Shoskes DA (2013) Clinical phenotyping of urologic pain patients. Curr Opin Urol 23(6):560–564. doi:10.1097/MOU.0b013e3283652a9d

Krieger JN, Nyberg N, Nickel JC (1999) NIH consensus definition and classification of prostatitis. JAMA 282(3):236–237

Krieger JN, Stephens AJ, Landis JR, Clemens JQ, Kreder K, Lai HH, Afari N, Rodríguez L, Schaeffer A, Mackey S, Andriole GL, Williams DA, MAPP Research Network (2015) Relationship between Chronic Nonurological Associated Somatic Syndromes and Symptom Severity in Urological Chronic Pelvic Pain Syndromes: Baseline Evaluation of the MAPP Study. J Urol 193(4):1254–1262, http://dx.doi.org/10.1016/j.juro.2014.10.086

Meyrier A, Fekete T (2015a) Chronic bacterial prostatitis. UpToDate. http://www.uptodate.com/contents/chronic-bacterial-prostatitis?topicKey=ID%2F86802&el…

Meyrier A, Fekete T (2015b) Acute bacterial prostatitis. UpToDate. http://www.uptodate.com/contents/acute-bacterial-prostatitis?topicKey=ID%2F8062&elaps…

Nguyen N (2014) Treating prostatitis effectively: a challenge for clinicians. US Pharmacist 39(4): 35–41

Nickel JC, Shoskes DA (2010) Phenotypic approach to the management of the chronic prostatitis/chronic pelvic pain syndrome. BJU Int 106(9):1252–1263. doi:10.1111/j.1464-410X.2010.09701.x

Nickel JC, Shoskes DA, Wagenlehner FM (2013) Management of chronic prostatitis/chronic pelvic pain syndrome (CP/CPPS): the studies, the evidence, and the impact. World J Urol 31(4):747–753. doi:10.1007/s00345-013-1062-y, Epub 2013 Apr 9

Nickel JC, Stephens A, Landis JR, Chen J, Mullins C, van Bokhoven A, Lucia MS, Melton-Kreft R, Ehrlich GD, MAPP Research Network (2015) Search for microorganisms in men with urologic chronic pelvic pain syndrome: a culture-independent analysis in the MAPP Research Network. J Urol 194(1):127–135, http://dx.doi.org/10.1016/j.juro.2015.01.037

Pontari M (2015) Chronic prostatitis/chronic pelvic pain syndrome. UpToDate. http://www.uptodate.com/contents/chronic-prostatitis-chronic-pelvic-pain-syndrome?topicK…

Pontari M, Giusto L (2013) New developments in the diagnosis and treatment of chronic prostatitis/chronic pelvic pain syndrome. Curr Opin Urol 23(6):565–569. doi:10.1097/MOU.0b013e3283656a55

Riegel B, Bruenahl CA, Ahyai S, Bingel U, Fisch M, Löwe B (2014) Assessing psychological factors, social aspects and psychiatric co-morbidity associated with Chronic Prostatitis/Chronic Pelvic Pain Syndrome (CP/CPPS) in men – A systematic review. J Psychosom Res 77(5):333–350. doi:10.1016/j.jpsychores.2014.09.012, Epub 2014 Sep 30

Schiller DS, Parikh A (2011) Identification, pharmacologic considerations, and management of prostatitis. Am J Geriatr Pharmacother 9(1):37–48. doi:10.1016/j.amjopharm.2011.02.005

Sharp V, Takacs E, Powell C (2010) Prostatitis: diagnosis and treatment. American Family Physician 82(4):397–406. http://www.aafp.org/afp/2010/0815/p397.html

Shoskes D, Nickel JC (2013) Classification and treatment of men with chronic prostatitis/chronic pelvic pain syndrome using the UPOINT system. World J Urol 31(4):755–760. doi:10.1007/s00345-013-1075-6, Epub 2013 Apr 16

Stein A, May T, Dekel Y (2014) Chronic pelvic pain syndrome: a clinical enigma. Postgrad Med 126(4):115–122. doi:10.3810/pgm.2014.07.2789

Wagenlehner F, Pilatz A, Bschleipfer T, Diemer T, Linn T, Meihardt A, Schagdarsurengin U, Dansranjavin T, Schuppe HC, Weidner W (2013a) Bacterial prostatitis. World J Urol 21:711–716. doi:10.1007/s00345-013-1055-x

Wagenlehner F, van Till J, Magri V, Perletti G, Houbiers J, Weidner W, Nickel JC (2013b) National Institutes of Health Chronic Prostatitis Symptom Index (NIH-CPSI) symptom evaluation in multinational cohorts of patients with chronic prostatitis/chronic pelvic pain syndrome. Eur Urol 63(5):953–959. doi:10.1016/j.eururo.2012.10.042, Epub 2012 Nov 2. http://www.ncbi.nlm.nih.gov/pubmed/23141933

Kidney Stones

8

Suzanne T. Parsell

Contents

> **Objectives**
> 1. Determine patients at risk for renal calculi and instruct regarding controlling risk factors.
> 2. Discuss management for patients with active renal calculi disease.
> 3. Demonstrate knowledge of appropriate testing and imaging.

S.T. Parsell, ANP-BC, CUNP
Division of Endourology, Department of Urology, University of Michigan Health System,
Ann Arbor, MI, USA
e-mail: sneboysk@med.umich.edu

© Springer International Publishing Switzerland 2016
M. Lajiness, S. Quallich (eds.), *The Nurse Practitioner in Urology*,
DOI 10.1007/978-3-319-28743-0_8

Introduction

Kidney stones: for many, these two small words can trigger a horrific response. For some, the memory will be of unbearable pain similar to labor pains; others will recall surgery and time off work. The incidence of experiencing a kidney stone in one's lifetime is increasing, from 3 % in 1976 to 29 % in 2000 (Scales et al. 2012). Research is being done to increase the quality of life for kidney stone patients and minimize their chance for recurrence. Research has been conducted on calcium supplements for women and has supported that calcium supplements do not contribute to renal calculi formation. Ongoing research is also investigating the effect of obesity and sugar and the roles they play in renal calculi formation.

Incidence

The prevalence of stone disease has increased in every age group and gender. The incidence of stone disease peaks in the fourth to sixth decades and is rare before age 20. Males have been historically at a higher risk for developing stones than their female counterparts, but recent data suggest that the gender gap is narrowing (Scales et al. 2007). Risk factors for stone formation also include increasing age and Caucasian race.

Anatomy

There are patient-specific conditions that increase the risk for stone formation. This includes the presence of a solitary kidney. Renal stones are considered a metabolic upper tract obstruction, although in large enough size they lead to mechanical obstruction of the urinary tract.

Risk Factors

Different areas of the United States can put individuals at an increased risk, such as the "stone belt," which is located in the Southeastern states, followed by the East, Midwest, and the West. This is influenced, to some extent, by exposure to excessive heat or other conditions that promote dehydration, such as a specific work environment. Additional risk factors include metabolic disease, i.e., gout, RTA, malabsorption disease, and Crohn's disease; there is also an increased incidence of stone disease seen with increasing body size, type II diabetes, family history, and metabolic syndrome. Obesity is a risk factor for stone formation; an increase in BMI in both males and females increases the chances of forming stones. SCI, spina bifida and non – ambulatory patients are at risk for stone formation.

There are a number of factors that can be controlled; dietary factors are one of them. Limiting salt and protein, mainly red meat, can decrease the risk for kidney stones. Staying well hydrated is key in preventing stone disease; drinking 2.5–3 l per day is optimal. Low urine volume is an independent risk factor for stone formation. Low or high urine pH and high urinary excretion of calcium, oxalate, or uric acid also influence stone formation (Table 8.1). Diabetic patients are more likely to have uric acid stones due to low urine volume and acidic urine.

Table 8.1 Factors that influence stone formation

Hypercalciuria	Urinary calcium excretion >4 mg/kg/day or >200 mg/day on a calcium and sodium-restricted diet
	Increased risk of both stone disease and osteoporosis
	Can result from issues with calcium handling in the gastrointestinal tract, kidney, or bone
	Renal hypercalciuria results from reabsorption of calcium from the proximal and distal renal tubules; creates calcium loss in the urine, increased PTH secretion, and stimulation of synthesis of 1,25 di-hydroxy vitamin D which increases intestinal calcium absorption and bone resorption
	Commonly due to primary hyperparathyroidism
Hyperuricosuria	Urinary uric acid excretion >700 mg/day
	Urine pH <5.5
	Promotes calcium oxalate stone formation
	Excessive purine intake from animal protein most common etiology
	More likely to be seen with chronic diarrhea, myeloproliferative disorders, gout
	Can be addressed by moderating sodium intake and a low purine diet
Hyperoxaluria	Can be the result from excessive intake of oxalate-rich foods (nuts, chocolate, spinach, beets, liver, brewed tea) or vitamin C (ascorbic acid)
	Can be due to vitamin B6 deficiency
	80 % of cases are due to primary hyperoxaluria, an autosomal recessive disorder
	Intestinal malabsorption leads to enteric hyperoxaluria (ulcerative colitis, Crohn's disease, celiac disease)
	Presentation includes low urine volume, low urinary pH, decreased urinary calcium, elevated sodium and citrate in the urine
	Treated with pyridoxine, low oxalate diet, low fat diet, increased fluid intake, calcium supplementation
Hypocitraturia	Urinary citrate excretion <320 mg/day
	Risk factor for one in ten stone formers acidic urine increases citrate metabolism and reduces citrate excretion, such as that seen with renal tubular acidosis
	Can also be a factor in chronic diarrhea, due to bicarbonate loss
	Thiazide diuretics also induce hypo-anemia and intracellular acidosis
	Cause is usually idiopathic
	Treated with potassium citrate

(continued)

Table 8.1 (continued)

Low urine pH	Urinary pH <5.5
	Calcium oxalate stones may form
	Primary factor leading to uric acid stones
Hypomagnesiuria	Magnesium inhibits calcium stone formation, as it binds oxalate
	Associated with low urinary hypocitraturia
	Can be treated with a magnesium supplement
Cystinuria	Urinary cysteine <400 mg/day
	Autosomal recessive defect resulting in impaired renal reabsorption of four amino acids
	Elevated urinary cysteine
	Cystine stones form in acid urine and may result in staghorn stones
	Treated with increased hydration, low sodium diet, low methionine diet (decreases cysteine production; limited intake of meat, eggs, wheat, milk, cheese)
	Oral potassium citrate can be added to alkalize the urine
	Cystine stones can be resistant to ESWL and are often treated with dissolution therapy

Cystine stones can form in patients with an autosomal recessive trait leading to a defective renal and intestinal transport of amino acids. Struvite stones can form in alkaline urine environments, as a result of the urease enzyme secreted by some bacteria (*Proteus mirabilis, Klebsiella pneumoniae, Staphylococcus aureus,* and *Staphylococcus epidermidis*).

History

Patients presenting to a urology office with kidney stones can present with a plethora of signs and symptoms. The "typical" renal calculus patient can present with flank discomfort, and a patient with a ureteral calculus may present with sharp flank/abdominal pain and N/V. Many patients may have already been seen by their PCP for hematuria before presenting to a urology office; others may have made a visit to the ED and will bring results of labs and imaging with them to their appointment. A detailed history should aim to determine the presence of any risk factors for stone disease (Box 8.1). The location of the stone, i.e., the kidney or ureter, obstructive or nonobstructive, and the creatinine results will help determine whether the patient will need surgery or if the stone pass without surgery.

Physical Examination

Conducting a physical exam on a patient with a kidney stone is largely unremarkable. Palpating the CVA region may elicit a positive response. Assess for fever, as this may be a sign of a possible infection. The patient may find it difficult to find a comfortable position; this can be a sign of active renal colic.

Box 8.1: Risk Factors for Urolithiasis
Bowel disease/intestinal malabsorption
Diabetes mellitus Type II
Family history of stone disease
Gout
History of bowel surgery (resection, gastric bypass/bariatric surgery, ileal
   conduit)
Hyperthyroidism
Obesity
Osteoporosis
Personal history of stone disease
Stone-provoking medications/supplements
* Furosemide
* High-dose vitamin C
* High-dose vitamin D
* Probenecid
* Protease inhibitors
* Salicylates
* Triamterene

Diagnostic Testing

Laboratory Evaluation

Labs and imaging assist with verifying the diagnosis of renal calculus. CBC and comprehensive panel may reveal elevated WBCs and elevated creatinine which could indicate an emergent situation. Additional lab tests include serum electrolytes, creatinine, calcium, and uric acid. Parathyroid hormone levels may be considered.

Urinalysis can also be helpful in this context and help rule out a simple urinary tract infection. Patients may experience gross hematuria where approximately 85 % of all patients demonstrate at least microhematuria. Urinalysis will also provide additional clues to the type of stones based on crystals within the urine. Urine pH can also be a clue as to what type of stones may be present. Urine culture may be helpful in the case of suspected infection; patient is febrile on presentation or if there is concern for infection by a urease splitting organism.

If the patient has been able to screen the urine and capture the stone, the stone should be sent for analysis. This will help establish any underlying pathophysiologic cause for their stone disease.

Recurrent stone formation should also be evaluated with 24-h urine testing, which can help distinguish among the potential causes for stone formation, which closely mirror the risk factors seen a Box 8.1, but include pathologic fractures, gout, young age at onset of stone disease, and recurrent calcium stone formation.

Imaging

Each patient suspected of having kidney stones has a baseline imaging study, in order to better quantify potential stone burden and estimate metabolic activity. Ninety percent of kidney stones are radiopaque and can be demonstrated on imaging studies. This may include a KUB (rapid screening test but can miss many stones), ultrasound, or CT renal stone. If the patient was seen in the emergency department, commonly, a non-contrast CT renal stone is ordered; this is the most accurate test to evaluate for the presence of urolithiasis and in detail the collecting system anatomy. A renal ultrasound can identify hydronephrosis or can be used with patients that cannot tolerate a CT scan.

A CT urogram or IVU can identify the presence of stone and suggest whether obstruction exists. The CT urogram is considerably more detailed than the IVU.

Management

Once imaging has established the existence of a renal/ureteral calculus, the decision to treat the stone with surgery or provide medication for MET (medical expulsive therapy) is contemplated. The decision for surgery or MET depends on the size and location of the stone and the surgeon and the patient agreeing with the plan. MET with tamsulosin hydrochloride is commonly prescribed in the ED for patients with ureteral calculus. Patients will need prompt intervention for complete or high-grade unilateral urinary obstruction, bilateral urinary obstruction, obstruction in a solitary kidney, obstruction in the context of infection or sepsis, obstruction with an elevated creatinine, inability to tolerate oral intake, or pain that is not controlled by oral medications.

If the patient is asymptomatic, and the stone is non-obstructing, the patient will be observed and encouraged increase fluid intake to promote passage of the stone, if the stone is less than 10 mm. Stones are more likely to pass when they are located in the distal ureter and are small. Approximately 60 % of stones less than 5 mm will pass spontaneously, usually within 40 days of symptom onset.

In the absence of these conditions, a referral is completed for the patient to be seen urgently by a urology provider. During the patient's urology visit, surgery is arranged in case the ureteral calculus does not pass with MET. But prior to beginning any treatment, any urinary tract infection should be adequately treated. Tamsulosin hydrochloride can decrease BP, so it is imperative to tell the patient regarding this risk and to take the medication at night.

Surgical Management

If passage of the stone is not possible, the patient should be scheduled for a ureteral stent or nephrostomy tube placement to relieve the obstruction and prevent kidney damage. Open or removal is rarely indicated for renal stones. A ureteroscopy with laser and possible stent is scheduled within 2 weeks. The details of the surgery are communicated with the patient; it is an outpatient and the patient will need a driver. The potential problems with a ureteral stent placement necessitate a brief discussion on the value of maintaining a patent ureter. Potential side effects include, pain, dysuria, and hematuria; these can be controlled with medication.

For stones approximately 1 cm, outside of the lower pole and proximal calculus, shockwave lithotripsy is the procedure of choice. This surgery is quite successful, with a rate of 74–90 %. This surgery is also outpatient, and requires a driver, as the patient receives sedation. The patient must pass the fragments; tamsulosin hydrochloride is prescribed postoperatively to facilitate passage of stone debris. *Steinstrasse* describes obstructing stone fragments in the ureter following SWL and correlates with increased stone burden. It is seen in up to 10 % of patients undergoing SWL (Matlaga and Lingeman 2010).

Percutaneous nephrolithotomy is recommended for patients with large lower pole renal calculi, staghorn calculi, or struvite calculi. The patient will have a general anesthetic and an overnight stay in the hospital. As with all surgeries, updated labs and additional testing may be ordered, i.e., CXR and EKG.

Postoperatively, instructions are reviewed during the initial clinic visit, and handouts are provided. Instructions that are provided during the initial visit and reviewed may decrease the number of post op phone calls. Medications that control pain, bladder spasms, and those that expedite stone passage need to be prescribed prior to discharge. Experienced urology phone triages RNs are crucial to the successful management of postoperative kidney stone patients.

Patients need education about their postoperative course that includes the expectation of hematuria and that small clots are to be expected, pain/discomfort if a stent is left in the ureter, and diet instruction short-term, especially to increase fluid intake to promote passage of stone fragments. Specific instructions are tailored to the individual and are based on both the procedure and stone burden.

Postoperative return visits commonly happen 4 weeks after surgery. It is during this visit that the provider can examine the patient's need for metabolic evaluation. Every patient needs to be reminded that drinking 2.5–3 l/day and adhering to low salt/protein diet will now be a principal part of their everyday life. A modest calcium diet, 800–1200 mg daily is also recommended.

Long-Term Management

There is a lack of high-quality data that evaluates the utility of diet or pharmacologic therapy within the context of stone disease. However, patients are encouraged to maintain a high fluid intake. Patients at increased risk for forming additional renal calculi should be encouraged to complete a metabolic evaluation. Patient will feel empowered if they can assist with controlling their renal calculi disease. Serum labs include PTH, uric acid, phosphorus, Vitamin D, and a basic chemistry panel. Outside labs can arrange for a 24-h urine kit to be mailed to the patient's home. Twenty-four-hour urine results can assist with controlling stone disease through diet modifications and/or medications. Repeat 24-h urine may be suggested to assess changes that were implemented. Hard to control renal calculi patients are referred to nephrology. Some nephrology departments have an RD who can assist the patient with portion size and how to read labels.

Patients with recurrent renal calculi are seen every 6 months or every year with appropriate imaging, i.e., KUB, ultrasound, or CT renal stone. During this visit, a urinalysis can be completed, and a review of his medications can be assessed for compliance. The frequency of follow-up can also be tailored to the frequency of stone formation.

NPs in rural areas may not have pamphlets and teaching materials to provide for their patients. AUA and SUNA provide specific information and guidelines regarding urology problems. Patient handouts can be extremely beneficial for patients; they are available in other languages. They can serve as a reminder to patients regarding diets and recommendations. Patients must recognize that recommendations for one individual may not pertain to them; they should listen to the suggestions of their provider. SUNA allows for networking with other NPs for assistance. It can be puzzling for the mid-level provider when searching the Internet as various articles will share dissimilar views. The AUA and SUNA can and may have different guidelines than those set up by various organizations, i.e., USPTF and ACS.

Clinical Pearls
- Greater than 60 % of stones less than 5 mm will pass spontaneously, usually within 40 days of symptom onset.
- Providers should be mindful of potential effects of ionizing radiation in patients undergoing repeated CT imaging, such as recurrent stone formers.
- Evaluation:
  - Obtain PTH level as part of screening evaluation if hyperparathyroidism is suspected.
  - Metabolic testing of one or two 24-h urine collection should be performed in the high risk, recurrent stone former, patients with a solitary kidney, young patients who present with bilateral renal calculi and family history, or interested first-time stone formers
  - Nephrology can be beneficial, if available, for patients whose stone disease can be challenging to manage.
- Diet:
  - Fluid intake should be increased to 2.5 l a day.
  - Limit sodium intake.
  - Calcium stone formers should consume 1,000–1,200 mg per day of dietary calcium. It is okay for female patients to continue with their calcium supplements as evidence-based articles have proven that calcium supplements do no play a role in forming renal calculi.
  - Calcium oxalate stone formers with high urinary oxalate intake should limit intake of oxalate-rich foods.
  - Low urinary citrate patients increase fruits and vegetables while decreasing nondairy animal protein

- High urinary uric acid should limit intake of nondairy animal protein.
- Cystine stone patients should limit sodium and protein intake.
- Obesity is linked to increase stone disease; advise patients on weight reduction.
- Research into the link between sugar intake and renal calculi is being investigated.
- Follow-up:
  - 24-h urine specimen should be obtained 6 months after beginning a new treatment.
  - Yearly 24-h urine specimen can be considered for surveillance.
  - Periodic blood testing is recommended for those on pharmacologic therapy.
  - Recheck stone analysis to ensure appropriate treatment is being given or for patients who continue to form stones with treatment.
  - Sources of infection should be prevented in patients with struvite stones.
  - Imaging can be obtained occasionally for assessment and discovery of stones in the form of low-dose CT, plain abdominal imaging, or renal ultrasound.

Resources for the Nurse Practitioner

European Association of Urology 2014, Guidelines on Urolithiasis. http://uroweb.org/wp-content/uploads/22-Urolithiasis_LR.pdf

AUA Guidelines: Medical Management of Kidney Stones, 2014 http://www.auanet. org/education/guidelines/management-kidney-stones.cfm

National Institute of Diabetes and Digestive and Kidney Diseases (NIDDK) www. niddk.nih.gov

National Kidney Foundation: www.nkfm.org

Resources for the Patient

National Institute of Diabetes and Digestive and Kidney Diseases (NIDDK) Diet for kidney stone prevention: http://www.niddk.nih.gov/health-information/health-topics/urologic-disease/diet-for-kidney-stone-prevention

www.urologyhealth.org
www.kidney.org
www.auanet.org/education
www.nkfm.org

References

Curhan GC (2007) Epidemiology of stone disease. Urol Clin North Am 34(3):287–293. doi:10.1016/j.ucl.2007.04.003

Ferrandino MN, Pietrow PK, Preminger GM (2011) Evaluation and medical management of urinary lithiasis. In: Wein AJ (ed) Campbell-Walsh urology. WB Saunders Elsevier, Philadelphia, p 1287

Matlaga BR, Lingeman JE (2010) Chapter 48. Surgical management of upper urinary tract calculi. In: Wein AJ, Kavoussi LR, Novick AC, Partin AW, Peters CA (eds) Campbell-Walsh urology, vol 2, 10th edn. WB Saunders Elsevier, Philadelphia

Scales CD, Curtis LH, Norris RD, Springhart WP, Sur RL, Schulman KA, Preminger GM (2007) Changing gender prevalence of stone disease. J Urol 177(3):979–982

Scales CD, Smith AC, Hanley JM, Saigal CS, Urologic Diseases in America Project (2012) Prevalence of kidney stones in the United States. Eur Urol 62(1):160–165

Semins MJ et al (2010) The association of increasing body mass index and kidney stone disease. J Urol 183(2):571–575

Idiopathic and Traumatic Male Urethral Strictures

9

Silvia S. Maxwell and Richard A. Santucci

Contents

Abbreviations

RUG	Retrograde urethrogram
VUCG	Voiding cystourethrogram
PFUDD	Pelvic fracture urethral distraction defect
PVR	Post-void residual
DVIU	Direct vision internal urethrotomy

S.S. Maxwell, ACNP-BC (✉)
Detroit Medical Center, Department of Urology, Detroit, MI, USA
e-mail: maxwellss@yahoo.com

R.A. Santucci, MD, FACS, HON FC Urol(SA)
Urology, Detroit Medical Center, Detroit Receiving Hospital,
The Center for Urologic Reconstruction™, Michigan State College
of Medicine, Detroit, MI, USA

© Springer International Publishing Switzerland 2016
M. Lajiness, S. Quallich (eds.), *The Nurse Practitioner in Urology*,
DOI 10.1007/978-3-319-28743-0_9

159

Overview

Incidence

Urethral stricture is defined as a narrowing of the urethra which obstructs the flow of urine from the bladder to the urethral meatus as a result of fibrotic tissue. Scar tissue buildup from traumatic injury, instrumentation, congenital malformations, malignancy, or infection can cause a narrowing of the urethral lumen. Although the actual incidence is unknown, urethral stricture disease represents a significant economic burden on the healthcare system. The economic burden of urethral stricture in the United States was last evaluated for the year 2000. The annual costs exceeded over $200 million and resulted in over 1.5 million office visits (Barbagli et al. 2014). Urethral stricture actually results in more office visits and procedures than more seemingly common urologic problems such as kidney stones.

True urethral stricture disease is considered to be a rare entity in females. Despite this fact, surgical procedures including urethral dilations and direct visualization and incision of urethra (DVIU) has historically been performed on women to treat a variety of lower urinary tract symptoms (LUTS) such as urinary urgency, frequency, recurrent urinary tract infection (UTI), and bladder pain. The diagnosis of female urethral stricture disease increases cost of health care per individual by more than $1,800 per year (Santucci et al. 2008). As this is rare, this chapter will focus on male urethral stricture disease.

Anatomy

The urethra is an approximately 20 cm hollow tube that allows urine to empty from the bladder to the urethral meatus. It is broken down into four sections: (1) posterior (prostatic) from bladder neck to the sphincter, (2) membranous including only the sphincter, (3) bulbar from the membranous urethra to the base of the penis, and (4) pendulous from the base of the penis to the tip of the penis.

Etiology

Most acquired urethral strictures are due to trauma, iatrogenic, or infectious processes, although truly the etiology of strictures (not Pelvic Fracture Urethral Distraction Defects – PFUDD) is perhaps unimportant. The symptoms and treatments are usually the same no matter what the cause (Santucci et al. 2007). In at least 50 % of patients with stricture, the cause of the stricture is completely unknown.

Iatrogenic causes accounted for over 45 % of all urethral strictures. Instrumentation from previous transurethral procedures such as a TURP, radical prostatectomy, removal of kidney stones, previous urethral dilations, and traumatic urethral catheterization can cause urethral injury resulting in stricture. Most idiopathic and inflammatory urethral strictures occur in the bulbar urethra for reasons that are not known (Siegel et al. 2014).

Urethral catheterization is one of the most commonly performed procedures by health care providers. It may be an important cause of urethral stricture, especially when a Foley catheter balloon is inadvertently inflated in the bulbar urethra. Some researchers believe that prolonged catheterization can cause inflammation and urethral ischemia, which eventually leads to urethral stricture (Lumen et al. 2009).

Less common causes of urethral stricture include:

- Gonococcal urethritis, or *Chlamydia* may cause scarring, which results in a stricture formation, possibly years after the original infection. Post-inflammatory urethritis continues to be a common cause of urethral strictures in developing countries (Lumen et al. 2009).
- Lichen sclerosis (LS) is an inflammatory skin condition which can cause extensive genitourinary scarring. Strictures related to LS not only have a higher degree of treatment-related complications but also disease recurrence (Liu et al. 2014).

Radiation damage can be an important cause of strictures, but these special cases require unusual treatments and are beyond the scope of this chapter.

There is a special category of urethral obstruction which is often referred to as a "stricture" but in fact results from complete distraction/breakage of the urethra usually due to severe pelvic fracture trauma. These have been classically called "posterior urethral strictures" but are neither always posterior in location nor strictures at all, since the urethra is not narrowed as much as absent. Modern nomenclature refers to these as: (PFUDDs). Pelvic trauma due to "straddle" injuries or pelvic fractures due to high-energy trauma such as motor vehicle accidents may partially or completely sever the posterior, membranous, or bulbar urethra.

Symptoms

Depending on severity of the stricture, patients may be completely asymptomatic or suffer extreme pain due to bladder distention or hydronephrosis. Most common symptoms include:

- Decreased force of stream
- Spraying with urination
- Urinary retention
- Urinary frequency
- Nocturia
- Recurrent urinary tract infections
- Dribbling
- Intermittency
- Bladder stones

Physical Exam

A physical exam may show the following:

- Decreased urinary stream
- Discharge from the urethra
- Enlarged bladder
- Enlarged or tender lymph nodes in the groin
- Enlarged or tender prostate
- Hardness on the under surface of the penis
- Redness or swelling of the penis

Sometimes, the exam reveals no abnormalities.

Diagnostic Testing

- Uroflow: Generally, patients with severe stricture will have a decreased flow rate <10 ml/s. Instead of a bell-shaped curve, the flow pattern will be flat (Mundy 2006) (Fig. 9.1). http://www.medindia.net/articles/manual-urodynamics.asp
- Post-void residual (PVR): To determine if patient is retaining urine. The "correct" PVR varies from patient to patient and arbitrary limits for concern are PVRs >200mls. Some patients with large, floppy, distended bladders from long-standing urethral stricture may have huge bladder capacity >1200 cc but are able to void large volumes >700 cc and leave large PVRs >400 cc without symptoms or problems.
- The existence of a stricture can be quickly determined by gently placing an 18 F urethral catheter. If the catheter passes into the bladder, significant stricture is not present. Cystoscopy can be used to determine the presence of stricture but does not indicate length. The definitive test for urethral stricture is the retrograde urethrogram (RUG) which will indicate length, location, and severity of any strictures present. Retrograde urethrogram is considered the "gold standard" for accurately diagnosing the true extent and location of the urethral stricture.
- Renal/bladder ultrasound may show thickening of the bladder wall or hydronephrosis due to outflow obstruction but is not diagnostic for stricture. Some

Fig. 9.1 Uroflow pattern of patient with urethral stricture

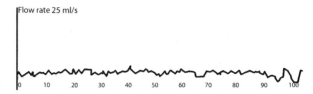

experts use urethral ultrasonography to determine the length and location of (mostly) bulbar urethral stricture preoperatively.

- Before any curative surgical procedure can be performed, the entire urethra must be evaluated. This can be done either radiographically or during previous urethroscopy, usually associated with direct vision internal urethrotomy (DVIU).

Management

Urethral strictures are an anatomical anomaly. There is no suitable medical treatment for this condition.

For centuries, urethral dilation and urethrotomy have been used to treat urethral strictures. Both of these procedures have been found to be effective mostly in the short term. The stricture recurrence rate after a single dilation is 88 % and after an initial DVIU is about 50 %. Only very short strictures ≤ 1.5 cm can expect cure from either procedure (Mundy 2006). Urethral dilation is the most common procedure for treating urethral strictures. It involves the use of progressively larger plastic or metal dilators to stretch the stricture and enlarge the urethral lumen (Mundy 2006). Urethral dilation is very useful, especially in emergency or complete urinary retention situation, but urethral dilation has a very high stricture recurrence rate that approaches 100 % in long or recurrent (previously dilated) strictures (See Table 9.1).

DVIU is another commonly performed procedure for the treatment of strictures. It is utilized to open the strictured area by cutting through the scar tissue without creating additional scarring. After the contracture is released, the urethral lumen is enlarged. A catheter is left in place for at least 3 days until healed (Santucci and Broghammer 2006). Some practitioners leave a Foley catheter longer than 3 days. There is no evidence that placement of a 16 F Foley for greater than 72 h after DVIU is superior.

Unfortunately, repeat DVIU/dilation or DVIU/dilation on longer strictures has a very poor success rate, and in these cases, curative urethroplasty must always be considered. Recent research has shown that the initial success rate of DVIU may be as low as 8 %. Repeated procedures eventually fail 100 % of the time. Furthermore, repeated treatments may actually contribute to increased scar formation, creating longer, more dense stricture (Santucci and Eisenberg 2010). According to

Table 9.1 Complications from stricture disease

Short term (moderate)	Long term (rare)
LUTS	Acute urinary retention
Recurrent UTI	Renal failure
Need for repeat procedures	Urethral carcinoma
	Fournier's gangrene
	Bladder failure

Table 9.2 Postoperative
complications of urethrotomy

Complication	Rate
Bleeding	4–6 %
Infection	8–9 %
Incontinence	1 %
Impotence	1 %
Failure after repeat procedure	Up to 100 %

Adapted from Santucci et al. (2007)

Anger et al. (2011), "repeat urethrotomy or dilation for urethral stricture is neither curative nor cost effective in the long term" (see Table 9.2).

Some patients who are unable or unwilling to undergo urethroplasty procedures may choose to perform intermittent self-catheterizations in an attempt to keep the urethral lumen open. Unfortunately, the strictures will always recur once patients stop self-catheterizing (Broghammer et al. 2014), and patients generally find this procedure painful, annoying, and difficult.

The only technique with the potential to cure urethral stricture in many cases is urethroplasty: a series of surgical techniques using tissue transfer to cure urethral stricture. There are more than 30 described techniques for urethroplasty. They fall into several major categories:

• Buccal mucosal
• Johanson (a two-stage technique where the urethra is split open in the first stage and closed again in the second stage)
• Fasciocutaneous
• Anastomotic

Anastomotic repair involves the complete excision of the fibrotic urethral stricture and joining the two healthy ends together. This technique is used for short <2 cm bulbar urethral strictures or PFUDD. This procedure has a 90 % success rate for inflammatory/idiopathic stricture and a slightly lower success rate for PFUDD. Anastomotic repair is deservedly popular, although recent data suggests that even in expert hands, it can be associated with unacceptable sexual complications such as chordee (ventral bend in the penis), erectile dysfunction, and poor glans blood flow (Barbagli et al. 2007).

Buccal urethroplasty can be used anywhere in the urethra and is the treatment of choice for longer strictures >2 cm. Although non-hair-bearing tissue from the postauricular, penile shaft or foreskin has been used, buccal mucosa is the preferred graft material today. A 2.5 cm-wide by up to 7 cm-long graft can be harvested from the inner cheek. This tissue is resistant to infection and trauma, "takes" well after placement, and is rich in elastin which decreases contraction of the graft. After incising the stricture (either ventrally – that is, the surface of the urethra closest to the skin, or dorsally – the surface of the urethral closer to the penis), the graft is then sutured to the edge of the urethra mucosa, creating a larger urethral lumen. This procedure has a variable reported success rate, generally accepted to be about 90 % (Santucci et al. 2007). A newer modification of this procedure, using a dorsal buccal graft has been described for even very long strictures, and it has an unusually good success rate of 80 % despite being used against the worst and longest strictures (Santucci and Eisenberg 2010)

Two-stage Johanson urethroplasty has proven useful over the decades since its popularization in the 1950s but is generally now best used for specific strictures. That is, penile urethral strictures resultant from the childhood repair of hypospadias. In hypospadias, the urethra is not formed properly, and the urethral meatus ends on the penile shaft, scrotum, or perineum. The Johanson urethroplasty can also be used for patients who have failed several other repairs and have extensively damaged urethral tissue. The first stage involves the incising of the scar tissue and converting the tubular urethra into a flat "urethral plate" which is then sewn to the surrounding skin. Buccal grafts may be sewn into the urethral plate to enlarge it and make the second stage tubularization of the plate more successful. The second stage involves the tubularization of the urethral plate, restoring the patient to a normal urethral appearance. This is done after all healing is complete and all postoperative inflammation is resolved, usually 5–6 months after the first stage (Zimmerman and Santucci 2011).

While the Johanson urethroplasty is used to cure urethral stricture, some patients elect not to have a second stage procedure, as the first stage generally allows unobstructed urination. This may require sitting to void forever. In some patients such as the extreme elderly, unwell, or unwilling to undergo urethroplasty, a form of the Johanson urethroplasty called a perineal urethrostomy may be performed. With the perineal urethrostomy, the patient is able to void without difficulty in a sitting position. This procedure has a high degree of satisfaction and success, at the cost of permanent modification in the patient's body (Burks and Santucci 2010).

Fasciocutaneous urethroplasty, a reliable but technically demanding form of urethroplasty, uses a penile skin fasciocutaneous (skin plus underlying tissue) flap to enlarge the urethra. The foreskin can be used, although most Americans lack a foreskin due to childhood circumcision. This technique is generally used for long, penile strictures but appears to have higher perioperative complication rates than other techniques. The high success rates and technical simplicity of the buccal urethroplasty has caused the buccal technique to largely replace the fasciocutaneous technique (Zimmerman and Santucci 2011).

PFUDD was introduced as a special case of urethral obstruction which is not truly a "stricture" or narrowing of the urethra but generally a torn urethra with a wall of scar formed in between the torn ends. The major treatment of this is an anastomotic urethroplasty where the wall of scar is cut out and the two ends are sewn together. This procedure is technically demanding and may require transfer to a center of excellence for urethroplasty (Burks and Santucci 2010).

Postoperative Care

See details of immediate postoperative management in Box 9.1.

Box 9.1. Postoperative Management for Urethral Stricture
Patient teaching:
Pain/Swelling

- Avoid sitting directly on perineal area. Sitting at a 45° angle in a reclining chair is best.
- To decrease the pain and swelling, place an ice pack on the surgical area (between your legs) for 24 h. Leave the ice pack in place for 20 or 30 min every 2 h (a bag of frozen peas works well and can be refrozen between uses).
- When sitting or lying down, place a rolled-up hand towel under the scrotum. Elevating the scrotum also helps decrease the pain and swelling.
- If graft is taken from cheek, you will need to apply an ice bag to your face for 24 h.
- Use Peridex Swish and Spit after each meal and at bedtime for 3 days.
- No sexual intercourse for 6 weeks after surgery.

Hygiene

- The dressings and jock strap may be removed after 48 h. If they get soaked or very dirty, they may be removed early. No further dressings are needed.
- It is *OKAY* to bathe or shower after 48 h,
- No soaking in tub for 6 weeks.

The patient should anticipate VCUG 3 days after an anstomotic urethroplasty or 7 days after a buccal mucosal urethroplasty to check for healing at the anastomotic site. If no extravasation of fluid is suspected, the Foley catheter may be removed permanently. If leakage of fluid is seen, the Foley catheter is reinserted and left in place for another week (Hosam et al. 2005).

Long-term management includes a uroflow, PVR, and symptom check every 4 months for the first year and yearly after that.

Clinical Pearls
Reassure patient some bruising and swelling is normal after surgery
Give patient "emergency" contact information to use when office is closed
Reinforce all pre-op/post-op teaching regarding catheter and use of overnight and daytime drainage bags

Normal activity is allowed, but no heavy lifting/strenuous activity until surgical site is healed

Teach patient to use correct dilation technique with 14 Fr. or 16 Fr. Catheter will keep urethra open with the least discomfort

Lubricate urethra well

Allow patient to choose catheter type

Give patient samples (obtained from Sales Reps) of different styles of catheters Lubricious, Silicone, or

Assist patient with ordering needed supplies

Follow up with patient periodically to assure he is continuing with plans activity until surgical site is healed

Resources for the Nurse Practitioner

Litwin MS, Saigal CS, editors. Urologic Diseases in America. Society of Urologic Nurses and Associates www.suna.org. McAninch JW, Lue TF, editors. General Urology. Newman DK, Wein AJ, editors. Managing and Treating Urinary Incontinence. American Urology Association www.auanet.org

Resources for the Patient

Society of Urologic Nurses and Associates www.suna.org. International Continence Society www.ics.org. National Institutes of Health www.nih.gov

References

Anger JT, Buckley JC, Santucci RA, Elliott SP, Salgal CS (2011) Trends in stricture management among male medicare beneficiaries: underuse of urethroplasty? Urology 77(2)

Barbagli G, De Angelis M, Romano G, Lazzeri M (2007) Long-term follow up of bulbar end-toend anastomosis: a retrospective analysis of 153 patients in a single center experience. J Urol 178(6):2470–2473. Epub 2007 Oct 15

Barbagli G, Kulkarni S, Fossati N, Larcher A, Sansalone S, Guzzoni G, Lasseri M (2014) Longterm followup and deterioration rate of anterior substitution urehtroplasty. J Urol 192:808–813

Burks FN, Santucci RA (2010) Complicated urethroplasty: a guide for surgeons. Nature Reviews Urology 7:521–528

Broghammer JA, Santucci RA, Schwartz BF (2014) Urethral strictures in males treatment & management. Medscape.com. Accessed 8/14/14

Hosam HSQ, Cavalcanti A, Santucci RA (2005) Early catheter removal after anterior anastomotic (3 days) and ventral Buccal mucosal only (7 days) urethroplasty. Int Brazilian J Urol 31(5):459–464

Liu JS, Walker K, Stein D, Prabhu S, Hofer MD, Han J, Yang XJ, Gonzalez CM (2014) Lichen Sclerosus and isolated bulbar urethral stricture disease. J Urol 192:775–779

Lumen N, Hoebeke P, Williamsen P, De Troyer B, Pieters R, Oosterlinck W (2009) Etiology of urethral stricture disease in the 21st century. J Urol 182:983–987

Mundy AR (2006) Management of urethral strictures. J Postgrad Med 82:489–493

Santucci R, Broghammer J (2006) Medscape Reference –Urethral Strictures … Retrieved 14 Aug 2014

Santucci RA, Eisenberg L (2010) Urethrotomy has a much lower success rate than previously reported. J Urol 183:1859–1862

Santucci R, Geoffry J, Wise M (2007) Male urethral stricture disease. J Urol 177:1667–1674

Santucci RA, Payne CK, Saigal CS (2008) Office dilation of the female urethra: a quality of care problem in the field of urology. J Urol 180:2068–2075

Siegel J, Tausch TJ, Simhan J, Morey AF (2014) Innovative approaches for complex penile urethral strictures. Transl Androl Urol 3(2):179–185

Zimmerman WB, Santucci RA (2011) Buccal mucosa urethroplasty for adult urethral strictures. Indian J Urol 3:364–370

Diagnosis and Management of Urinary Tract Infections and Pyelonephritis

10

Laura J. Hintz

Contents

L.J. Hintz, FNP-BC, CUNP
Midwest Prostate and Urological Institute, Saginaw Center for Female Urology,
Saginaw, MI, USA
e-mail: laurahintz@mpui.org

© Springer International Publishing Switzerland 2016
M. Lajiness, S. Quallich (eds.), *The Nurse Practitioner in Urology*,
DOI 10.1007/978-3-319-28743-0_10

Diagnosis and Management of Urinary Tract Infections

The purpose of this chapter is to assist nurse practitioners, particularly those specializing in urology, on how to recognize and manage urinary tract infections. Unfortunately, the lack of knowledge in assessing both a urine specimen correctly and the inability to correlate this information with a patient's presenting signs and symptoms is cause for frequent misdiagnosis of urinary tract infections. In addition, the misuse and overuse of antibiotics in today's society has made treating urinary tract infections more complicated. This chapter will review the different types of infections, the diagnostic testing required, as well as population-specific guidelines for proper management.

Definitions

Urinary tract infection (*UTI*) is an inflammatory response of the urothelium to bacterial invasion that is typically associated with bacteriuria and pyuria. The term acute cystitis is often used interchangeably.

Bacteriuria is the presence of bacteria in the urine and it may be symptomatic or asymptomatic.

Asymptomatic bacteriuria (*ASB*) is the isolation of bacteria from the urine in significant quantities that would be consistent with infection but in the absence of local or systemic urinary tract symptoms.

Pyuria is the presence of white blood cells in the urine. This typically indicates an inflammatory response secondary to an infectious process caused from bacteria. Pyuria without bacteriuria warrants evaluation for tuberculosis, stones, or cancer. Pyuria in the presence of bacteriuria is indicative of "true" infection.

Acute pyelonephritis is the presence of bacteriuria and pyuria, in addition to the presence of specific symptoms (i.e., fever, chills, and flank pain), indicating an interstitial inflammation of the renal parenchyma.

Incidence and Epidemiology

Urinary tract infections (UTIs), also referred to as acute cystitis, are the most common bacterial infection and are responsible for between four and eight million clinic visits (Hanno 2014). Therefore, this ranks UTIs as the most common cause for ambulatory care visits in the United States. The direct costs are more than $1.6 billion per year (Hanno 2014).

Urinary tract infections affect men, women, and children. In women, the incidence is higher in the younger population, typically at the onset of sexual activity. The risk factors relevant to the premenopausal woman are the use of spermicides and sexual frequency. The incidence will increase slowly again after menopause due to the changes in the vaginal tissues and the increased pH of the vagina as a result of estrogen deficiency.

Of the millions of UTIs reported, women account for approximately 85 % of them. Eleven percent of women will report having had a UTI during any given year (Hanno 2014). Fifty percent of all women will report having had at least one infection in their lifetime. By the age of 24, one in three women will have had a urinary tract infection. UTIs in men are less common until after the age of 50 when the incidence of enlarged prostate increases, contributing to bladder outlet obstruction and urinary retention.

Nearly 25 % of women with a first UTI will have a second episode within 6 months. Nearly 50 % of women will report a second UTI within a year of experiencing their first UTI (Hanno 2014). Whether the infection is left untreated, or treated with short-term, long-term, or prophylactic antibiotic therapy, the risk of reoccurrence remains unchanged. Therefore, the symptomatic episodes are more of a nuisance than a health threat in the healthy population.

Asymptomatic bacteriuria (ASB) occurs in 3 % of women in their early twenties (Hanno 2014). It increases 1 % at the onset of intercourse, which typically occurs during the late teenage years. It will also increase 1 % per decade of life. In the pregnant population, the implications are more concerning, even though the incidence is similar to that of the nonpregnant population. This is due to the increased risk for pyelonephritis, in those harboring bacteria in the urinary tract. During pregnancy, it is of increased concern during the second and third trimester. Based on some studies, it is suggested that there is a 20–40 % incidence of pyelonephritis, if ASB is left untreated, in the pregnant population (Hanno 2014).

Other populations at risk are those suffering from diabetes and multiple sclerosis. Female diabetic patients have a higher incidence of UTI than do male diabetics. UTIs are also considered complicated in the ambulatory diabetic patient, and there is an increased risk for pyelonephritis, as well as other complications, if left untreated. When UTIs occur in multiple sclerosis patients, increased exacerbations and progression of the disease may be observed. As for the elderly, non-catheterized patient population, 11–25 % percent can develop transient ASB (Hanno 2014). In turn, it is difficult to eradicate the persistent colonization that can occur in up to 50 % of the elderly population. In the 65 years and older population, as many as 20 % of women and 10 % of men will have bacteriuria, and routine treatment is considered unjustified, unless special circumstances exist.

Catheter-associated urinary tract infection (CAUTI) has also become of great concern over the past several years. They are the most common cause of nosocomial infection (Stamm and Norrby 2001). The end result is an increased risk for falls, delirium, and immobility in the older population and an increased financial burden on the health care system. Most of the uropathogens responsible for CAUTIs gain access by extraluminal (direct inoculation when inserted) or intraluminal (reflux of uropathogens from failure to maintain a closed system). As soon as the catheter is inserted, bacteria will start to develop colonies known as biofilms (living layers). These biofilms are collections of microorganisms with altered phenotypes that adhere to a medical device, such as the catheter and/or collection bag. The biofilm is protective against antimicrobials and the host immune response. The risk of colonization increases in relation to the duration of catheterization and reaches nearly 100 % at 30 days (Hanno 2014).

Risk factors for UTIs
Sexual intercourse
A new sex partner within the past year
Use of spermicides
Use of diaphragm/cervical cap
Estrogen deficiency
Previous UTI
History of UTI in first degree female relative
Urinary retention
Benign prostatic hyperplasia
Steroid use

Subpopulations at increased risk
Infants
Pregnant women
Elderly
Spinal cord injury
Indwelling catheters
Diabetes
Muscular sclerosis
Acquired immunodeficiency disease
Underlying urological abnormalities

Pathophysiology

The model for uncomplicated UTIS is that bacterial virulence is crucial for overcoming normal host defenses (Hanno 2014). However, in complicated UTIs the paradigm is reversed; the bacterial virulence is not as critical as the host factors. UTIs are typically initiated by a potential urinary pathogen migrating from the bowel. In some cases the pathogens arise from the vaginal flora, as a direct result of inoculation during sexual activity. These pathogens then begin to colonize the vagina and perineum with enteric organisms. As the organisms move to the periurethral mucosa, they ascend through the urethra into the bladder (urethritis and/or cystitis) and in some cases through the ureter to the kidney (pyelonephritis).

Most infections in women represent an ascending infection, and this process of infection is related to the relatively short length of the female urethra. UTIs are less common in the younger male, with the incidence increasing in the aging male. The male urethra is considerably longer than the female, which makes ascending infections less common. Most UTIs in older men are typically related to a voiding dysfunction that puts them at risk for acquiring an infection (i.e., urinary retention secondary to an enlarged prostate), or they may acquire it after some form of instrumentation.

In relation to the pediatric population, UTIs may be responsible for a significant source of morbidity; this is particularly true when there are associated anatomic abnormalities. The most common abnormality in children is vesicoureteral reflux. The risk associated with reflux is renal scarring, as a result of ascending UTIs, causing pyelonephritis. In this population, when any UTI is suspected, it is recommended that a complete workup be performed. The diagnosis and treatment of UTIs in the pediatric population is a topic that needs to be reviewed in depth, in a separate discussion. For the purpose of this book, we will only focus on the adolescent and adult population.

Classification

Urinary tract infections may be classified by several different categories: complicated or uncomplicated, upper tract or lower tract, and first infection, unresolved bacteriuria, or recurrent infection. Recurrent infections can be separated into two separate classifications of "reinfection" or "bacterial persistence." On occasion, UTIs may be classified by the type of organism.

Uncomplicated UTIs may be defined as a UTI in the setting of a functionally and structurally normal urinary tract, in a patient that is typically afebrile. This type of infection typically occurs in women, and the uropathogen is one that is susceptible to and eradicated by a short course of an inexpensive oral antimicrobial therapy. Complicated UTIs are typically defined as pyelonephritis and/or a structural or functional abnormality that decreases the efficacy of antimicrobial therapy. In most cases, complicated UTIs are caused by bacteria that are resistant to many antimicrobials. CAUTIs are classified as complicated and the rate of infection averages about 5 % per day (Bernard et al. 2012).

The diagnosis of upper UTI refers to an infection of the kidney (pyelonephritis). The lower urinary tract (LUT) refers to infections of the bladder (cystitis) or urethra (urethritis). As for the organism responsible for the infection, it may be caused by bacterial, fungal, viral, or parasitic organisms.

E. coli, a gram-negative bacillus, accounts for 75–90 % of community-acquired cases of acute uncomplicated cystitis. It accounts for 50 % of the nosocomial infections (Hanno 2014). In women, another 5–15 % are caused by *Staphylococcus saprophyticus*, a gram-positive coccus (Ellsworth and Onion 2012). The remaining UTIs are typically caused by *Enterobacteriaceae*, such as *Klebsiella pneumoniae*, and gram-positive bacteria such as *Enterococcus faecalis* and *Streptococcus agalactiae* (group B streptococcus). However, the two latter gram-positive organisms often represent contamination of the voided specimen, when isolated from a voided urine.

UTIs categorized as first infections are typically new or an isolated infection that is separated by a previous infection of at least 6 months, such as the "honeymooners' UTI." Unresolved bacteriuria occurs during therapy and implies that the urinary tract is not sterilized during the treatment period. Recurrent UTIs are subdivided into *reinfection* and *bacterial persistence*. Reinfection accounts for up to 80 % of the cases and is typically a direct result of recurrence caused from a new organism outside of the urinary tract. In the majority of these cases, there is no underlying anatomic issue. Bacterial persistence typically refers to a recurrent infection caused by the same uropathogen, despite the sterilization of urine with therapy. This category of recurrence is less common and is most likely a result of something specific within the urinary tract (i.e., calculus or obstructive prostate). The long-term goal for treating recurrent UTIs should be to improve quality of life, while minimizing antibiotic exposure.

Among the younger and healthier female population, the reinfection rate is 25 % within 6 months after the first urinary tract infection (Hooten 2012). In this healthier population and in the majority of patients, about two-thirds of the cases are "recurrent" involving the same bacteria that is believed to have caused the first infection. The term reinfection is said to occur when a patient presents with new signs and symptoms of a UTI after a previous infection has been eradicated and in the presence of a "new" organism.

Presentation

In most patients, the presenting signs and symptoms may include dysuria (pain with urination), frequency, urgency, nocturia (nighttime voiding), suprapubic pain, gross hematuria, malodorous urine, and low back pain. Fever with an uncomplicated UTI is unusual. Therefore, acute pyelonephritis should be considered when fever, tachycardia, and/or costovertebral angle pain are present. In addition, patients with suspected pyelonephritis may present as ill appearing and seem uncomfortable.

Uncomplicated UTI	Pyelonephritis
Dysuria	Fever (temp > 38 °C)
Urgency	Chills
Frequency (voiding smaller amounts)	Nausea
Gross hematuria	Vomiting
Cloudy urine	Flank pain
Malodorous urine	Any combination of uncomplicated UTI signs and symptoms
Low back pain	Costovertebral angle tenderness with palpation
Suprapubic pain and tenderness with palpation	

History and Physical Examination

The patient's history is the most important tool for diagnosing an uncomplicated UTI. Always include an evaluation of the patient's current urinary tract symptoms, past history of urinary tract infections, and any other urinary tract problems or conditions. Follow that with a routine family history, social history (specifically looking at smoking history), and any antibiotic use in the previous 6 months. In addition, one should also inquire into the patient's sexual history, with a special focus on any known history of sexually transmitted infections (STIs). Finally, one should support the detailed history with a focused physical exam and urinalysis.

Female Examination
- Temperature
- Check post void residual
- Evaluate the possibility of pregnancy and history of reproductive issues
- Include pelvic exam, assessing for cystocele, and if symptoms indicate a possible pelvic infection or urethritis
- Examine low back, abdomen, and suprapubic area for tenderness, pain, or abnormalities

Male Examination
- Temperature
- Check post void residual
- Evaluate any history of prostate problems
- Examine genitals, low back, and abdomen for tenderness, pain, or abnormalities
- Examine rectum and prostate for prostate enlargement, growths, inflammation, or pain

Abnormal Findings
- Pain or discomfort in response to pressure on the lower back, abdomen, or the area above the pelvic bone (10–20 % of patients have suprapubic tenderness in uncomplicated UTIs)
- Costovertebral angle tenderness is typically indicative of pyelonephritis
- Growths or abnormalities detected during the pelvic or rectal exam
- Enlarged or tender prostate gland (men only)
- Discharge from the urethra

Differential Diagnosis

Among the female population, interstitial cystitis (IC) and sexually transmitted infections (STIs) are the most common diagnoses that present with similar symptoms. Dysuria is common with cystitis, urethritis, and vaginitis. However, cystitis is more likely when the signs and symptoms also include frequency, urgency, and/or hematuria. If the symptoms are of severe or sudden onset and in the absence of vaginal irritation and/or discharge, then cystitis is also more likely. The probability of acute UTI is greater than 50 %, in women with any one of the signs or symptoms. It increases to more than 90 % when there is a combination of symptoms, such as dysuria and frequency, without vaginal irritation or discharge. A urine culture is typically positive with bacterial cystitis.

Urethritis is typically caused by *Chlamydia trachomatis*, *Neisseria gonorrhoeae*, or the herpes simplex virus. Vaginitis is caused by *Candida* species or *Trichomonas vaginalis*. Pyuria is commonly seen in cystitis and urethritis but is less likely in vaginitis. The symptoms of urethritis also tend to be mild, gradual in onset, and include vaginal discharge. Vaginal irritation or discharge, if present, is a symptom suggestive of vaginitis and reduce the likelihood of the diagnosis of bacterial cystitis by 20 %. In a patient that has a documented history of bacterial cystitis, as evidenced by a positive urine culture, and they present again, with similar symptoms, the likelihood of true infection approaches 90 % (Hanno 2014).

In the male population, prostatitis, epididymitis, and STIs are the most common diagnoses that present with similar symptoms when compared to acute cystitis. However, with acute bacterial prostatitis, in addition to the typical dysuria, frequency, urgency, and nocturia, additional constitutional symptoms, such as fever, chills, and malaise, may also occur. Patients may also report complaints of perineal and/or low back pain. On exam, the prostate may feel enlarged and boggy, with acute tenderness. Epididymitis occurs more commonly in the adolescent and elderly male population but can affect men of all ages. In the population of men under the age of 35, the form of transmission is sexual and is typically caused by *C. trachomatis* and *N. gonorrhoeae* pathogens. In the elderly population, *E. coli* and *Pseudomonas* are the most common offending pathogens. Indwelling catheters, in the elderly population, are also responsible for the development of epididymitis, through a retrograde mechanism. In patients, with epididymitis, the presenting symptoms may include a tender hemiscrotum, in addition to a swollen epididymis. The scrotum may be warm, erythematous, and swollen. Fever, chills, voiding symptoms, and pain that radiates to the ipsilateral flank may also occur.

Diagnostic Testing

Commercially available dipsticks that test for leukocyte esterase (an enzyme released by leukocytes), and for nitrites (which is reduced from nitrates by some bacteria), are an appropriate alternative to urinalysis and urine microscopy, to diagnose cases of acute uncomplicated cystitis. When obtaining a urine specimen for evaluation, it is recommended that in order to avoid contamination, the patient should obtain a midstream, clean-catch urine specimen. Since nitrites and leukocyte esterase are the most accurate indicators of uncomplicated cystitis in symptomatic patients, the urine dipsticks are convenient and cost effective. However, critical evaluation of each individual patient's case needs to be evaluated cautiously since even negative results for both tests do not reliably rule out the presence of infection.

Urine sediment after centrifuge will show microscopic bacteriuria in 90 % of infections with 10^5 colony-forming units (CFU/mL). Microhematuria is evident in 50 % of infections and pyuria in about 80–90 %. However, pyuria can also be the result of several other inflammatory conditions of the urinary tract. The normal vaginal flora can appear to be gram-negative bacteria on urinalysis which can lead to a false-positive result. Alternatively, if the urine is diluted from a high fluid intake, in a symptomatic patient who is voiding frequently, which prevents the bacteria from multiplying to the high counts associated with UTI, then the urine result may be a false negative. Based on a recent meta-analysis, a urine dipstick that is positive for nitrituria will increase the odds of a positive culture by a factor of 11 (Hanna 2014). The same analysis demonstrates that the finding of leukocyte esterase increases the likelihood of a positive culture by a factor of 3 (Hanna 2014). Colony counts of midstream urine specimens ranging from 10^2–10^4 CFU/mL that are caused by *E. coli*, *S. saprophyticus*, or *Proteus* sp. occur in one-third of patients who present with acute symptomatic cystitis. Therefore, a pure culture must be considered significant, regardless of the colony count in the presence of symptoms.

Urine cultures are recommended for those patients with suspected acute pyelonephritis; patients with unresolved symptoms or those with symptoms that recur within 2–4 weeks after the completion of treatment. In addition, a urine culture should be performed on patients who present with atypical symptoms. The benefit of a urine culture is to confirm the presence of bacteriuria and the antimicrobial susceptibility of the infecting uropathogen.

There are studies that have compared voided urine specimens and bladder-aspirate specimens in women with cystitis. The studies indicate that the traditional criterion for a positive culture of voided urine (10^5 colony-forming units per milliliter) is less sensitive for bladder infection. In addition, 30–50 % of women with cystitis have colony counts of 10^2–10^4 colony-forming units per milliliter in voided urine (Hooten 2012). Therefore, according to one source, in the presence of typical signs and symptoms, a colony count greater than or equal to 10^3 colony-forming units per mL, of a uropathogen, is diagnostic of acute uncomplicated cystitis and does represent a positive culture (Colgan and Williams 2011). Most laboratories do not quantify bacteria below a threshold of 10^4 colony-forming units per milliliter from voided urine specimens. Therefore, with a culture report of "no growth," caution should be used when interpreting the results, in a patient who presents with signs and symptoms of cystitis. Routine posttreatment urinalysis or urine cultures are not necessary in asymptomatic patients, except in those where hematuria was initially present. If hematuria persists, then cystoscopy and additional testing should be performed to rule out other urological pathology.

Imaging

Typically, no further studies beyond urinalysis and urine cultures are needed to diagnose acute uncomplicated cystitis. In those patients that present with atypical symptoms of acute uncomplicated cystitis, those who do not respond to initial anti-microbial therapy, those with a history of recurrent UTIs, or those with suspected pyelonephritis may need imaging studies to rule out complications and other disorders. A brief description of the recommended testing follows, along with a generic cost analysis of each test.

Ultrasound (U/S) Ultrasonography is the recommended initial screening tool if testing is indicated. It is noninvasive, is cost effective, has no risk of contrast reaction, and has no risk of radiation exposure. Ultrasonography is able to identify calculi, obstruction of the upper urinary tracts, abscess, and other congenital abnormalities. Renal ultrasounds are the most cost-effective treatment option.

Intravenous Pyelogram (IVP) IVP is essential for visualizing the ureters, the details of calyceal anatomic structures and the presence of calyceal dilatation, and the presence of stricture, stones, or obstruction. The calyceal details are necessary for diagnosis of reflux nephropathy as well as papillary necrosis.

Imaging studies should be considered in the following
Women with febrile infections
Men
If urinary tract obstruction is suspected and with history of
Calculi
Ureteral tumor
Ureteral stricture
Congenital ureteropelvic junction obstruction
Previous urologic surgery or instrumentation
Diabetes
Persistent symptoms despite several days of appropriate antibiotic therapy
Rapid recurrence of infection after apparently successful treatment

Computed Tomography (CT Scan) CT scan offers the best anatomic detail but its cost prevents it from being used for screening. It is more sensitive than ultrasound in the diagnosis of acute focal bacterial nephritis and renal and perirenal abscess (it may demonstrate stones or obstruction).

Patients with known pyelonephritis should have a CT scan with contrast or a U/S to assess the presence of foci of pyelonephritis in the renal cortex or cortical or perinephric abscesses. Immediately after a CT scan with contrast, it is possible to obtain the equivalent of an IVP by taking a KUB (X-ray of kidney, ureter, and bladder) film of the patient in the prone position and observe the anatomic structures of the collecting system and ureters, as the contrast is cleared into the bladder.

Magnetic Resonance Imaging (MRI) MRI provides much greater contrast between different soft tissues than a CT scan. It relies on obtaining a radiofrequency

(RF) signal from alignment and subsequent relaxation of protons in hydrogen atoms in water in the body. It should never be utilized in routine practice or as a first-line diagnostic test. It is typically used in follow-up when the ultrasound has already been performed and has been unable to fully answer the diagnostic question. The CT and magnetic resonance imaging (MRI) provide the best anatomic data as well as the cause and extent of the infection.

Comparison of the Cost of Radiologic Testing

Test	Cost $
Renal ultrasound (US)	$
Intravenous pyelogram (IVP)	$$
Computed tomography (CT) scan (with and without contrast)	$$$
Magnetic resonance imaging (MRI)	$$$$
*Medicare allowable charges	

Risk Factors

Some of the risk factors for UTIs, along with the causes of bacterial persistence, and the factors that increase the risk of complications from UTIs are shown in tables below.

Causes of bacterial persistence
Infected stones
Chronic bacterial prostatitis
Unilateral infected atrophic kidney
Vesicovaginal fistula
Intestinal fistula
Ureteral anomalies
Infected diverticula
Foreign bodies (stent or catheters)
Infected urachal cyst
Infected medullary sponge kidney
Infected papillary necrosis
Ureteral stump after nephrectomy

Factors that increase the risk of complications from UTIs
Urinary tract obstruction
Infection from urea-splitting bacteria
Diabetes
Renal papillary necrosis
Neurogenic bladders

Factors that increase the risk of complications from UTIs
Pregnancy
Congenital urinary tract anomalies
Elderly patient with acute bacterial prostatitis
End-stage renal disease on hemodialysis
Immunosuppression after a renal transplant

Management of Urinary Tract Infections

Behavioral Modifications
The majority of behavioral interventions are aimed at prevention. There are many different sources, including research done by Dr. Thomas Hooton, that report avoiding the use of spermicide or diaphragm/spermicide use is beneficial. In addition, decreasing the frequency of coitus and the practice of urination after may reduce the risk of infection. Finally, one should encourage women to utilize proper cleansing technique following voiding, using a front to back motion when wiping. The use of bubble baths has also been questioned. The practice of pushing fluids and maintaining a high intake of water is also recommended. Patients should also be encouraged to void every 2–3 h and to take their time to empty completely.

Oral Supplements
There have been several studies looking at the use of cranberry juice to prevent urinary tract infections. Cranberry juice does inhibit bacterial attachment to epithelial cells. Based on a meta-analysis done in 2012, it was concluded that adults that consumed cranberry juice on a regular basis were 38 % less likely to develop symptoms of UTI. In addition, the cranberry may reduce the symptoms of UTI by suppressing the inflammatory response. It remains unclear which ingredients in cranberry products may be responsible for the overall benefit. Cranberry is essentially safe and inexpensive and is recommended for the prevention of UTI. However, it is not currently recommended as a treatment for acute cystitis.

Treatment

The management of UTIs has become quite complicated due to the increasing prevalence of antibiotic-resistant uropathogens. Complicated nosocomial UTIs were primarily responsible for antibiotic resistance in the past. However, as things change the resistance has spread to uncomplicated community-acquired UTIs. It is important to try and understand the antibiotic resistance rates within the area that one is practicing. Urine levels are more important than serum levels in relation to the efficacy of antibiotics treating UTIs. When an antibiotic appears to be a poor choice based on sensitivity data-related serum levels, they may actually be a good choice if they have a high urinary excretion rate.

Ampicillin has the highest rate of resistance and should not be used for empiric treatment (Hanno 2014). It is followed by fluoroquinolones (broad spectrum) which have around a 30 % resistance rate, and trimethoprim has only about a 20 % resistance rate (Hanno 2014). Once the culture and sensitivity results are available, the least expensive and the most limited spectrum antibiotic is preferred. However, it is important to interpret antibiotic susceptibility carefully because the tests are typically based on serum levels of a drug. It is also of benefit if one keeps in mind the local antibiotic resistance rates. This information is more likely to be available in hospital settings, which reflects cultures of inpatients, or those with complicated and/or recurrent infections and may overestimate the rates of resistance in relation to patients diagnosed with uncomplicated UTI.

The recommended treatment option for the majority of uncomplicated UTIs is a single dose to a 5-day course of antibiotics, depending on the antibiotic preference. Sulfas have become the most widely prescribed antibiotic for uncomplicated outpatient UTIs, along with nitrofurantoin, and have an estimated overall clinical cure rate of 85 % (Bastani 2001). Unfortunately, in the ambulatory care setting, US surveys demonstrate that fluoroquinolones are the most commonly used antimicrobials for UTIs (Hooten 2012).

Sulfas are broad spectrum and they effectively reduce the fecal, vaginal, and periurethral colonization. The side effects of this drug class are typically skin rash and gastrointestinal (GI) upset. They are also considered potentially lifesaving antibiotics. The overuse of this class raises the risk for resistance in the future.

First-generation cephalosporins are appropriate in treating uncomplicated UTI. However, the second and third generation cephalosporins should be reserved for infections requiring a broader coverage. In general, cephalosporins have poor activity against *Enterococcus*.

There is one natural occurring antibiotic, fosfomycin, that can be administered as a single dose therapy. It gives a very high urinary concentration that kills bacteria rapidly, reducing the opportunity for mutant selection. It may be less efficacious in some situations; however, even when the urine is sterile, the patient may report persistent symptoms for an average of 48 h after. In turn, the patient may be concerned as to whether the infection is really eradicated and may cause them to ask for additional antibiotic therapy. In this situation, the use of urinary analgesics may be beneficial.

Choose antibiotics based on the following:
1. Likelihood that it will be active against enteric bacteria that commonly produce UTIs
2. High concentration level of the antibiotic in the urine
3. Tendency not to alter the bowel or vaginal flora
4. Selection for resistant bacteria
5. Limited toxicity
6. Available at a reasonable cost/covered by patient insurance

If treating with nitrofurantoin, one should consider that it is *not* recommended in the elderly population or those with renal impairment. Routine monitoring of patient's renal function is recommended in all patients over 65 years of age. In those patients with moderate to severe renal impairment, the therapeutic urinary concentration of nitrofurantoin may not be achieved. These patients are also at risk for peripheral neuropathy. Nitrofurantoin is well tolerated, has good efficacy, and does tend to be effective against *Pseudomonas* and *Proteus* species. If symptoms persist after 2–3 days of therapy, one can always consider changing the antibiotic to a more expensive, broad-spectrum antibiotic. However, the recurrence of symptoms after the initial short-course therapy would indicate the need for culture and sensitivity testing, and retreatment should be for a 7–10-day period.

Fluoroquinolones have a very broad spectrum of activity against the majority of uropathogens, including *Pseudomonas*. However, it is not recommended to use this drug class in treating uncomplicated UTIs. This class has limited gram-positive activity and is not effective in treating *Enterococcus*. Fluoroquinolones are very expensive agents and should be reserved for the treatment of complicated UTI, pseudomonal infections, or treatment of resistant organisms.

Antimicrobial Agents for the Management of Uncomplicated UTI

Tier	Drug	Dosage	Pregnancy category
First	Fosfomycin (Monurol)	3-g single dose	B
	Nitrofurantoin (macrocrystals)	100 mg BID for 5 days	B
	Trimethoprim-sulfamethoxazole (Bactrim/Sulfa)	160/800 BID for 3 days	C
Second	Ciprofloxacin (Cipro)	250 mg BID for 3 days	C
	Ciprofloxacin, extended release (Cipro XR)	500 mg QD for 3 days	C
	Levofloxacin (Levaquin)	250 mg QD for 3 days	C
Third§	Ofloxacin	200 mg QD for 3 days Or 400 mg single dose	C
	Amoxicillin/clavulanate (Augmentin)	500/125 mg BID for 7 days	B
	Cefdinir (Omnicef)	300 mg BID for 10 days	B
	Cefpodoxime	100 mg BID for 7 days	B

Adapted from Colgan and Williams (2011)

Recurrent Bacterial Cystitis

It is critical to obtain a detailed culture history when attempting to differentiate whether a recurrent bacterial infection is caused from a site of bacterial persistence inside or outside of the urinary tract. Ninety-five percent of recurrent infections are caused from a source outside the urinary tract (Hanno 2014). However, when the cause is considered to be from outside the urinary tract, then a full urological workup is necessary. Therefore, it is crucial to identify the bacteria responsible for the infection. In a case, where one has treated the UTI successfully, identified by antimicrobial eradication (negative culture) and reinfection occurs by a varying strain of *Enterobacteriaceae*, this is specific in indicating reinfection. The only other factor that may cause a similar scenario is reinfection from an enterovesical fistula. In the case of a fistula, the urine is never sterilized, and the infection may be with multiple organisms, which should raise the suspicion for a fistula.

If urinary symptoms persist or recur within 1–2 weeks after completing treatment, then this suggests infection with an antimicrobial-resistant strain. A culture *should* then be performed and therapy should be initiated utilizing a broad-spectrum antibiotic (fluoroquinolones). As urological specialists, it is acceptable to start with a broad-spectrum antibiotic, with the expectation that treatment may need to be altered based on the final culture and sensitivity results. In individuals that experience episodes of cystitis that recur at least 1 month after successful treatment, then treatment should be initiated utilizing a first-line course regime. If recurrence is within 6 months, then consideration should be given to a first-line antimicrobial other than the one that was initially used. Due to high resistance rates, this is especially true when considering the use of trimethoprim-sulfamethoxazole.

If it is determined that a recurrent infection is caused by gram-negative introital colonization, prophylaxis should be considered. In relation to postcoital cystitis, also called "honeymoon cystitis," it is recommended to have the patient void after intercourse and to use a single low-dose antibiotic. The typical recommended antibiotic dose for these patients, which has remained effective over the years, would be TMP-SMZ (one dose of double strength), cephalexin (250 mg), or nitrofurantoin 50–100 mg) after intercourse (Bastani 2001). This regimen tends to work well in patients who are having less frequent intercourse. If the patient is having intercourse more than four times per week, then it is better to only treat symptomatic infections with a short course of antibiotics to reduce the overall antibiotic use.

Over the years, patients have also been treated with long-term prophylactic use of antibiotics. This therapy may have been utilizing nitrofurantoin (50–100 mg every night) or TMP-SMZ (1/2 tab every other night). Typically after 6–12 months, the therapy could be stopped in the hopes that the colonization with uropathogenic gram-negative organisms has resolved. Over the next 6 months, if a patient develops 2–3 episodes of UTI, then another course of prophylaxis would be initiated (Hanno 2014).

The current goal in treating UTIs is to decrease the overall use of antibiotics while maintaining a quality of life. Several studies have looked at different strategies that can be used to achieve this goal. One of these strategies is the "self-start" strategy. This relies on the patient to make the clinical diagnosis of UTI, which is typically not difficult for these patients, when the previous infections have been confirmed by a positive culture. These patients are given a prescription for an antibiotic (i.e., TMP-SMZ, cephalexin, or nitrofurantoin), to be taken for 2–3 days at the onset of symptoms. If symptoms persist or reoccur beyond this initial therapy, then an office visit is recommended for culture and sensitivity testing. Self-start therapy works very well in the patient who has been well educated.

Special Situations

There are certain populations in which an otherwise uncomplicated UTI requires more attention. There are physiologic changes that take place during pregnancy that have important implications in regard to ASB and the progression of infection. During pregnancy there is an increased renal size, altered renal function, hydroureteronephrosis, and anterosuperior displacement of the bladder. The rate of pyelonephritis in pregnant females is much higher than that of the nonpregnant female and a 20–40 % increase in acute pyelonephritis if ASB is left untreated in the pregnant population (Hanno 2014). In turn, it is associated with higher rates of prematurity and perinatal mortality. In a pregnant woman with acute uncomplicated UTI, one could consider treating with amoxicillin (250 mg every 8 h), ampicillin (250 mg every 6 h), nitrofurantoin (100 mg every 6 h), or even an oral cephalosporin. As previously noted, amoxicillin and ampicillin are no longer first-line recommendations due to their ability to interfere with the fecal flora.

Young healthy men with no complicating risk factors may be treated with a 7–10-day course of antibiotics. The recommended course of treatment is TMP-SMZ (double strength every 12 h), trimethoprim (100–200 mg every 12 h), or a fluoroquinolone, and a pretreatment culture and sensitivity is recommended in this population. In the middle-aged and elderly population, who are sexually active, no further workup is needed if the infection is eradicated with antibiotic therapy. However, in the younger, nonsexually active, population or when there is a high clinical suspicion, then further workup can be done to look for an abnormality of the urinary tract. One might obtain imaging studies to assess the kidneys, ureters, and bladder, a cystoscopy, and a post void residual.

Patients with indwelling catheters, whether short term or long term, pose a risk for infection. It should be noted that for every day that a catheter is left indwelling, the risk of infection raises 3–10 % per day (Bernard et al. 2012). The Center for Disease Control (CDC) has completed studies evaluating the majority of circumstances where an indwelling catheter may be utilized. The recommendations can be reviewed at http://www.cdc.gov/hicpac/pdf/CAUTI/CAUTIguideline2009final.pdf and a brief summary of the recommendations are as follows:

- Limit long-term use, especially for the treatment of incontinence, unless the patient has a stage 3 decubitus
- Limit use in nursing home patients and consider intermittent or external catheters if possible
- Only use for specific surgical procedures when necessary, not as a routine surgical intervention and remove the catheter within 24 h or as soon as possible

In addition, the CDC guidelines support the use of indwelling catheters when attempting to promote comfort and quality of life for the terminal patient and those patients whom will be experiencing prolonged immobilization (i.e., spinal surgery or traumatic injuries, such as pelvic fractures).

Pyelonephritis

Incidence

Acute uncomplicated pyelonephritis is much less common than cystitis. There is an estimated ratio of 1:28 cases of pyelonephritis to that of cystitis, with an annual incidence of 25 cases per 10,000 women between the ages of 15–34 years (Hooten 2012).

Presentation

As previously shown in table (__), the classic symptoms of pyelonephritis are any combination of cystitis symptoms, accompanied by bacteriuria, pyuria, fever, chills, flank pain, and/or nausea and vomiting. One should remember that patients with flank pain and UTI do not necessarily have pyelonephritis, and the reverse is true in that patients may actually have a case of pyelonephritis in the absence of local and systemic symptoms. The majority of patients with acute pyelonephritis will be ill appearing and may have additional symptoms such as malaise or hypotension. It should create a high level of suspicion if a patient has any of the known risks factors, listed in the table below.

Risk factors for pyelonephritis
Vesicoureteral reflux
Obstruction of the urinary tract (congenital ureteropelvic junction obstruction, stone disease, pregnancy)
Genitourinary tract instrumentation
Diabetes mellitus
Voiding dysfunction
Age (renal scarring rarely begins in adulthood; this is typically related to reflux in children)
Female gender

Classification

Pyelonephritis may be caused by several different routes:

1. Ascending: Bacteria reach the renal pelvis through the collecting ducts at the papillary tips and then ascend through the collecting tubules. The presence of urinary reflux from the bladder or increased intrapelvic pressures caused by lower urinary tract obstruction can also cause upper urinary tract infection.
2. Hematogenous: This tends to be the result of *Staphylococcus aureus* septicemia or *Candida* in the blood stream. Hematogenous causes are uncommon.
3. Lymphatic: This is an intraperitoneal infection (i.e., abscess) caused by an unusual form of extension to the renal parenchyma.

The majority of acute uncomplicated pyelonephritis cases can be managed in the outpatient setting. However, if one has diabetes, a renal stone, hemodynamic instability, or is pregnant, then they should be hospitalized for the initial 2–3 days of parenteral therapy. Pyelonephritis can lead to sepsis, hypotension, and even death, especially if the infection is caused by an unrecognized upper tract obstruction.

Flank tenderness is a prominent finding on physical exam. In addition, an infected urine with large amounts of granular or leukocyte casts in the sediment is also indicative for the diagnosis. Eighty percent of the cases of pyelonephritis are caused by *E. coli*. In patients who have undergone a form of urinary tract instrumentation, who have had a previous indwelling catheter, or those that have developed a nosocomial infection, the microorganism responsible for the infection in these situations is typically *Pseudomonas, Serratia, Enterobacter, and Citrobacter*. In patients with stone disease, one should suspect *Proteus* or *Klebsiella*. Both of these microorganisms contain the enzyme urease, which has the ability to split urea with the production of ammonia and an alkaline environment. This leads to the precipitation of the salt struvite (magnesium ammonium phosphate), which form branched calculi. These calculi harbor bacteria in the interstices of the renal calculi. These types of stones are referred to as staghorn calculi, which can lead to chronic renal infection.

Diagnostic Testing

Laboratory testing and radiology studies can assist in differentiating the cause. One should order both urine and blood cultures to rule out sepsis. An intravenous urogram may demonstrate normal results or it may show renal enlargement secondary to edema. It is necessary to distinguish whether focal enlargement is a result of a renal mass or abscess. A delayed appearance of the pyelogram or a diminished nephrogram may be caused by inflammation. When assessing an imaging study, the most important thing to rule out is the presence of obstruction and/or urolithiasis. Both of which could lead to a life-threatening situation if left undiagnosed and untreated. Ultrasound is useful in some cases; however, CT may demonstrate the patchy decreased enhancements that suggest focal renal involvement.

Complications

Abnormal findings and complications associated with pyelonephritis are:

(a) Xanthogranulomatous pyelonephritis (XGP) – severe and chronic renal infection that destroys the kidneys.
(b) Chronic pyelonephritis – rare in the absence of an underlying functional or structural abnormality of the urinary tract.
(c) Renal insufficiency – rare complication.

(d) Hypertension – is noted in over 50 % of patients.
(e) Renal abscess – collection of purulent material confined to the renal parenchyma.
(f) Infected hydronephrosis – bacterial infection of a hydronephrotic kidney and can often be associated with destruction of the renal parenchyma.
(g) Perinephric abscess – typically results from a rupture of a cortical abscess or hematogenous seeding from another infection site.
(h) Emphysematous pyelonephritis – acute necrotizing parenchyma and perirenal infection caused by gas-forming uropathogens.

Management

In the majority of cases, acute uncomplicated pyelonephritis can be treated on an outpatient basis. However, the patient should be hospitalized in the following situations:

- Nausea or vomiting
- Dehydrated
- Pregnant
- History of non-adherence to medical therapies
- Evidence of septicemia

Urine cultures should be obtained on all suspected cases of pyelonephritis. On all hospitalized patients, one should obtain blood cultures and baseline labs to check renal functioning. The results of the blood cultures tend to be positive in approximately 15–20 % of patients (Bastani 2001).

Initial treatment for uncomplicated pyelonephritis should be started using a fluoroquinolone pending cultures results. It is becoming a more common practice to administer a single parenteral dose of ceftriaxone (1 g), a consolidated 24 h dose of an aminoglycoside (i.e., gentamicin), or a fluoroquinolone before initiating oral antibiotics (Hanno 2014).

Clinical Pearls
- In uncomplicated UTIs, there is no association between recurrent infections and renal scarring, hypertension, or renal failure.
- Methenamine or hexamine hippurate are used as urinary antiseptics for chronic therapy, which reduces the risk of antibiotic resistance and efficacy may be increased if used as adjuvant therapy to cranberry supplements.
- Asymptomatic bacteriuria, in the elderly population, may be unjustified and is typically ineffective.

- It is a challenge clinically to differentiate between upper and lower UTI; however, it is most often not necessary because management and treatment are similar.
- Recurrent UTI tends to be biological in nature and not necessarily related to personal hygiene.
- When investigating UTIs, the best overall screening tool remains the retroperitoneal ultrasonography.
- Due to the risk of pulmonary fibrosis with nitrofurantoin use, it is not recommended as a long-term prophylactic antibiotic of choice. However, it remains an excellent option for short-course treatment of recurrent UTI.
- If a male patient has no culture documented history of a UTI, then it is unlikely that he will have a diagnosis of chronic bacterial prostatitis.

In the outpatient setting, it is recommended to treat with a 10-day course of antibiotics using a fluoroquinolone or trimethoprim-sulfamethoxazole. In the presence of sepsis, it is recommended to treat for 14 days. According to the Infectious Disease Society of America (IDSA), the recommendation is to treat with ciprofloxacin 500 mg BID for 7 days or levofloxacin 750 mg QD × 5 days (2011). If the patient demonstrates improvement within 72 h, then continue the oral antibiotic therapy and obtain a repeat urine culture at 4 days on and 10 days off of the medication. If no improvement is noted, then the patient should be hospitalized and one should review the culture and sensitivity results. In the presence of an obstruction or abscess, treatment and/or drainage of the causative factor would be recommended. Complicated cases of pyelonephritis requiring hospitalization or a procedure may also require up to 3 weeks of antibiotic therapy.

Bibliography

Bass-Ware A, Weed D, Johnson T, Spurlock A (2014) Evaluation of the effect of cranberry juice on symptoms associated with a urinary tract infection. Urol Nurs 34(3):121–127

Bastani B (2001) Urinary tract infections. In: Noble J, Greene HL II, Levinson W, Modest GA, Mulrow CD, Scherger JE, Young MJ (eds) Textbook of primary care medicine, 3rd edn. Mosby, Inc., Missouri, pp 1364–1371

Bernard MS, Hunter KF, Moore KN (2012) A review of strategies to decrease the duration of indwelling urethral catheters and potentially reduce the incidence of catheter-associated urinary tract infections. Urol Nurs 32(1):29–37

Center for Disease Control and Prevention (2005) Urinary tract infections [Disease Listing]. Retrieved from http://www.cdc.gov/ncidod/dbmd/diseaseinfo/urinarytractinfections_t.htm

Center for Disease Control and Prevention (2009) Guideline for prevention of catheter associated urinary tract infections 2009. Retrieved from http://www.cdc.gov/hicpac/pdf/CAUTI/CAUTIguideline2009final.pdf

Colgan R, Williams M (2011) Diagnosis and treatment of acute uncomplicated cystitis. Am Family Phys 84(7):771–776, Retrieved from http://www.aafp.org/afp/2011/1001/p771.html

Ellsworth P, Onion DK (2012) The little black book of urology, 3rd edn. Jones & Bartlett Learning, Sudbury, pp 68–71

Goldman HB (2001) Evaluation and management of recurrent urinary-tract infections. In: Kursch ED, Ulchaker JC (eds) Office urology: the clinician's guide. Humana Press Inc., Totowa, pp 105–111

Gould CV, Umscheid CA, Agarwal RK, Kuntz G, Pegues DA, Healthcare Infection Control Practices Advisory Committee (HICPAC) (2009) Guideline for catheter associated urinary tract infections 2009. Center for Disease Control and Prevention. Retrieved from http://www.cdc.gov/hicpac/pdf/cauti/cautiguideline2009final.pdf

Gupta K, Hooton TM, Naber KG, Wullt B, Colgan R, Miller LG, Moran GJ, Nicolle LE, Raz R, Schaeffer AJ, Soper DE (2011) International Clinical Practice Guidelines for the Treatment of Acute Uncomplicated Cystitis and Pyelonephritis in Women: A 2010 Update by the Infectious Diseases Society of America and the European Society for Microbiology and Infectious Diseases

Hanno PM (2014) Lower urinary tract infections in women and pyelonephritis. In: Hanno PM, Guzzo TJ, Malkowicz SB, Wein AJ (eds) Penn clinical manual of urology, 2nd edn. Elsevier Saunders, Philadelphia, pp 110–132

Harlow HF (1983) Fundamentals for preparing psychology journal articles. J Compar Physiol Psychol 55:893–896

Hooten TM (2012) Uncomplicated urinary tract infection. N Engl J Med 366:1028–1037, Retrieved from http://www.nejm.org/doi/full/10.1056/NEJMcp1104429

Macfarlane MT (2013) Urology, 5th edn. Lippincott Williams & Wilkins, Philadelphia, pp 86–110

Sandock DS, Kursh ED (1995) Urinary tract infections in adult females. In: Resnick MI, Novick AC (eds) Urology secrets. Hanley & Belfus, Inc., Philadelphia, pp 205–207

Society of Urological Nurses Association (2010) Prevention & Control of Catheter-Associated Urinary Tract Infection (CAUTI) [Clinical Practice Guidelines]. Retrieved from https://www.suna.org/sites/default/files/download/cautiGuideline.pdf

Stamm WE, Norrby SR (2001) Urinary tract infections: disease panorama and challenges. J Infect Dis 183(Suppl 1):S1–S4. Retrieved from http://www.ncbi.nlm.nih.gov/pubmed/11171002

Uphold CR, Graham MV (1998) Clinical guidelines in family practice, 3rd edn. Barmarrae Books, Gainesville, pp 601–607

Urodynamics

11

Christine D. Koops

Contents

Objectives
1. Provide a basic understanding and overview of urodynamics.
2. Introduce the components of urodynamic testing and discuss the indications for specific urodynamic tests.
3. Discuss tips for interpreting and documenting urodynamic results.

C.D. Koops, RN, BSN
Owner and President, Dynamic Measurements LLC Mobile Urodynamics, Grand Rapids, MI, USA
e-mail: christinekoops@gmail.com

© Springer International Publishing Switzerland 2016
M. Lajiness, S. Quallich (eds.), *The Nurse Practitioner in Urology*,
DOI 10.1007/978-3-319-28743-0_11

Introduction

Urodynamics are a collection of tests used to measure bladder, urethral, and pelvic floor muscle function in order to diagnose disorders of the lower urinary tract (Chapple et al. 2009). These tests include simple, noninvasive tests such as uroflowmetry and more complex multichannel filling and pressure flow studies, which can include electromyography and fluoroscopy. Learning the complexities of urodynamics can seem overwhelming but every test can be simplified to the study of two basic lower urinary tract functions: *storage* and *emptying*.

Step-by-step instructions on how to perform urodynamics are beyond the scope of this chapter, but additional resources appear at the end of the chapter.

The terminology, methods, and units used throughout this chapter conform to the standards recommended by the International Continence Society (ICS) and the International Urogynecological Association (IUGA) (Abrams et al. 2003; Hayden et al. 2010).

Indications for Urodynamics

There is a lack of consensus in current literature regarding precise indications for urodynamic testing, but in general, urodynamics are indicated when the results and information provided from the tests will guide treatment management decisions. The purpose of urodynamics is to answer well-defined *questions* about specific functions of the urinary tract. These questions are formulated after the initial history and physical have been completed and information from other tests such as urinalysis, voiding diaries, symptom questionnaires, and pad tests has been attained. The goal of urodynamics is to reproduce and characterize urinary symptoms in order to uncover underlying cause(s) of lower urinary tract *storage* or *emptying* dysfunction. Urodynamic testing is not considered a standard evaluation for all patients, with lower urinary tract symptoms, but should be considered when:

(a) *Neurological involvement is suspected*:
   (i) Male or female patient presents with OAB symptoms and has recently been diagnosed with MS.
(b) *There is a history of previous pelvic surgery*:
   (i) Female patient presents with simple stress incontinence symptoms and has had a bladder suspension 8 years ago.
(c) *Upper urinary tract compromise is suspected, due to elevated storage pressure*:
   (i) Male or female spinal cord injury patient on four times daily intermittent self-catheterization presents with elevated creatinine levels.
   (ii) Urodynamics are done to determine bladder volumes safe for preservation of the upper urinary tracts.

(d) *Urodynamic data is needed to evaluate the effectiveness of an intervention*:
   (i) Male or female spinal cord injury patient in "c" is placed on new anticholinergic medication.
   (ii) He or she should be evaluated to determine effectiveness and new safe bladder capacity, in order to prescribe catheterization regime.
(e) *History is complicated*:
   (i) 32-year-old female patient presents with mixed urinary incontinence symptoms and has two documented post void residual volumes that exceed 200 ml.
(f) *Physical exam or preliminary findings do not match history or patient's symptoms*:
   (i) 68-year-old female patient, who denies bladder leakage, presents with grade 4 uterine prolapse with suspected urethral compromise and post void residual exceeding 100 ml.
   (ii) Urodynamics will evaluate for occult stress incontinence so patient can be counseled appropriately regarding surgical options.
(g) *Urodynamic data will help in counseling the patient about their treatment options*:
   (i) 68-year-old male patient is seen and treated in the ER with urinary retention and was catheterized for volume exceeding 2 l. This patient has known history of BPH.
   (ii) Urodynamics can be used, in this scenario, to determine bladder contractility, which will be helpful when counseling the patient regarding his treatment options and expected outcomes.

Clinical expertise in deciding when, why, and how to perform urodynamic studies is critical to the accurate interpretation and ultimate clinical utility of the test. Before embarking on urodynamic testing, the clinician must be certain the indications are clear. Outlining the *urodynamic question*(s) is imperative to attaining meaningful urodynamic results (Chapple et al. 2009; Winters et al. 2012).

Components of Urodynamics

Urodynamics can include simple noninvasive uroflow testing with post void residual measurements, multichannel filling cystometry, leak point pressure testing, urethral pressure testing, multichannel pressure flow studies, and sphincter electromyography and can include fluoroscopy (see Table 11.1 for full list of components of urodynamics). Some of these tests might be performed independent of one another, but most often they are performed as a group or collection. Some of the tests overlap or are considered components of one another and should be coded as such according to CPT coding guidelines (see Appendix). For example, leak point pressure and urethral pressure tests are done during the filling phase of cystometry (see Appendix). Urodynamic findings themselves would be insufficient for formulating diagnoses and treatment plans but, as previously mentioned, must be used in conjunction with complete history and physical and combined

Table 11.1 Components of urodynamics

Name, abbreviation	Description	Primary function being evaluated	Indications & aims
Uroflow	Electronic measurements of urine flow rates and voided volume	Global voiding function	Used to identify voiding patterns when voiding dysfunction associated with LUTS is suspected
Post void residual, PVR	Amount of urine remaining in bladder after void. Measured by catheterization or ultrasound	Global voiding function	Used to evaluate sufficiency of bladder emptying when voiding dysfunction associated with LUTS is suspected
Cystometry, CMG Also known as filling cystometry	Commonly used to describe the filling phase of urodynamics. This is a measurement of infused volume, pressures, and sensation	Storage function and sensation of the bladder	Used to identify abnormalities in bladder capacity, compliance, stability, and sensation in patients with LUTS, particularly when history of previous pelvic surgery, suspected neurological involvement, failure of conservative treatment, or complicated history is present
Leak point pressure, LPP Abdominal leak point pressure (ALPP) Detrusor leak point pressure, DLPP	*LPP* is a general term that is used to describe bladder pressure that results in transurethral loss of urine. *ALPP* is the intravesical pressure at which urine leakage occurs due to an increased abdominal pressure in the absence of a detrusor contraction. *DLPP* is defined as the lowest detrusor pressure at which leakage occurs in the absence of either a detrusor contraction or increased abdominal pressure	*ALPP* – urethra competence *DLPP* – urethral competence in regard to elevated storage pressures	*ALPP* – used to determine urethral competence and quantify urethral incompetence when stress incontinence is suspected *DLPP* – along with associated cystometric filling volume, DLPP is used to determine safe bladder volumes, typically in patients with suspected neurogenic urinary tract dysfunction, for the purpose of protecting the upper tracts from sustained elevated storage pressures

Urethral pressure profile, UPP	Pressure measurements taken from all points along the urethra which are reproduced in the form of a profile. These measurements can be taken at rest or during stress (coughing or straining)	Urethral competence and closing functions	Generally performed by gynecologists and urogynecologists to determine urethral competence and rule out intrinsic sphincter deficiency when evaluating symptoms of incontinence
Pressure flow study, PFS	Simultaneous measurements of bladder pressure and flow rates taken during the voiding phase of multichannel urodynamics	Detrusor contractility and bladder outlet during the voiding phase	Used to determine cause of inadequate evacuation or urine or abnormal urine flow (obstruction vs. detrusor underactivity) and sometimes to evaluate the cause of urgency symptoms
Electromyography, EMG	A graphic representation of the electrical activity of the urethral sphincter or pelvic floor muscles during multichannel urodynamics	Coordination of pelvic floor contraction during filling and stress and relaxation of pelvic floor during void	Used to determine coordination between the detrusor function and the pelvic floor during bladder filling and during the voiding phase when detrusor sphincter dyssynergia or neurological involvement is suspected with regard to LUTS or to evaluate the integrity of the pelvic floor
Fluoroscopic urodynamics	Combines and links radiographic imaging with urodynamic pressure, flow, and EMG tracings	Simultaneous observation of the morphology and function of the lower urinary tract	Used to identify abnormalities in bladder storage or outlet when complicated pathology is expected or when diagnosis is unclear after simpler tests have been performed
Ambulatory urodynamics	Functional tests of the lower urinary tract, utilizing natural filling and reproducing the patient's everyday activities. Monitors pressures, leakage, and flow for a period of 4–24 h	Behavior of bladder (and urethra) mechanisms and leakage during activities of daily living	Used to identify abnormalities in bladder storage or outlet when complicated pathology is expected, when diagnosis is unclear after simpler tests have been performed, or when initial treatment regimens have failed

with data from other associated tests such as urinalysis, cystoscopy, VCUG or pad tests and assessment tools such as bladder diaries, and LUTS questionnaires (Table 11.2).

Preparing for Urodynamics, Urodynamics Equipment

Since the objective data obtained during urodynamic testing can be influenced by patient anxiety, the unnatural conditions of the testing environment, and the knowledge and experience of the clinician performing the studies, it is imperative for both the clinician and the patient to be well prepared prior to embarking upon testing:

Table 11.2 Tests and tools associated with urodynamics

Name	Description	Indications & aims
Urine dip stick	A basic diagnostic tool used to determine pathological changes in a patient's *urine*	To determine presence of absence of UTI
Urinalysis with or without culture	An electronic tool used to determine pathological changes in a patient's *urine*	To determine presence of absence of UTI
Bladder diary	Chart used by patient to record volume and time of each void, fluid intake, pad usage, and incontinence episodes	To evaluate voiding patterns, quantify severity of symptoms, and add objectivity to the history in evaluating patients with LUTS
LUTS questionnaires	Patient-completed questionnaires for evaluating lower urinary tract symptoms and their impact on quality of life	To summarize LUT symptoms and the impact of the symptoms, to evaluate effectiveness of treatment, to facilitate patient-clinician discussion, and used in epidemiological surveys
Supine stress test	During physical exam, or after retrograde filling of the bladder, the patient is asked to cough while the examiner visualizes the urethral meatus and notes presence or absence of leakage	To confirm evidence of stress incontinence
Q-Tip test	Measures the change in angle of a patient's urethra during a Valsalva maneuver using a lubricated cotton swab and a protractor measuring device. Urethral hypermobility is considered if the change in angle from relaxed to Valsalva is >30°	To confirm the presence or absence of urethral hypermobility in evaluating the possible cause of stress incontinence

Table 11.2 (continued)

Name	Description	Indications & aims
Pad test	Measures the volume of leakage during a specific period of time based on pad weight. 1 ml = 1 g	Used to detect and quantification urine loss
Pyridium pad test	The patient is given Pyridium prior to pad test to determine if moisture is indeed urine leakage	Used to detect and quantification urine loss
Tampon test/double-dye test	Oral Pyridium is given to the patient, methylene blue and sterile water are instilled into the bladder, and a tampon is placed vaginally. The tampon is later inspected for the presence and color of dye	Used to identify extra urethral leakage and to determine the source of extra urethral leakage (e.g., vesicle/vaginal fistula or urethral/vaginal fistula)
Cystoscopy	Cystoscopy is an endoscopic procedure that uses a flexible scope inserted through the urethra to visualize the lower urinary tract – the urethra, the external sphincter, the prostate, and the bladder	Used to evaluate cause of hematuria, irrigative bladder symptoms, or frequent UTIs. Used to diagnose urethral strictures or bladder cancer. Used for procedural purposes such as to remove bladder tumors, bladder stones, and ureteral stones or to place or remove ureteral stints
Cystography, cystourethrography, voiding cystourethrography (VCUG), and urethrography (antegrade and retrograde)	These radiographic studies involve imaging of the bladder, urethra, ureters, and/or kidneys after administration of contrast. These studies may be done at rest or during voiding	To diagnose structural abnormalities of the bladder, urethra, or ureters or to evaluate the integrity of these structures after trauma or injury. Also used to document the presence of vesicoureteral reflux

1. Provide written instructions at the time their appointment is being scheduled:
   (a) Include the date and time.
   (b) Approximate length (1 h) of the procedure.
   (c) A phone number they can call should questions arise prior to the appointment.
   (d) A brief description of what to expect.
   (e) The written instructions should clearly state that the patient is to arrive with a full bladder and should include instructions on completing a voiding diary and medication use prior to testing if appropriate.

If a uroflow study is planned prior to the cystometrogram, the patient should be instructed to consume 16 oz of fluid 1 h before arriving for the test. Remind the patient this is total fluid intake, not 16 oz over and above what they would normally consume during that hour. Overhydration could result in diuresis during testing, which will alter volume results. Be sure to educate clinic staff and receptionists regarding these instructions to ensure compliance.

Voiding diaries (see Chapter 14) should be required prior to urodynamic testing, as this information will be helpful in formulating urodynamic questions and in determining expected cystometric capacities:

2. Preparing the clinic to ensure the testing environment is as comfortable as possible will help to alleviate patient anxiety and ensure more accurate test results. Urodynamic clinics can be sterile and unaccommodating:
   (a) Controlling the temperature
   (b) Offering privacy
   (c) Covering or hiding unnecessary medical equipment and providing soothing background music

> **Clinical Pearl**
> Urodynamics is an interactive test, so communication during the procedure is important and will also help to ease patient's anxieties. Be sure the patient is aware at all times of what is happening and how it is relevant to the procedure. Talking with the patient about their job, hobbies, families, or the weather can be a helpful distraction and make the patient feel more comfortable.

Urodynamic Equipment

In order to prepare for urodynamics, the clinician must be familiar with the necessary equipment. Determining what urodynamic equipment is best for a clinic will depend on the purpose of the testing. Most equipment will provide the same basic functions with slightly different editing options and report formats. Some urodynamics equipment can interface directly with fluoroscopy equipment to allow for capturing images, simultaneous with pressure readings, which is necessary when performing video urodynamics. Other urodynamics equipment will have software, which can be customized to meet the specific needs of a clinic or interface with electronic medical records.

Special procedure chairs are often used for urodynamic testing. These chairs serve both as exam table and commode. They are ergonomically accommodating but not absolutely necessary for performing urodynamics. One of the advantages of the specialty chair is easier access to, and visualization of, the perineal area, which is particularly useful when performing urodynamics on female patients. Another advantage of the specialty chair is that it allows the patient to remain in one place for preparation, filling, and voiding phases of the urodynamic test, eliminating the risk of catheters falling out or getting misplaced during transfer or ambulation. One of the disadvantages of the specialty chairs is that voiding on the procedure chair is unnatural and difficult for some patients.

Clinical Pearls

When using a urodynamic procedure chair for the voiding phase of the study, it is important to position the patient sitting as upright as possible with their feet on the ground or securely in the foot pedals of the chair. Make sure the voiding funnel, or catch basin, is positioned up against the underside of the chair to avoid loss of fluid during the flow. Some clinicians prefer to move their patients to an adjacent commode for more accurate flow studies.

There are three styles of urodynamic pressure catheters. The first is a disposable water pressure catheter system, which requires external transducers. This type of manometry system was the first type used in urodynamic testing, is the most widely used method internationally, and is recognized as the gold standard by the International Continence Society. One advantage of the water pressure catheters is the availability of several different sizes and styles, which is particularly helpful in pediatric urodynamics. The second type of urodynamics catheter is a non-disposable electronic microtip catheter. This system has the pressure transducer built into the catheter itself. The third style of urodynamic catheter is the T-DOC air-charged catheter.

The preparedness of the clinician performing the urodynamics is a key factor in obtaining meaningful urodynamic results. Though much of the data obtained during urodynamics is objective, the ultimate interpretation of the data is subjective and requires the clinician to have an understanding of how the patient's symptoms, history, and physical findings relate to the urodynamic questions to be answered. Formulating meaningful urodynamic questions prior to embarking upon urodynamics is absolutely necessary. Using Dr. Alan Wein's framework for categorizing symptoms will be helpful in formulating your urodynamic questions (Table 11.3).

For normal storage and emptying to occur, the bladder and bladder outlet must function in a proper and coordinated fashion. According to Wein (1981), all lower urinary tract dysfunction can be classified under the following rubrics:

- Is there a "failure to store" (incontinence), a "failure to empty" (retention), or a combination of both?
- Is the problem due to a dysfunction of the "bladder," a dysfunction of the "outlet" (urethra), or a combination of both?

Uroflow with Post Void Residual

Uroflow is an electronic measurement of urine flow rates and urine volume (Chapple et al. 2009), and used for initial screening or to monitor response to medication or treatment. It is usually followed by a post void residual

Table 11.3 Wein's classification of voiding dysfunction

Failure to store	Failure to empty

Due to the bladder:
  Urge incontinence/detrusor overactivity
  Overflow incontinence
  Poor compliance
	Due to the bladder:
	  Underactive bladder (hypotonic, atonic)

Due to the outlet:
  Stress incontinence
	Due to the outlet:
	  Obstruction (BPH, strictures, prolapse)
	  DSD (detrusor sphincter dyssnergia)

measurement. Urine is measured in milliliters per second (ml/s), which is plotted against time and the data is then converted to a graph tracing. Uroflow, along with and post void residual measurements, can be used to evaluate the general effectiveness of voiding, but the data is not sufficient to determine the cause of lower urinary tract or voiding dysfunctions. Ideally, voided volume should be greater than 150 ml for accurate uroflow data acquisition; however, some patients with incontinence will not be able to tolerate this volume. In these instances, smaller volume uroflows will need to be interpreted and can be compared to voiding diary volumes for further incite.

The following parameters should be measured and reported during uroflow testing:

1. Voided volume
2. Total voiding time (including times of interruption)
3. Flow time (not including times of interruption)
4. Maximum flow rate (expressed in ml/s as Q_{max})
5. Time to maximum flow
6. Average or mean flow rate (expressed as Q_{mean} and is volume voided divided by flow time)
7. Post void residual
8. Flow pattern (described as continuous or intermittent, smooth arc shaped curve or fluctuating curve) (Figs. 11.1, 11.2 and, 11.3)

Multichannel Urodynamics

Multichannel urodynamics measure pressure/volume relationship of the bladder during the filling and voiding phases of micturition and include filling cystometry, leak point pressure tests, urethral pressure testing, and pressure flow studies. During the filling and voiding phases of urodynamics, pressure is measured inside the bladder or vesical cavity (referred to as P_{ves}) and outside the bladder within the abdominal cavity (referred to as P_{abd}). A third channel represents the detrusor muscle activity (referred to as P_{det}). The P_{det} value is derived from subtracting abdominal pressure from vesical pressure ($P_{ves} - P_{abd} = P_{det}$). The clinician must keep in mind that, though this channel is often referred to as "true detrusor," the P_{det} channel is a calculated math channel, which actually represents the subtraction of the abdominal

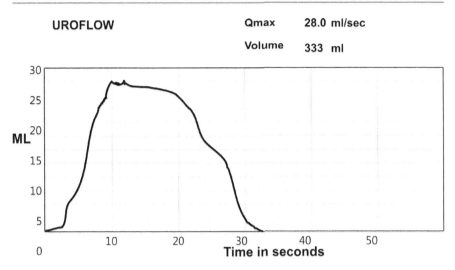

Fig. 11.1 Normal uroflow. This was a 71-year-old man without voiding symptoms. The patient voided 333 ml and his maximum flow rate (Q_{max}) was 28.0 ml/s

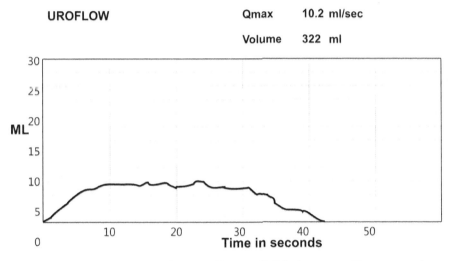

Fig. 11.2 Decreased flow rate. This was an 82-year-old diabetic woman with recurrent urinary tract infections and a residual urine volume of 175 of 150 ml. The uroflow demonstrated a voided volume of 322 ml and a maximum flow rate (Q_{max}) of only 10.2 ml/s. The low uroflow is abnormal, but it cannot differentiate among progressive impaired detrusor contractility with aging or diabetes

pressure from the vesical pressure. Artifact from either the P_{abd} or the P_{ves} channels will be reflected in the P_{det} channel and must be interpreted as such.

Urethral pressure (referred to as P_{ura}) may also be measured during multichannel urodynamics. Urethral pressure is often accompanied by another calculated math channel, urethral closure pressure (represented by P_{clo}). This value is derived when vesical pressure is subtracted from urethral pressure ($P_{ura}-P_{ves}+P_{clo}$). Additional channels often represented in multichannel urodynamics are EMG for monitoring

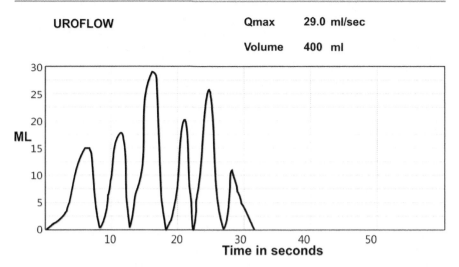

Fig. 11.3 Straining uroflow. The maximum flow rate was normal (Q_{max} 29.0 ml/s) and this 69-year-old woman did not have any residual urine. However, the uroflow pattern is consistent with abdominal straining. The urinary stream occurs in spurts with complete interruption between the spurts. This pattern of "Valsalva voiding" points out the value of looking at the uroflow pattern in addition to just the numeric readout

sphincter activity, volume infused (VH20) for representing the amount of fluid has been introduced into the bladder, flow representing the ml/s being expelled from the urethra, and volume voided representing the amount of fluid voided during the test. The order of channels is most typically displayed as in the example below but can be customized within most urodynamic software programs (Fig. 11.4).

When preparing for, performing, and interpreting multichannel urodynamics, keep in mind the two basic functions being evaluated, storage, and evacuation. It is helpful to conceptualize the study in two phases: the *filling* phase and the *voiding* phase. The filling is generally referred to as filling cystometry or CMG and can also include leak point pressure tests and urethral pressure profile studies. The voiding phase is formally referred to as the pressure flow study.

Filling Cystometry

Filling cystometry is the method by which the pressure/volume relationship of the bladder is measured during bladder filling (Winters et al. 2012). Measurements obtained during filling cystometry include capacity, compliance, sensation, and stability (Table 11.4). Additionally, competency (of the urethral sphincter) is measured by way of abdominal leak point pressure or urethral pressure testing, often performed during the filling phase of urodynamics. During the filling cystometry and ALPP or UPP testing, clinician should consider five essential questions in attempt to generate meaningful urodynamics results:

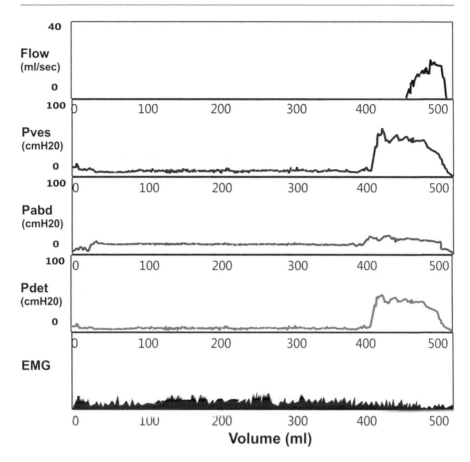

Fig. 11.4 Illustration of normal multichannel urodynamics. The patient did not have involuntary detrusor contraction during filling to a capacity of approximately 420 ml where she voided with a normal uroflow and maximum detrusor voiding pressure of 50 cmH₂O

1. What is the bladder's *capacity*?
2. Is the bladder wall *compliant*?
3. Is the urethral sphincter *competent*?
4. What are the *sensations* during bladder filling?
5. Is the detrusor muscle *stable* during filling?

These questions or concepts can be remembered as the three *C*'s and the two *S*'s of urodynamics. In reference to Wein's (1981) classification system, *capacity*, *compliance*, *sensations*, and *stability* are all functions of the bladder and *competency* is a function of the urethra, or outlet, as it relates to storage.

Cystometric *capacity* is defined as the bladder volume at the end of the filling cystometry (Abrams et al. 2003). Normal cystometric capacity for adults ranges from 300 to 600 ml. Capacity can be calculated using a number of different methods based on age and weight for pediatric patient. Capacity occurs during CMG filling

Table 11.4 Summary of the five essential functions and their associated reportable urodynamic findings

Function	Urodynamic findings
Capacity	Large (>600 ml)
	Normal (300 ml to 600 ml)
	Small (<300 ml)
Compliance	Normal bladder wall compliance (>30 ml/cmH₂O)
	Low bladder wall compliance (<10 ml/cmH₂O)
Competency	Competent urethral sphincter mechanism (no abdominal leak point pressure)
	Incompetent urethral sphincter mechanism (measurable leak upon urodynamic stress test and/or maximum urethra closure pressure ≤ 20 cmH2O)
Sensations	Increased (sensations of bladder filling occur at low volumes)
	Reduced (delayed or diminished sensations of bladder filling)
	Absent sensations (no sensation of bladder filling)
Stability	Stable/normal (no overactive detrusor contractions during bladder filling)
	Detrusor overactivity (one or more detrusor contractions with or without associated urge and with our without associated leak during bladder filling)

when the patient is given permission to void or when the patient experiences a bladder contraction that results in bladder emptying (terminal detrusor overactivity).

Clinical Pearl

Since urodynamic filling is typically much faster than a natural filling rate, the patient's anatomic capacity, which can be estimated by bladder diary information, should be compared to the cystometric capacity when interpreting urodynamic data. The clinician should consider the patient's naturally accumulating urine volume, in addition to the cystometric volume infused, as true capacity. This can be determined after the voiding phase of urodynamics by combining the volume voided and the measured post void residual.

Common causes for high bladder capacity are bladder outlet obstruction and poor detrusor contractility. Common causes for low bladder capacity are detrusor overactivity, increased sensation, or low bladder wall compliance.

Bladder *compliance* describes the relationship between the change in bladder volume and the change in detrusor pressure during the filling CMG (Abrams et al. 2003). Compliance refers to the distensibility of the bladder wall. Bladder compliance can be determined by visually inspecting the slope of the detrusor (P_{det}) during filling CMG. Detrusor tracings in a healthy compliant bladder will not change much from the beginning to the end of fill. Conversely, detrusor tracings in a bladder with low compliance will demonstrate a gradual increase in slope. Bladder compliance can also be expressed as a value and can be calculated by change in bladder volume, divided by change in detrusor pressure from the beginning to the end of fill or $C = \Delta V / \Delta P_{det}$. When using this formula, a value less than or equal to 10 ml/cm would be considered low compliance. An alternative method for quantifying bladder wall compliance is to document infused volume associated with specific detrusor pressures throughout filling, usually documented at P_{det} 20 cmH$_2$O, P_{det} 30 cmH$_2$O, and P_{det} 40 cmH$_2$O (Houle et al. 1993). There are several other methods of calculating compliance that are specific to pediatric urodynamics that are beyond the scope of this chapter.

Low bladder compliance is associated with a variety of conditions such as interstitial cystitis, post radical prostatectomy, and pelvic irritation, but most often it is identified with neurogenic bladder disorders. Low bladder compliance is clinically relevant, particularly when associated with a high detrusor leak point pressure (which will be discussed later in the chapter) as this can cause upper urinary tract distress leading to ureteral reflux, hydronephrosis, upper urinary tract infections, renal scaring, and sometimes loss of renal function (Fig. 11.5).

Sensations during filling CMG are subjective feelings reported by the patient and should be documented as:

1. FS – first sensation of bladder filling (when the patient first becomes aware of bladder filling)
2. FD – first desire to void (when the patient feels the need to pass urine at the next convenient moment but would be able to postpone void)
3. SD – strong desire to void (persistent desire to void)

Further urodynamic documentation regarding sensation can be documented as:

1. Normal   aware of bladder filling and increasing sensation up to a strong desire to void
2. Increased – early and persistent desire to void
3. Reduced – diminished sensation or no definite desire to void throughout bladder filling
4. Absent – no sensation of bladder filling or desire to void
5. Urgency – a sudden compelling desire to void
6. Painful

Sensations during filling CMG are subjective and can be influenced by patient anxiety. When interpreting urodynamics, it is necessary to compare sensation observations with data provided by the patient's bladder diary. Increased, urgency, or painful sensations during filling CMG can be an indication of inflammation, infection, detrusor overactivity, neuralgia, and more. Reduced or absent sensations are most often indicative of neuralgia, but can also be the result of overextension (Abrams et al. 2003).

Stability refers to detrusor function during filling cystometry. Normal detrusor function allows bladder filling with little or no change in pressure. Detrusor overactivity is a urodynamic observation characterized by involuntary contractions of the detrusor muscle during the filling phase of urodynamics (Abrams et al. 2003). Detrusor overactivity during filling CMG should be reported as:

1. With or without leak
2. With or without sensory awareness
3. Spontaneous or provoked

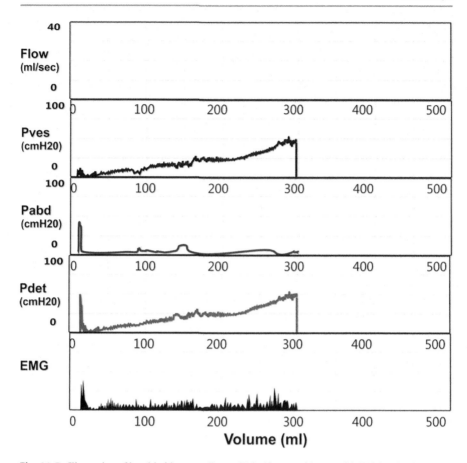

Fig. 11.5 Illustration of low bladder compliance. This 42-year-old man with T12 level spinal cord injured leaked at a detrusor leak point pressure of 50 cmH₂O at 300 ml despite maximal antimuscarinic bladder medications

4. Neurogenic or idiopathic in cause
5. Phasic or terminal (Phasic detrusor overactivity is characterized by wave form, usually occurs multiple times throughout filling, and may or may not lead to incontinence. Terminal detrusor overactivity is a single detrusor contraction that happens at cystometric capacity, which results in incontinence and usually complete bladder emptying.)

Detrusor overactivity can be associated with a number of specific neurological disorders such as multiple sclerosis (MS), Parkinson's disease, spinal bifida, spinal injury, or stroke. It can also be caused by many non-neurological disorders such as cystitis, BPH, or other obstructive disorders. The cause of detrusor overactivity can be idiopathic or undetermined (Fig. 11.6).

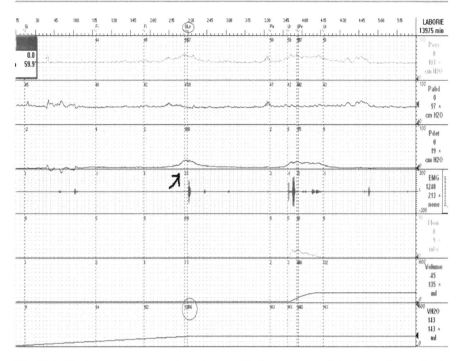

Fig. 11.6 Urodynamic study urge incontinence with detrusor overactivity. *Arrow* denotes involuntary detrusor contraction with leakage

Competency is a function of the urethral sphincter, measured during the filling phase of urodynamics by method of abdominal leak point pressure testing, detrusor leak point pressure testing, or urethral pressure testing during urodynamics.

Abdominal Leak Point Pressure Test

Abdominal leak point pressure test (ALPP) is done during the filling phase of urodynamics, most typically at an infused volume of 200 ml. ALPP can also be referred to as "urodynamic stress test." Although the test is named "abdominal" leak point pressure, it is actually the change in vesicle pressure caused by an intentional increase in abdominal pressure from a cough or Valsalva maneuver that is recorded. The goal of ALPP testing is twofold. One is to determine if the patient has any measurable leakage during ALPP, indicating testing a diagnosis of urodynamic stress incontinence. The second is to determine the actual pressure of the leak. Low-pressure leak point pressures, generally less than 60 cmH$_2$O, are diagnostic of intrinsic urethral sphincter deficiency or urethral incompetence, which will be clinically managed different than higher pressure incontinence, usually associated with urethral hypermobility.

ALPP example below shows cough ALPP of 87 cmH$_2$O (124 minus baseline P_{ves} of 37) and Valsalva ALPP of 76 cmH$_2$O (113 minus baseline P_{ves} of 37) (Fig. 11.7).

These techniques may be useful when performing or interpreting ALPP or urodynamic stress tests:

1. If a patient is being evaluated for a known sign of stress incontinence, but does not demonstrate leakage with cough of Valsalva at 200 ml, the ALPP should be repeated every 100 ml during filling until urodynamic stress incontinence is observed.
2. In effort to diagnose or rule out "occult" SUI when evaluating patients with significant uterine prolapse or large cystocele, the prolapse must be reduced before performing the ALPP test.

Clinical Pearls

Reduction can be accomplished using two large OB swabs, posterior ½ of a speculum, a pessary, or by other methods. Efforts should be made to avoid anterior pressure upon the urethra during reduction.

---

3. Position the patient upright, sitting or standing, for VLPP testing.
4. The urethral meatus *MUST* be visualized during *VLPP* testing in order to determine if leakage is present.
5. Detrusor pressure should be noted immediately following cough and Valsalva maneuvers. These maneuvers can occasionally induce a detrusor contraction and ultimately leakage, which would be considered Valsalva-induced detrusor overactivity, NOT stress incontinence.

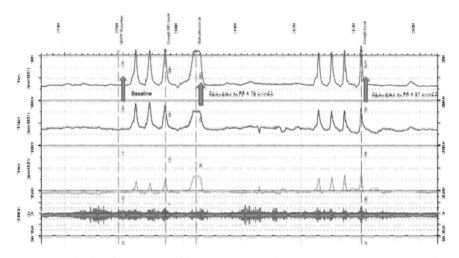

Fig. 11.7 Cystometrogram demonstrating abdominal leak point pressure test, showing valsalva ALPP of 76 cmH$_2$O (113 minus baseline P$_{ves}$ of 37) and cough ALPP of 87 cmH2O (124 minus baseline P$_{ves}$ of 37).

Detrusor Leak Point Pressure Test

Detrusor leak point pressure test (DLPP) is another urodynamic test for evaluating urethral competency. This leak point pressure test is *NOT* done for the purposes of quantifying or measuring incontinence but rather for evaluating storage pressures as they relate to low bladder compliance. DLPP is defined as the lowest detrusor pressure at which urine leakage occurs in the absence of either a detrusor contraction or increased abdominal pressure (Abrams et al. 2003). The higher the DLPP, the more likely that upper urinary tract damage could occur as a result of intravesical pressure being transmitted to the kidneys. Patients with neurogenic conditions such as spina bifida, spinal cord tumors, spinal cord injury, etc. often require urodynamics with DLPP testing for a baseline assessment and often on a routine basis to evaluate ongoing treatment and to ensure upper tract preservation (Fig. 11.5).

Urethral Pressure Test (UPP)

The last way to determine urethral competence during urodynamics is by measuring *urethral pressure*. There are several different techniques and measurements clinicians use for measuring urethral pressures, all of which are subject to artifact and inconsistencies. These measurements should be used with observation of urine loss during ALPP, in order to diagnose urodynamic stress incontinence (Hayden et al. 2010). Common urethral pressure measurements are:

1. Urethral pressure is the pressure needed to open the urethra.
2. Urethral pressure profile (UPP) is a graph indicating the intraluminal pressure along the length of the urethra.
3. Maximum urethral pressure (MUP) is the maximum pressure measured in the urethra.
4. Maximum urethral closure pressure (MUCP) is the maximum difference between the urethral pressure and the intravesical pressure ($P_{ura}-P_{ves}$).
5. Functional profile length is the length of the urethra along which the urethral pressure exceeds the intravesical pressure. This can be tested at rest or under stress.
6. The pressure "transmission" ratio is the increment in urethral pressure on stress as a percentage of the simultaneously recorded increment in intravesical pressure.

When reporting urethral mechanism following urodynamics, the ICS and IUGA recommend using the following terms (Hayden et al. 2010):

1. *Normal urethral closure mechanism* – when no incontinence was demonstrated during ALPP tests and positive urethral closure pressure was maintained during bladder filling, even in the presence of increased abdominal pressure.
2. *Incompetent urethral closure mechanism* – leakage was observed during ALPP or during activities that raise the intra-abdominal pressure.

3. *Urethral relaxation incompetence* ("urethral instability," formerly referred to as intrinsic sphincter deficiency) – leakage due to urethral relaxation observed during urodynamics in the absence of raised abdominal pressure (ALPP) or a detrusor contraction. This generally coincides with maximum urethral closure pressures less than 20 cmH_2O.
4. *Urodynamic stress incontinence* – the involuntary leakage of urine during filling cystometry, associated with increased intra-abdominal pressure (ALPP), in the absence of a detrusor contraction.

Clinical Pearl

uterine prolapse, cystocele, enterocele or large rectoceles should be reduced (without putting pressure on or obstructing the urethra) when performing upp studies.

Pressure Flow Studies

The pressure flow study (PFS), or voiding cystometry, measures the relationship between pressure in the bladder and urine flow rate during emptying. This phase of urodynamics begins when the clinician instructs the patient to void or when terminal detrusor overactivity leads to complete bladder emptying. Using Wein's (1981) classification system, the pressure flow study is performed to answer questions about bladder contractility and urethral resistance as they relate to the emptying phase of micturition (Fig. 11.4; Table 11.3).

Voiding is a complex function that requires neural circuits of the brain and spinal cord to function in a coordinated manor. The bladder must contract adequately, the urethra must relax to lower resistance, and the urethral must be free of anatomic obstruction for normal bladder emptying to occur. The ICS defines normal detrusor function as a voluntarily initiated continuous contraction that leads to complete bladder emptying within a normal time span (Abrams et al. 2003). The amplitude and duration of the detrusor contraction is dependent upon outlet resistance. Due to the structural differences, male patients normally require higher detrusor pressure to complete bladder emptying than female patients. The maximal detrusor pressure for adult male patients ranges from 15 to 40 cmH_2O, and the maximal detrusor pressure for adult female patients ranges from 8 to 30 cmH_2O. It is not uncommon for the maximum detrusor pressure to increase with age in men due to prostatic changes, but typically high detrusor pressure with low flow on PFS is an indicator of BPH or other anatomical urethral obstruction. It is not uncommon for female patients with very low urethral resistance (or low-pressure SUI) to void with extremely low detrusor pressures.

The following data should be obtained and reported during pressure flow studies:

1. Maximum flow rate (expressed as Q_{max}).
2. Average flow rate (expressed as *Qmean* or Q_{ave} and is volume voided divided by flow time) 15 ml/s or greater is the normal average flow rate for female patients and 12 ml/s or higher is the normal average flow rate for male patients.

3. Flow time.
4. Voiding time.
5. Voiding volume.
6. Maximum detrusor pressure (expressed as $P_{det/max}@Q_{max}$ and is maximum detrusor pressure measured during flow).
7. Detrusor pressure at maximum flow (expressed as $P_{det/max}@Q_{min}$ and is detrusor pressure measured at the time of maximum flow).
8. Urethral opening pressure (expressed as P_{det}/open and is the detrusor pressure measured at the start of flow).
9. Post void residual.
10. Flow pattern (described as continuous or intermittent, smooth arc shaped curve or fluctuating curve)
11. The detrusor contractility should be documented as normal, acontractile, or underactive.

- Normal detrusor is defined as a contraction that is able to complete bladder emptying in the absence of obstruction.
- Acontractile detrusor is when no contraction is demonstrated during pressure flow study. This must be correlated with a clinical diagnosis. If a patient is unable to void due to psychosocial factors of the test, this would not be considered "acontractile."
- Underactive detrusor is a contraction of inadequate magnitude and/or duration to complete bladder emptying.

Several nomograms have been developed using pressure flow variables, which are used to identify and categorize male obstruction. The most commonly accepted are the Griffiths, the LinPUrr, and the ICS nomograms.

Pressure flow studies can be used to distinguish bladder outlet obstruction (BOO), versus detrusor hypocontractility, or acontractility, as the cause of voiding dysfunction. Pressure flow studies are appropriate for evaluating neurogenic bladder conditions. They can be helpful in determining treatment options and evaluating response to treatment for urinary retention, hydronephrosis, pyelonephritis, or complicated UTIs in patients with neurogenic pathology. PFS can also be helpful for evaluating detrusor contractility in patients with BPH that have history of large volume PVR, complete retention, or coexisting neurologic pathology.

PFS is not a standard procedure for all female patients being evaluated for stress incontinence surgery, but should be considered when there is history of urinary retention or coexisting neurologic pathology. PFS can also be helpful in detecting habitual Valsalva voiding patterns, which would require counseling prior to anti-incontinence surgery. There is a lack of criteria for measuring anatomical urethra obstruction in females, since this condition is rare. Despite the lack of standardization for measuring obstruction in females, PFS can be helpful, particularly in situations where urgency or retention develops post anti-incontinence surgery. Figure 11.8 is an example of pressure flow study showing bladder outlet obstruction characterized by high detrusor pressure, low flow rate, and incomplete emptying.

Clinical Pearl

Pressure flow studies can be subject to inconsistencies due to many factors such as size of the urodynamic catheter, discomfort from the urodynamic catheter, position of the patient, discomfort from the urodynamic catheter, position of the patient, testing anxiety, and many other psychosocial factors. Consistency of equipment used, limiting the size of urodynamic catheter to 8 fr or smaller and providing a comfortable, and a private testing environment are suggested to help minimize the inconsistencies during pressure flow testing. These variables must be considered during interpretation and the data acquired should always be compared to the flow pattern, rates, and PVR of the patient's un-instrumented uroflow study.

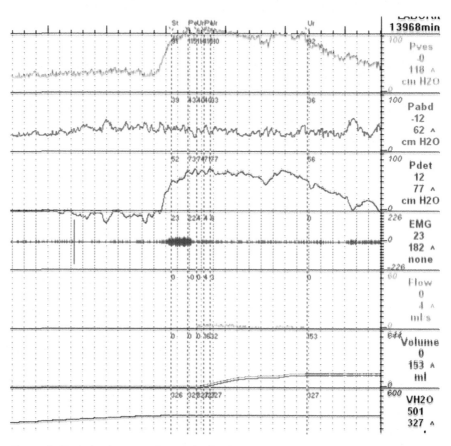

Fig. 11.8 Example of pressure flow study showing bladder outlet obstruction characterized by high detrusor pressure, low flow rate, and incomplete emptying

Electromyogram

Electromyogram (EMG) studies the bioelectric potentials of muscles. The goal of EMG during urodynamics is to determine whether the pelvic floor muscles (levator ani) and the external urethral sphincter are coordinated or discoordinated with the bladder during filling and emptying. A normal response to bladder filling is a gradual increase in EMG recruitment. There should also be an increase in EMG response during cough, Valsalva, or other provocative maneuvers. Normally, the pelvic floor muscles and urethral sphincter should relax during void, which would be observed as silence on the EMG tracing.

Urodynamic EMG can be performed using surface electrodes, wire electrodes, or concentric needles. Surface electrodes are the most common in standard urodynamics, as this method is the least invasive and allows the patient to move about during the urodynamic study. Surface electrodes record EMG activity of the pelvic floor, which usually mimics the activity of the urethral sphincter. In specialized situations where neurogenic dysfunction is being evaluated, concentric needles, which are placed periurethrally, are the most precise and often preferred. In addition to graphic representation, concentric and wire EMG can include audible signals. Wire and concentric EMG tests require a urologist, urogynecologist, neurologist, or specially trained EMG specialist to be present in the room during urodynamic testing.

Clinical Pearls
1. EMG recordings are highly subject to artifacts. External electrical signals can be depicted on EMG from:
   (a) Fluorescent lights
   (b) Nearby appliances
   (c) Electrical equipment
2. EMG artifacts related to the patient can be created by:
   (a) Electrical activity of nearby muscle groups
   (b) Pacemakers or implantable electrical devices
   (c) Water flowing over surface patches during void
   (d) Surface patches falling off
3. Some of these artifacts can be avoided by following proper technique; others are unavoidable and should be noted as artifact to avoid misinterpretation.
4. Proper placement of the surface electrodes is essential to obtaining a quality EMG reading:
   (a) Surface electrodes should be applied directly across from each other, or at 2 o'clock and 8 o'clock, on the anal margin or the pigmented skin immediately surrounding the anal orifice.

    (b) Third grounding electrode placed over a bony prominence.
    (c) The skin should be thoroughly dried before placement.
    (d) An EKG skin prep is helpful to remove oils from the skin and hair removal is occasionally necessary to ensure efficient contact.
5. Another technique to ensure reliability of the EMG signal is to assess the response to a cough or voluntary pelvic floor contraction (Kegel) at the beginning and throughout the urodynamic study. There should be an increase in EMG recruitment during these provocative maneuvers.

EMG is useful in diagnosing detrusor sphincter dyssynergia (DSD) with neurogenic disorders. In this scenario, EMG tracing would show intermittent recruitment with simultaneous intermittent increases in detrusor pressure and mirroring pattern of intermittent flow, often referred to as the "shark tooth" pattern. In nonneurogenic situations EMG can be useful in determining voiding dysfunctions that could include voluntary contraction of pelvic floor or abdominal straining during void (Fig. 11.9).

Video Urodynamics

Video urodynamics combine routine urodynamics with X-ray imaging. Radiographic solution is used for the filling agent, and fluoroscopic equipment is used to capture images and video loops during the filling and voiding phases of CMG. Video urodynamics are helpful in evaluating patients with complicated lower urinary tract dysfunction, particularly when neurogenic pathology is present or primary bladder neck obstruction without neurogenic or obvious anatomic cause is suspected. Video urodynamics can differentiate between functional cause of obstruction and dysfunctional voiding. Documentation of

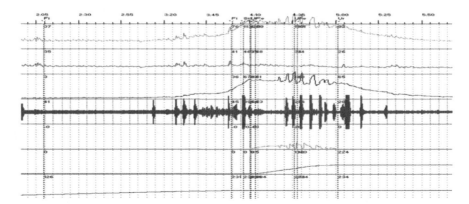

Fig. 11.9 EMG pattern demonstrating detrusor sphincter dyssynergia (DSD) with the classic shark tooth pattern

incompetent bladder neck, inadequate urethral closure during filling, decent of the bladder base, location of urethral obstruction, bladder diverticula, and ureteral reflux are some of the advantages of video urodynamics. Radiation exposure, less comfortable conditions for the patient, and higher initial and running costs are some of the disadvantages of video urodynamics. Further discussion regarding technique and interpretation of video urodynamics is beyond the scope of this chapter.

Summary

Urodynamics are the only means of objectively assessing lower urinary tract function and dysfunction and should be performed whenever detailed knowledge of the lower urinary tract function is needed to determine treatment, predict or monitor treatment outcomes, or to understand reasons for treatment failure. Urodynamic investigations themselves are inadequate for determining the cause of lower urinary tract dysfunction and must be used in conjunction with history and physical, symptom questionnaires, voiding diaries, and other similar tools. If the clinician has not answered all of the posed urodynamic questions prior to termination of the study, parts of test may need to be repeated. Urodynamics should be done in accordance with standard methods, using ICS terminology and good urodynamic practices to ensure reliability of the tests.

Additional Resources and Urodynamic Education Opportunities

No publication or course can provide all the tools necessary to become an expert in urodynamics. These skills can only be acquired over time and from real patient experiences. It is highly recommended that all new urodynamics clinicians work closely with an experienced urodynamics mentor to guide and educate them through the processes of patient selection, performing studies, and interpreting results. Likewise, once proficiency is attained, continuing education is necessary in order to stay current with accepted techniques and terminology.

The Society of Urological Nurses and Associates (SUNA) organization provides a basic urodynamic training course, which is currently held each spring, in conjunction with their annual symposium. *Urological Nursing* includes many articles related to urodynamics, including Mikel Gray's comprehensive 13-part series "Making Sense of Urodynamics Testing." Another key resource helpful for all clinicians new to urodynamics is the SUNA manual for urodynamics titled *A Practical Guide to Performing Urodynamics*. In addition to SUNA, the American Urological Association (AUA), the American Urogynecologic Society (AUGS), and the International Continence Society (ICS) also provide guidelines, publications, conferences, and courses related to urodynamic testing.

Resources for the Nurse Practitioner

www.suna.org

www.auanet.org

www.auga.org

www.ics.org

Resources for the Patient

https://www.kramesstore.com

http://www.kidneyurology.org/Library/Urologic_Health.php/Urodynamic_Testing.php

References

Abrams P et al (2003) The standardisation of terminology in the lower urinary tract function: report from the standardisation sub-committee of the International Continence Society. Urology 61:37–49

Chapple C, MacDiarmid S, Patel A (2009) Urodynamics made easy, 3rd edn. Churchill Livingstone, Edinburgh/New York

Gray M. (2012) Making sense of urodynamics testing-part 9: evaluation of detrusor response to bladder filling. J Urol Nurs 32:1

Hayden B et al (2010) Standardization and Terminology Committees IUGA and ICS, Joint IUGA ICS Working Group on Female Terminology. Neurourol Urodyn 29(1):4–20

Houle AM, Gilmour RF, Churchill BM, Gaumond M, Bassonnette B (1993) What volume can a child normally store in the bladder at a safe pressure. J Urol 149(3):561–564

Winters JC, Dmochowski RR, Goldman HB, Herndon CD, Kobashi KC, Kraus SR, Lemack GE, Nitti VW, Rovner ES, Wein AJ (2012) Adult urodynamics: AUA/SUFU guidelines.

Wein AJ (1981) Classification of neurogenic voiding dysfunction. J Urol 125(5):605–609

Neurogenic Bladder/Underactive Bladder

12

Michelle J. Lajiness

Contents

Objectives
1. Discuss the definition and incidence of underactive bladder (UAB).
2. Describe assessment techniques in UAB.
3. Discuss appropriate interventions for the treatment of UAB.

M.J. Lajiness, FNP-BC
Department of Urology and Department of Infectious Disease,
Beaumont Health System, Royal Oak, MI, USA
e-mail: Michelle.Lajiness@beaumont.org

© Springer International Publishing Switzerland 2016
M. Lajiness, S. Quallich (eds.), *The Nurse Practitioner in Urology*,
DOI 10.1007/978-3-319-28743-0_12

217

Definition, Incidence, and Epidemiology

Underactive bladder (UAB) is a chronic, complex, and debilitating disease that is not well known and has few options for treatment. UAB is closely related to detrusor underactivity (DU), a urodynamic definition; however, few clinicians, scientist, or researchers agree on a definition (Chancellor and Diokno 2014). UAB is more correctly defined as a constellation of clinical symptoms that include the symptoms and signs of DU. The International Continence Society (ICS) defines DU as "a contraction of reduced strength and/ or duration, resulting in prolonged bladder emptying and/or failure to achieve complete bladder emptying" (Abrams et al. 2002). UAB is a multifactorial condition that may be caused by myogenic (muscle denervation) and/or neurogenic (nerve denervation) conditions, aging, and medication side effects.

Lower urinary tract dysfunction is especially prevalent in the elderly. As the population continues to age, the number of affected people and the associated costs will escalate (Chancellor and Diokno 2014). Solid epidemiology is dependent on accurate and precise definitions of a disease studied. As a result UAB is thought to be misrepresented (Chancellor and Diokno 2014).

Prevalence of UAB varied across clinical studies and patient populations. Diokno et al. (1986) concluded that 22 % of men and 11 % of women over 60 years had difficulty emptying their bladders. A study by Taylor et al. in 2006 found detrusor underactivity in two-thirds of incontinent institutionalized patients. Valente et al. (2014) did an epidemiological study and had 633 subjects return questionnaires. It was determined that 23 % of the respondents reported difficulty emptying his/her bladder and only 11 % had ever heard of the term underactive bladder.

Pathophysiology

The exact cause of UAB is not always known; known causes include myogenic, neurogenic, and medication side effects. Theories have been postulated to account for the signs and symptoms associated with UAB (see Table 12.1). These

Table 12.1 Signs/symptoms of UAB

Hesitancy
Weak stream
Interrupted urine flow
Straining to void
Feeling of incomplete emptying
Frequent small volume urination
Urinary tract infections
Nighttime leakage
Flank pain (bilateral, rare—related to hydronephrosis)
Incontinence
Diminished stream
Rely on abdominal straining to urinate

hypotheses include but are not limited to overactive bladder (OAB) to UAB model and the aging bladder model (Miyazato et al. 2013). Comorbidities can also increase the risk of OAB (see Table 12.2).

A myogenic basis for DU may result from abnormality of the myocytes to generate contractile activity in the absence of external stimuli, or the problem may lie with the extracellular matrix, resulting in impaired contractility. Bladder outlet obstruction (BOO)-related DU has been well studied in numerous animal models where sequential changes were described leading to decompensation of bladder contraction (Osman et al. 2014). Disruption to the efferent nerves may result in reduced neuromuscular activation that may manifest as an absent or poor detrusor contraction. This is typically seen with diseases causing direct neuronal injury such as multisystem atrophy and other autonomic neuropathies. In DU of non-neurogenic origin, the exact contribution of efferent dysfunction is unknown. The decline in autonomic nerve innervation in normal human bladders with aging, as well as BOO, may contribute to insufficient activation for adequate contraction to occur in individuals without overt neurologic disease (Osman et al. 2014).

DHIC, or detrusor hyperactivity with impaired contractility, was first characterized by Resnick and Yalla in 1987 in a series of women with both urge urinary incontinence and elevated post-void residual volumes associated with poor bladder contractility. Men with DHIC or even pure detrusor underactivity may have their symptoms incorrectly attributed purely BPH alone and undergo unnecessary surgical procedures to relieve obstruction (Griebling 2015).

Neurogenic cause is well known to those working with UAB patients (see Table 12.3). Neurogenic bladder dysfunction happens when the efferent and/or afferent pathways or the lumbosacral spinal cord is damaged. The afferent system is integral to the function of the efferent system in the neural control of micturition during both the storage and voiding phases. The afferent system monitors the volumes during storage and also the magnitude of detrusor contractions during voiding. Urethral afferents respond to flow and are important in potentiating the detrusor contraction. Bladder and urethral afferent dysfunction may lead to DU by reducing or prematurely ending the micturition reflex, which may manifest in a loss of voiding efficiency (Osman et al. 2014).

Table 12.2 Comorbid conditions that predispose patients to retention and incomplete emptying	
	BPH
	Cognitive impairment
	Diabetes
	Mobility impairment
	Neurological diseases
	Pelvic organ prolapse
	Spinal cord injury
	Spinal stenosis
	Stroke
	Urethral stricture

Table 12.3 Predisposing/risk factors for neurogenic bladder

Neurogenic	Myogenic
Spinal cord injury	Excessive fluid intake with infrequent voiding
CVA	BOO
Parkinson's disease	Aging bladder
Multiple sclerosis	Diabetes
Spina bifida	
Diabetic neuropathy	
Guillain-Barre syndrome	
Multisystem atrophy	
Herniated disk	
Cauda equina syndrome	
Aids	
Neurosyphilis	
Herpes zoster/herpes simplex	
Pelvic radiation	
Pelvic/sacral fracture	
Pelvic surgery	

OAB may over time lead to the development of UAB. Chancellor (2014) postulates that in OAB the bladder wall thickens, and a rise in nerve growth factors occurs resulting in structural changes leading to alteration of the muscle and connective tissue structure and function that results in impaired contractility.

The causes of detrusor underactivity as a result of the typical aging process are not well understood. The bladder should remain adequately elastic and contractile despite a patient's age, and urinary incontinence should not be considered either an inevitable or normal part of aging (Griebling 2015). Animal studies suggest that as the bladder ages, there is a reduction in the strength of contraction; however, the few urodynamic studies done on older humans have differing results. There are age-induced morphology changes noted in the bladder which include a decrease in the ratio of detrusor muscle to collagen as well as a decrease in M3 receptors. This may all lead to decreased ability of the bladder to contract (Miyazato et al. 2013). The simple fact remains not every person over the age of 70 is affected by UAB. The true relationship between microscopic and cellular changes to clinically significant bladder behavior is unclear, and the associate between aging and detrusor underactivity is likely multifactorial (Griebling 2015).

History

An accurate assessment of voiding symptoms is essential in UAB (see Table 12.1). Include onset and duration of symptoms. A voiding diary, a daily record of the patient's bladder activity, is an objective documentation of the patient's voiding pattern, incontinent episodes, and inciting events associated with urinary incontinence and can be helpful in eliciting voiding patterns (see Chap. 14 for an example). For those who present with acute urinary retention, attempts should be made to obtain potential precipitating factors that led to urinary retention (see Table 12.2). For those who present with an indwelling Foley catheter, doing intermittent catheterization, or with significant voiding symptoms and a high post-void residual urine, attempt should be made to determine any predisposing/risk factors factor/s such as neurologic disorders including spinal cord injury and cerebrovascular accidents (see Table 12.3) that lead to the problem.

Obtain history of previous surgical intervention related to the GU tract. Obtain an accurate list of current medications to evaluate drugs that can lead to detrusor weakness (Table 12.4). However, the diagnostician must also be aware that UAB may be completely silent, meaning that the person with UAB may be totally asymptomatic (Diokno 2015).

Table 12.4 Medications that can cause detrusor weakness

Class	Drug
Antipsychotics (anticholinergic effects)	Chlorpromazine (Thorazine)
	Clozapine (Clozaril)
	Mesoridazine (Serentil)
	Olanzapine (Zyprexa)
	Promazine (Sparine)
	Quetiapine (Seroquel)
	Thioridazine (Mellaril)
Antiarrhythmics (anticholinergic effects)	Disopyramide (Norpace)
	Procainamide (Pronestyl)
	Quinidine (Quinaglute, Quinidex)
Antiemetics (anticholinergic effects)	Dimenhydrinate (Dramamine)
	Meclizine (Antivert, Bonine)
	Trimethobenzamide (Tigan)
	Prochlorperazine (Compazine)
Antihistamines (anticholinergic effects)	Azatadine (Optimine)
	Chlorpheniramine (Chlor-Trimeton)
	Clemastine (Tavist)
	Diphenhydramine (Tylenol PM, Sominex, Benadryl)
Hydroxyzine (anticholinergic effects)	Atarax, Vistaril
	Promethazine (Phenergan)
Antiparkinson agents (anticholinergic effects)	Benztropine (Cogentin)
	Biperiden (Akineton)
	Procyclidine (Kemadrin)
	Trihexyphenidyl (Artane)

(continued)

Table 12.4 (continued)

Class	Drug
Antispasmodics (anticholinergic effects)	Atropine (Sal-Tropine)
	Belladonna alkaloids (Donnatal, Bellatal, Barbidonna)
	Dicyclomine (Antispas, Bentyl)
	Flavoxate (Urispas)
	Hyoscyamine (Anaspaz, Levbid, Cystospaz, Levsin/SL)
	Oxybutynin (Ditropan)
	Scopolamine
	Tolterodine (Detrol)
	Solifenacin succinate (VESIcare)
	Darifenacin (Enablex
	Trospium (Sanctura)
	Fesoterodine (Toviaz)
Skeletal muscle relaxants (anticholinergic effects)	Carisoprodol (Soma)
	Chlorzoxazone (Parafon, Forte)
	Cyclobenzaprine (Flexeril)
	Methocarbamol (Robaxin)
	Orphenadrine (Norflex)
Tricyclic antidepressants (anticholinergic effects)	Amitriptyline (Elavil)
	Desipramine (Norpramin)
	Doxepin (Sinequan)
	Imipramine (Tofranil)
	Nortriptyline (Aventyl, Pamelor)
Opiate analgesics	Codeine (Atasol, Tylenol 2,3,4)
	Morphine
	Methadone
	Meperidine (Demerol)
	Hydromorphone (Dilaudid)
	Oxycodone (OxyContin, Percocet)
NSAIDs	

Physical Examination

A focused physical examination is essential in a comprehensive evaluation of a patient suspected of having an UAB. This should include an overall general assessment of the physical and cognitive ability of the patient. Include a functional assessment and a neurological assessment. Abdominal examination must include inspection and palpation of the suprapubic area to identify any signs of distended bladder. The lumbar area must also be palpated for any evidence of any masses or tenderness that may indicate hydronephrosis.

Genital and perineal examination is mandatory for suspected cases of UAB. The skin of the genitalia and the perineum may indicate significant irritation manifested by erythema or even excoriation and ulceration from chronic urinary leakage and wearing of undergarments/diapers. For men, the penis and scrotum and its content must be evaluated. Digital rectal examination should elicit the anal sphincter tone and the voluntary ability to contract the sphincter. The prostate is palpated to assess the size and evidence of any tenderness or masses/nodules. One must remember that the size of the prostate on digital rectal examination does not necessarily correlate to the voiding symptoms. A small-size prostate may present with more intense lower urinary tract symptoms than one with a large prostate palpated on digital examination (Diokno 2015).

For women, a vaginal inspection, including speculum examination and bimanual examination, must be performed. Inspection should identify the health of the vaginal mucosa to identify signs of atrophy and signs of skin irritation suggestive of atrophic vaginitis. Pelvic organ prolapse is identified visually for any organ protruding outside of the vaginal introitus and provoked by asking the patient to strain and cough to determine the extent of the prolapse. One must also look for evidence of urine leakage during coughing and straining. The lack of leakage does not eliminate urinary incontinence; however, the presence of urine leakage during straining or coughing is a positive sign for stress urinary incontinence. The vaginal speculum is used to inspect the cervix and the vaginal mucosa and to assess the level of the individual pelvic organ prolapse if one is present. The prolapsing organ must be identified such as cystocele (anterior), rectocele (posterior), uterus, or intestine/enterocele (central/vaginal vault). The severity of prolapse must be established (See Chap. 13) This is important because in severe vaginal prolapse, chronic obstruction from the prolapsing pelvic organ could lead to chronic urinary retention. Digital examination of the anal canal must also be performed to assess the anal tone and voluntary strength as well as assess the status of the recto-vaginal wall (Diokno 2015).

In both men and women, the perineal sensation must be tested for sensory deficiency by testing the ability to perceive a gentle pinprick applied to the saddle and the perianal area. Without performing this maneuver, one may miss saddle perineal anesthesia that may be the only neurologic sign that may suggest sacral cord lesions that may be contributing to an underactive bladder (Diokno 2015).

Diagnostic Testing

Urinalysis should look for signs of pyuria and bacteriuria and if infection is suspected, urine culture and sensitivity should be ordered. Urinalysis should also seek to check the presence of glucose as this may correlate to diabetes and its potential consequence, diabetic neuropathy, and for albumin for possible kidney disease. Specific gravity should also be tested to provide a hint of the ability of the kidney to concentrate the urine. Nephrogenic diabetes insipidus causing excessive diuresis can lead to chronic bladder overdistention and underactive bladder (Diokno 2015).

Urine Cytology

Carcinoma in situ of the urinary bladder causes symptoms of urinary frequency and urgency. Irritative voiding symptoms out of proportion to the overall clinical picture and/or hematuria warrant urine cytology and cystoscopy. Blood tests that may contribute to the overall assessment of UAB include the renal panel (BUN, creatinine, GFR rate), serum protein, electrolytes, and glucose/Hgb A1c levels.

Imaging Tests

The portable bladder scanner has made it easier to quickly measure post-void residual (PVR) urine volume and establish the efficiency of bladder emptying. It also obviates the risk of trauma, pain, and potential contamination with the use of catheter to measure the post-void residual urine (Diokno 2015). Other imaging techniques that have led to identifying large distended bladder are abdominal and/or pelvic ultrasound, CT, and MRI imaging.

Endoscopic Assessment

Cystourethroscopy is an optional procedure performed to confirm the presence or absence of anatomical obstruction including enlarged occluding prostate gland, bladder neck contracture, or presence of urethral strictures. The presence of obstruction may indicate that the underactive bladder may be secondary to the obstruction. Cystoscopy may confirm the presence of bladder wall trabeculations, and even diverticula formations, noted in cases of obstruction. Relieving the obstruction may allow the patient to void spontaneously. However if there is no evidence of any detrusor contractility, relieving the obstruction may not benefit the patient's ability to void. Endoscopy is helpful if the study revealed no evidence of any urethral stricture and the prostatic fossa appeared wide open especially after a previous TURP. Likewise, in UAB not caused by chronic obstruction, cystoscopy may reveal a large bladder with smooth lining (Diokno 2015).

Urodynamic Tests (See Chap. 11 for Definitions and Explanations of Tests)

Uroflowmetry can provide useful indirect information as to the strength of the detrusor contraction based on the measurement of the maximum or peak flow rate, the time it took to complete the act of voiding, and the average flow rate. However, it in itself will not be sufficient to make a diagnosis of underactive bladder (Diokno 2015).

Cystometry can provide a hint of underactive bladder with observation of a large capacity bladder, poor sensation or perception of bladder distention, abnormally high compliance, and lack of detrusor contractility. Although in underactive bladder, the post-void residual urine is usually abnormally elevated, the fact that the bladder is empty post-void does not rule out underactive bladder (Diokno 2015).

Combined pressure-flow test is the only legitimate test that can diagnose underactive detrusor and therefore confirm underactive bladder suspected on the basis of clinical symptoms (see Table 12.1). (Diokno 2015). The basic principle in this test is to simultaneously measure the intravesical pressure, the abdominal pressure, intraurethral pressure, bladder volume, urine flow rates, and post-void residual urine volume. When properly done, the detrusor pressure can be ascertained by subtracting the intravesical pressure from the abdominal pressure. The detrusor pressure at the height of the maximum urine flow rate will determine the presence of underactive, overactive, obstructive, or normal detrusor function. The most common accepted tenets of pressure-flow abdominal pressure diagnosis include the following results:

- Obstructed outlet when there is high detrusor pressure associated with poor urine flow rate.
- Underactive bladder when there is abnormal low or absent detrusor voiding pressure associated with poor urine flow rate.
- Overactive bladder may be diagnosed when involuntary detrusor contractions are noted during the filling phase of the study.
- Normal study when the detrusor pressure and the urine flow rate are within the limits of accepted normal rates.

Unfortunately, except for the obvious case of extreme pressures of high detrusor and poor flow or extremely low detrusor pressure and poor flow, there are many cases that are somewhere in between. This may be due to the severity of the dysfunction or technicalities of the procedure as performance of pressure-flow abdominal pressure test demands great precision and patient cooperation (Diokno 2015).

Behavioral/Conservative Therapy

The treatment for underactive bladder (UAB) is to protect the upper urinary tract, to improve continence and quality of life, and whenever possible to improve lower urinary tract functioning (Stohrer et al. 2009). Regular bladder emptying reduces intravesical bladder pressure and overdistention, which improves blood flow to the bladder and reduces the risk of infection (Lapides et al. 1972).

The objectives of conservative therapy in the underactive bladder are to provide low-pressure storage, preserve continence, avoid renal deterioration, minimize complications, and maintain quality of life. Conservative therapy in the underactive bladder patient includes behavioral management, incontinence products, and catheters.

Behavioral Treatment

There is a lack of information in the literature that discusses behavioral therapy for underactive bladder, other than discussing catheters and incontinence products. A PubMed search in March of 2015 utilizing the term "underactive bladder" revealed 134 articles available for review, utilizing "behavioral interventions" found in 149,240 articles available for review, but these terms combined yielded only two articles.

According to the European Association of Urology (EAU) guidelines on neurogenic lower urinary tract dysfunction, there are few prospective, randomized, controlled studies supporting conservative treatment. The guidelines state that lower urinary tract rehabilitation might be beneficial. Rehabilitation techniques include prompted voiding, timed voiding (bladder training), and lifestyle modifications (See Chapter 15) (Stohrer et al. 2009). The EAU guidelines do not recommend assisted bladder emptying such as Valsalva maneuver, crede, or triggered reflux. The authors state these procedures may create high pressures and are potentially hazardous.

Tubaro and colleagues (2012) completed a systemic review on the treatment of lower urinary tract symptoms in patients with multiple sclerosis. A meta-analysis could not be performed secondary to the multiple and differing outcome criteria. The authors concluded the nature of bladder dysfunction and the course of the disease make it difficult to standardize treatments or create guidelines.

Patil and colleagues (2012) completed an open arm pre-post study on 11 patients with multiple sclerosis (MS). The MS patients underwent a 21-day yoga intervention with statistical improvement noted in post-void residual, total micturition, and quality of sleep. Prior to that McClurg and colleagues (2006) compared electromyography (EMG) feedback and neuromuscular electrical stimulation , alone or in combination with pelvic floor muscle training, and were able to reduce the amount of leakage in the MS population. Later McClurg et al. (2008) taught 11 patients with MS pelvic floor training for lower urinary dysfunction and found the participants quality of life (QOL) was enhanced after completing the 9-week training course.

Behavioral therapy has been extensively studied in the overactive bladder population and authors have concluded that it may work in the UAB population. Other than those discussed above, no clinical studies are available to determine the effectiveness of behavioral therapy in the UAB population.

Incontinence Products

Patients may choose incontinence pads or diapers as their first initial method to remedy the loss of urine or may use them as a last resort. These items tend to be for long-term usage with UAB patients. The main goal of incontinence products is to minimize, conceal, and control urinary leakage. There are a variety of options available from pads to undergarments. Patient preference, comfort, and level of incontinence, shape, and contour of the product will determine which products to use (AUA 2014; Newman and Wein 2009). Patients should be counseled that incontinence products are *management strategies* and not treatment options (Newman and Wein 2009; Stohrer et al. 2009).

Catheterization

Intermittent Catheterization (IC) Versus Indwelling

The best treatment for neurogenic bladder remains controversial. Clean intermittent catheterization (CIC) was first introduced in 1972 by Lapides and colleagues. The authors concluded that CIC aids the treatment and prevention of urinary tract infections. Prevention is a direct result of reducing intravesical bladder pressure and improving blood flow to the bladder wall. Tubaro and colleagues (2012) in a comprehensive review discussed the importance of bladder emptying but were unable to make a recommendation on intermittent catheterization (IC) vs. indwelling catheter and felt the decision should be based on lifestyle.

Weld and Dmochowski (2000) retrospectively reviewed medical records, upper tract imaging, and video urodynamic of 316 posttraumatic spinal cord-injured patients looking at their rate of urologic complications. They compared indwelling catheters, IC, spontaneous voiding, and suprapubic catheterization. Their results indicated that IC is the safest management option for spinal cord injured patients.

Cochrane reviews concluded that there is a lack of compelling evidence from clinical trials that the incidence of UTI is affected by use of aseptic or clean technique, coated or uncoated catheters, single- (sterile) or multiple-use (clean) catheters, self-catheterization or catheterization by others, or by any other strategy. There is no evidence to support any method above another; however, patient preference is noted throughout the clinical trials. More well-designed trials are strongly recommended and should include analysis of cost-effectiveness data, because there are likely to be substantial differences associated with the use of different catheter designs, catheterization techniques, and strategies (Jamison et al. 2013; Prieto et al. 2014). Evidence-based guidelines suggest CIC is preferable to indwelling or suprapubic catheters for patients with bladder-emptying dysfunctions (AUA 2014).

Indwelling catheters can be used for short-term and long-term use; for the purposes of underactive bladder, only long-term use will be discussed. Indwelling catheters can be urethral or suprapubic. The complications of indwelling catheters include bacteriuria, catheter-associated urinary tract infections (CAUTI), catheter-associated biofilms, encrustations, urosepsis, and urethral damage (see Table 12.5). Indwelling catheters should be considered when anatomical, functional, or familial limitations prohibit intermittent catheterizations. A suprapubic tube is an attractive alternative to long-term urethral catheter use. The most common use of a suprapubic catheter is in individuals with spinal cord injuries and a malfunctioning bladder.

Table 12.5 Complications of indwelling catheterization

Complication	Prevention
Bacteriuria—Most patients with long-term catheterizations develop bacteriuria. The incidence is 3–8 % per day and duration of catheter is the most important risk factor	1. Ensure sterile technique
	2. Maintain a closed system
	3. Do not treat unless patient is symptomatic
Catheter-associated urinary tract infections (CAUTI)—Incidence varies based on definitions used. The Center for Disease Control (CDC) has come out with new definitions for use. http://www.cdc.gov/nhsn/PDFs/pscManual/7pscCAUTIcurrent.pdf	1. Ensure proper insertion technique (see Chap. 22)
	2. Use sterile technique
	3. Use ample lubrication
	4. Following aseptic insertion, maintain a closed drainage system
	5. Maintain unobstructed urine flow
	6. Practice good hand hygiene
Biofilms and encrustations—Biofilms are a result of colonization with uropathogens creating adhesions and adhering to the catheter wall. Encrustations are formed by organisms in biofilms and usually associated with alkaline urine. Encrustation can cause catheter blockage	1. Maintain natural pH
	2. Ensure sterile technique
	3. Maintain a closed system
	4. Change catheters when blockage occurs; it is not recommended to irrigate
Urethral damage—Occurs primarily in men. Risk increases with the length of catheterization	1. Ensure proper technique is used
	2. Ensure liberal lubrication
	3. Ensure stability of catheter to leg
	4. May use antibiotic ointment at tip of meatus

Both paraplegic and quadriplegic individuals have benefited from this form of urinary diversion. Suprapubic tubes should be changed once a month on a regular basis.

Suprapubic catheters have many advantages. With a suprapubic catheter, the risk of urethral damage is eliminated. Multiple voiding trials may be performed without having to remove the catheter. Because the catheter comes out of the lower abdomen rather than the perineal area, a suprapubic tube is more patient friendly. Bladder spasms occur less often because the suprapubic catheter does not irritate the trigone as does the urethral catheter.

Potential complications with chronic suprapubic catheterization are similar to those associated with indwelling urethral catheters, including leakage around the catheter, bladder stone formation, urinary tract infection, and catheter obstruction (Table 12.6).

Intermittent Catheterization (IC)

IC is the insertion of a catheter several times daily to empty the bladder. Once the bladder is empty, the catheter is immediately removed. There is no evidence that recommends frequency of IC, other than to prevent overdistention of the bladder. According to the EAU guidelines on neurogenic lower urinary tract dysfunction, the gold standard for management is intermittent catheterization. The guidelines

Table 12.6 Complications of clean intermittent catheterization

Complication	Prevention
Bleeding—More frequently seen in new patients and prevalence is about 1/3 of patients	1. Ensure patient is using proper technique (See Appendix)
	2. Encourage liberal lubrication
Urethritis—Prevalence varies widely but is below 8 %	1. Ensure patient is using proper technique (See Appendix)
	2. Change catheter material
Stricture—The incidence of stricture increases with longer follow-up with most events occurring 5 years after initiation. Prevalence is around 4 %	1. Ensure gentle introduction of the catheter
	2. Use of hydrophilic catheters may benefit
Creation of a false passage—Trauma especially in men can create false passages; however incidence is rare	1. Ensure patient is using proper technique (See Appendix)
	2. Gentle slow introduction of catheter
Epididymitis and prostatitis—Both are rare and can be related to recurrent UTI	1. Ensure patient is using proper technique (See Appendix)
	2. Ensure adequate hydration
	3. Ensure bladder is being emptied frequently to maintain residuals less than 500 cc
	4. Treat only when symptomatic
UTI—Prevalence is between 12 and 88 % secondary to definition used and patient populations	1. Ensure patient is using proper technique (See Appendix)
	2. Ensure adequate hydration
	3. Ensure bladder is being emptied frequently to maintain residuals less than 500 cc
	4. Treat only when symptomatic
Bladder stone—Incidence is very rare and is usually related to introduction of a foreign body into the bladder such as a pubic hair, loss of catheter in the bladder, bladder perforation, or necrosis	1. Ensure patient is using proper technique (See Appendix)
	2. Ensure adequate hydration

recommend using a 12–14 French catheter four to six times per day (Stohrer et al. 2009). CIC is also the preferred method of patients who have neurogenic bladder (Stohrer et al. 2009; Tubaro et al. 2012; Newman and Wilson 2011).

Newman and Wein (2009) stated that the advantages of CIC over indwelling included self-care and independence, reduced need for equipment, less barriers for intimacy and sexual activities, and potential for reduced lower urinary tract symptomology.

Sterile versus clean catheterization in this patient population remains a controversial topic; however, experts agree that clean intermittent catheterization (CIC) is appropriate for the majority of patients. Sterile catheterization is required for those with immunosuppression, those at risk for developing UTIs, and patients in acute or long-term care facilities (AUA 2014; Stohrer et al. 2009; Newman and Wein 2009).

The reuse of catheters remains controversial. The current standard of care is that catheters are for single use only. Several authors support this level of care (AUA 2014; Stohrer et al. 2009; Jamison et al. 2013).

Teaching patients CIC takes a knowledgeable practitioner and lots of patience. There are many patient handouts available; see resources for links on teaching patients.

Pharmacology

There are very few medications that are used to treat UAB. The main drug that is used is bethanechol (urecholine), a parasympathomimetic that provides direct stimulation of muscarinic receptors to allow a better detrusor contraction. Barendrecht and others (2007) did a systematic review and determined that the medication is not effective in the majority of patients studied.

Surgical Care

Sacral Nerve Stimulation

Sacral neuromodulation may be an effective minimally invasive intervention for some patients with underactive bladder. This is clinically indicated in some patients with nonobstructive urinary retention and incomplete bladder emptying. The therapy offers several potential benefits including avoidance of medications which could be associated with polypharmacy or drug-drug interactions. It may also be useful in those who either cannot perform or have not responded to other forms of behavioral therapy. Other patients with other neurological conditions who need regular magnetic resonance imaging (MRI) examinations may not be good candidates for neuromodulation.

Although the exact mechanisms of sacral neuromodulation are not known, its principles are based on the fact that the S2–S4 nerve roots provide the primary autonomic and somatic innervation to the lower urinary tract, including the pelvic floor, urethra, and bladder. Neuromodulation works on the principle that activity in one neural pathway can influence activity in another neural pathway. Yoshimura and Chancellor (2011) have suggested that SNS causes somatic afferent inhibition of sensory processing in the spinal cord. The S2–S4 nerve roots provide the primary autonomic and somatic innervation to the bladder, urethra, and pelvic floor. Thus, sacral neuromodulation somehow helps in dysfunctional voiding of UAB by stimulating these nerve roots.

Botulinum Toxin

Botulinum toxin has been extensively used in the neurogenic population to prevent urgency and urge incontinence. The main concern with patients who have UAB is that the patient will almost always require ISC and must be taught before the procedure.

Normally, muscle contraction occurs after acetylcholine is released at the neuro-muscular junction. Botulinum toxin blocks neurotransmission by binding to accep-tor sites on motor or sympathetic nerve terminals, entering the nerve terminals and inhibiting the release of acetylcholine. Without acetylcholine release, the muscle is unable to contract (AHFS Drug Information 2009). This inhibition occurs as the neurotoxin cleaves a protein (SNAP-25) necessary to the docking and release of acetylcholine from the vesicles within nerve endings. As a result Botulinum toxin acts as a temporary biochemical neuromodulator, meaning that muscle contraction will resume after the affects of the medication have worn off (usually 3–6 months) (Chancellor 2009).

Preventing and Treating Infections

As a result of impaired storage and voiding function, UTIs occur frequently in UAB patients. UTI is the leading cause for septicemia in these patients which is associ-ated with a significantly increased mortality (Pannek 2011). Symptomatic UTIs are often bothersome for the patients and are therefore related to a decreased quality of life. As UTIs are often recurrent and the bacterial strains are increasingly resis-tant to antibiotic treatment, UTIs are a clinical challenge for both patients and caregivers.

The EAU (Stohrer et al. 2009) and AUA white paper (2014) guidelines state that screening for and treatment of asymptomatic UTI in patients with UAB are not recommended (Stohrer et al. 2009). Patients should only be treated when there is symptomology, bacteriuria, and pyuria. Determining symptomology is based on infection in this population that can be challenging due to the overlap of symp-toms (see Table 12.7). If treatment is determined to be necessary, see Chap. 10.

Table 12.7 Signs and symptoms associated with UTIs in the neurologically compromised patient

Signs and symptoms associated with a UTI include
1. New onset or worsening of fevers
2. Rigors
3. Altered mental status changes
4. Malaise or lethargy with no other identified cause
5. Flank pain
6. Costovertebral angle tenderness
7. Acute hematuria
8. Pelvic discomfort
9. In patients with spinal cord injury
(a) Increased spasticity
(b) Autonomic dysreflexia
Pyuria is not diagnostic of a UTI in catheterized patients; however the absence of pyuria in a symptomatic patient suggests a diagnosis other than UTI
The absence or presence of odorous urine or cloudy urine should not be used to diagnose a UTI

Table 12.8 Preventing UTIs in patients undergoing catheterization

1. Treat only symptomatic UTIs
2. Do not do routine urinalysis or culture
3. Maintain good hygiene
4. Maintain adequate hydration
5. Do not routinely irrigate
6. Ensure adequate emptying of the bladder
(a) In CIC catheterize to maintain 500 cc or less in the bladder
(b) In indwelling catheters secure to leg and ensure no kinking of dislodgement of tubing
7. Although controversial acidification of the urine with use of cranberry pills has shown to be useful in preventing UTI. Cranberry pills cannot be used on patients with anticoagulant therapy
8. Change patient catheter based on patient tolerance

In this patient population, a urine culture should always be ordered if treatment is decided. The antibiotic ordered can then be changed or continued based on the susceptibility. Preventing infections in the UAB patient must be a part of the patient education. See Table 12.8 for suggestions.

Clinical Pearls

- There is no one magic number that can be used to declare the PVR volume to be abnormal in elderly patients; an elevated post-void residual volume alone should be handled with caution. Consider each patient individually: do they have bothersome symptoms and is their CR elevated? If the answer is no, consider watching the patient rather than intervening.
- Many patients respond well to conservative measures such as scheduled toileting, prompted voiding, or other treatments, particularly with the assistance of caregivers when needed. Double voiding, defined as urinating again after a brief delay from the initial void, can help to better empty the bladder in some patients.
- When a distended bladder is incidentally identified and reported by the radiologist, it is important to clarify with the patient whether he/she voided prior to the study. Also, a bladder scan should be performed post-void to confirm an elevated PVR.
- The impact of detrusor underactivity on older patients can range from minimal to severe. Bothersome nocturia may be improved by decreasing fluid intake several hours before retiring to bed.
- Patients with dependent edema in the lower extremities or an element of congestive heart failure may benefit from reclining with their legs elevated

for a time before going to bed for the night. Timing of diuretic use is important, and these medications should be taken in the morning or early afternoon rather than closer to bedtime.

- The risk of urinary retention associated with pain medications appears to be higher with the longer-activating pain medication. Similarly, general anesthetics promote smooth muscle relaxation and can contribute to postoperative urinary retention. The risk is even higher in those patients treated with epidural pain management.
- Asymptomatic bacteria should not be treated ever in a patient with UAB. If there are no significant white blood cells in the urine and the patient does not have symptoms, do not give an antibiotic.

Resources for the Patient
Teaching CIC:
http://www.cc.nih.gov/ccc/patient_education/pepubs/bladder/ciscwomen5_22.pdf
https://www.suna.org/download/members/selfCatheterization.pdf
Bladder Diary: http://www.niddk.nih.gov/health-information/health-topics/urologic-disease/daily-bladder-diary/Pages/facts.aspx
Nerve Disease and Bladdder control: http://www.niddk.nih.gov/health-information/health-topics/urologic-disease/nerve-disease-and-bladder-control/Pages/facts.aspx
Sexual and Urological problems of Diabetes http://www.niddk.nih.gov/health information/health-topics/Diabetes/sexual-urologic-problems-diabetes/Pages/index.aspx
Urinary retention: http://www.niddk.nih.gov/health-information/health-topics/urologic-disease/urinary-retention/Pages/facts.aspx

Resources for the Nurse Practitioner
http://www.auanet.org/common/pdf/education/clinical-guidance/Catheter-Associated-Urinary-Tract-Infections-WhitePaper.pdf
Managing and Treating Urinary Incontinence 2nd edition by Diane Newman and Alan Wein 2009 Health Professions Press
The Underactive Bladder Michael Chancellor and Ananias Diokno editors 2015 Springer
SUNA white paper on CAUTI: https://www.suna.org/resources/cautiWhitePaper.pdf
SUNA Practice Guidelines
Acute Urinary retention: https://www.suna.org/sites/default/files/download/indwellingCatheter.pdf
Female Catheterization:https://www.suna.org/sites/default/files/download/female-Catheterization.pdf

Male Catheterization: https://www.suna.org/sites/default/files/download/male-Catheterization.pdf

CAUTI: https://www.suna.org/sites/default/files/download/cautiGuideline.pdf

Supropubic cath change: https://www.suna.org/sites/default/files/download/suprapubic-Catheter.pdf

References

Abrams P, Cardozo L, Fall M, Griffiths D et al. Standardisation Sub-committee of the International Continence Society (2002) The standardization of terminology of lower urinary tract function: report from the Standardisation Sub- committee of the International Continence Society. Neurol Urodyn 21(2):167–178

AHFS Drug Information (2009) BOTOX®. Retrieved 2 Sep 2009. From http://ashp.org/ahfs/index.cfm

American Urological Association. White paper on catheter-associated urinary tract infections: definitions and significance in the urologic patient 2014. Downloaded from https://www.aua-net.org/common/pdf/education/clinical-guidance/Catheter-Associated-Urinary-Tract-Infections-WhitePaper.pdf. On 29 June 2015

Barendrecht MM, Oelke M, Laguna MP, Micheal MC (2007) Is the use of parasympathomimetics for treating an underactive bladder evidence based? BJU Int 99:749–752

Chancellor M (2009) Ten years single surgeon experience with botulinum toxin in the urinary tract: clinical observations and research discovery. Int Urol Nephrol J 42(2):383–391

Chancellor M (2014) The overactive bladder progression to underactive bladder hypothesis. Int Urol Nephrol 46(Suppl 1):523–527

Chancellor M, Diokno AC (2014) CURE-UAB shedding light on the underactive bladder syndrome. Int Urol Neph 46(Suppl 1):S1

Diokno A (2015) Evaluation and diagnosis of underactive bladder in The Underactive Bladder. In: Chancellor M: Diokino A (eds) pp 13–24

Diokno AC, Brock BM, Brown MB, Herzog AR (1986) Prevalence of urinary incontinence and other urological symptoms in the noninstitutionalized elderly. J Urol 136:1022–1025

Griebling T (2015) Geriatric Urology and Underactive Bladder in The Underactive Bladder. In: Chancellor M; Diokno A (eds) Springer Switzerland pp 177–188

Jamison J, Maquire S, Mcann J (2013) Catheter policies for management of long term voiding problems in adults with neurogenic bladder disorders (Review). Cochrane Libr 11:1–59

Lapides J, Diokno A, Silber S, Lowe B (1972) Clean intermittent self-catheterization in the treatment of urinary tract disease. J Urol 107(3):458–4613

McClurg D, Ashe RG, Marshall K, Lowe-Strong AS (2006) Comparison of pelvic floor muscle training, electromyography biofeedback and neuromuscular electrical stimulation for bladder dysfunction in people with multiple sclerosis: a randomized pilot study. Neurourol Urodyn 25:337–348

McClurg D, Ashe RG, Lowe-Strong AS (2008) Neuromuscular electrical stimulation and the treatment of lower urinary tract dysfunction in multiple sclerosis-a double blind, placebo controlled, randomised clinical trial. Neurourol Urodyn 27:231–237

Miyazato M, Yoshimura N, Chancellor M (2013) The other bladder syndrome: underactive bladder. Rev Urol 15(1):11–22

Newman D, Wein A (2009) Managing and treating urinary incontinence, 2nd edn. Health Professions Press, Baltimore, pp 365–483

Newman D, Wilson M (2011) Review of intermittent catheterization and current best practices. Urol Nurs 31(1):12–28

Osman N et al (2014) Detrusor underactivity and the underactive bladder: a new clinical entity? A review of current terminology, definitions, epidemiology aetiology and diagnosis. Eur Urol 65(2):389–398

Pannek J (2011) Treatment of Urinary Tract infection in persons with spinal cord injury: guidelines, evidence, and clinical practice. A questionnaire based survey and review of the literature. Journal of Spinal Cord Medicine, 34(1):11–15

Patil NJ, Nagaratna R, Garner C, Raghurman NV (2012) Effect of integrated yoga on neurogenic bladder dysfunction in patients with multiple sclerosis–a prospective observational series. Compliment Ther Med 20:424–430

Prieto J, Murphy CL, Moore KN, Fader M (2014) Catheterisation for long term bladder management (Review). Cochran Libr 9:1–97

Stohrer M, Blok B, Castro-Diaz D, Chartier-Kastler E, Del Popolo G, Kramer G, Pannek J, Piotr R, Wyandaele J (2009) EAU guidelines on neurogenic lower urinary tract dysfunction. Eur Urol 56:81–88

Tubaro A, Puccini F, De Nunzio C, Diggesu GA, Elneil S, Gobbi C, Khullar V (2012) The treatment of lower urinary tract symptoms in patients with multiple sclerosis: a systemic review. Curr Urol Rep 13:335–342

Valente S, Du Beau C, Chancellor D et al (2014) Epidemiology and demographics of the underactive bladder: a cross sectional survey. Int Urol Nephrol 46 (Suppl):S7–S10

Weld K, Dmochowski R (2000) Effect of bladder management on urological complications in spinal cord injured patients. J Urol 163:768–772

Yoshimura N, Chancellor MB (2011) Physiology and pharmacology of the bladder and urethra. In: Wein AJ, Kavoussi LR, Novick AC, Partin AW, Peters CA (eds) Campbells Urology, 10th edn. Elsevier, Philadelphia PA, USA

Stress Incontinence

13

Natalie Gaines, John E. Lavin, and Jason P. Gilleran

Contents

Objectives
1. Discuss the incidence and definition of stress urinary incontinence (SUI).
2. Review and provide tips for the assessment of SUI.
3. Discuss management of SUI.

N. Gaines, MD
Female Pelvic Medicine and Reconstructive Surgery, Department of Urology,
Beaumont Health System, Royal Oak, MI, USA

J.E. Lavin, MD
Department of Urology, Beaumont Health System, Royal Oak, MI, USA

J.P. Gilleran, MD (⊠)
Department of Urology, Oakland University William Beaumont School of Medicine,
Royal Oak, MI, USA
e-mail: Jason.Gilleran@beaumont.org

© Springer International Publishing Switzerland 2016
M. Lajiness, S. Quallich (eds.), *The Nurse Practitioner in Urology*,
DOI 10.1007/978-3-319-28743-0_13

Introduction

Incidence

Stress urinary incontinence (SUI) is defined as involuntary urinary leakage with any activities that increase abdominal pressure, such as coughing, laughing, sneezing, or even moving from a seated to a standing position. SUI is a very common problem affecting 15–80 % of women. In terms of financial burden, urinary incontinence of all types was estimated to cost over $19.5 billion dollars a year (Hu et al. 2004).

Unfortunately, incontinence has been considered by many as a normal, irreversible aspect of aging that is an indication of mental incompetence. It dramatically increases the risk that a patient will be institutionalized as the burden on the caregiver becomes too much to care for the patient at home. Because of the social stigma associated with its hygienic issues, incontinence is under-reported by patients; other patients do not self-report and minimize their symptoms as they feel that incontinence is not a legitimate medical issue. Because of these barriers in societal perception, only 1/4–1/2 of patients with incontinence are adequately managed.

Pertinent Anatomy, Physiology

The female urethra is approximately 4 cm in length from the bladder neck to the urethral meatus. In order to maintain continence, the urethra must remain closed at rest and also during any activity that may increase in abdominal pressure, such as coughing, bearing down, or sneezing.

Three structures are required to permit urethral closure. First, the urethral mucosa and submucosa must have a good vascular supply to help form a watertight closure. This is under the influence of estrogens. The second structure is the striated urogenital sphincter, also called the rhabdosphincter, which surrounds the urethra and keeps it closed at rest. Third, muscular and fascial tissues form a supportive hammock for the upper and mid-urethra. The largest connective tissue component, the endopelvic fascia, has two important connections which form the pubourethral and urethropelvic ligaments, connecting the urethra to the pubic bone and other strong tissues in the pelvis. The levator ani is a group of skeletal muscles that act as a pelvic support structure, with the pubourethral muscle being one portion of the levator ani arranged in a "sling" configuration around the proximal urethra. The levator ani complex also includes the puborectalis and pubococcygeus; this pelvic floor musculature has a significant role in supporting not only the pelvic organs but also the weight of the abdominal contents. Within the midline of these muscles is an exit aperture called the urogenital hiatus, where the urethra and vagina exit the pelvis. The predominant innervation to these muscle groups is via the pudendal nerve.

Pathophysiology

Stress urinary incontinence can occur in women as a result of two primary mechanisms. The most common etiology is urethral hypermobility (UH), which causes 80–90 % of cases. In normal anatomy, the endopelvic fascia and pelvic floor muscles (levator ani) stabilize the urethra within the pelvis. This support coapts the urethra against the vagina posteriorly, compressing the urethra during any increase in intra-abdominal pressure. This "hammock theory" was proposed by DeLancey in 1994 (DeLancey 1994).

In a woman with urethral hypermobility, the support structures no longer maintain the urethra in its normal anatomic position during stress maneuvers, which permits movement of the bladder neck and proximal urethra. Consequently, abdominal pressure is not distributed equally to the urethra, and when the bladder pressure is greater than the closure pressure of the urethra, urinary leakage occurs.

Common causes for urethral hypermobility include childbirth, stretching of the portions of the fascia which support the urethra, and injury to the structures which support the uterus, causing the urethra to pull down and away from the pubic bone. These conditions worsen with age and hormonal changes.

Intrinsic sphincter deficiency (ISD) is a less common cause of stress urinary incontinence, occurring in 10–20 % of SUI patients. In ISD, the urethral mucosa and submucosa coapt poorly despite adequate vaginal support. This can be caused by multiple previous surgeries, pudendal nerve injury (which causes decreased urethral resistance to leakage), radiation, or injury to the blood supply after pelvic or vaginal surgery. ISD is typically seen in the presence of urethral hypermobility, but can occur as an isolated finding, particularly in the geriatric population, or in women who have previously undergone a urethral support surgery.

History

Accurately recognizing the type of incontinence in a patient can be challenging and requires a detailed history. Pertinent points include when the leakage started, what situations or movements tend to exacerbate it, and the overall severity – is the patient leaking just a few drops or emptying her entire bladder? Leakage that occurs after cough, sneeze, standing up, or while straining to have a bowel movement is the hallmark of SUI, whereas leakage that occurs after the patient feels an intense need to urinate is characteristic of urge incontinence. However, patients may report leakage that occurs without awareness of the mechanism behind it, which is classified as unaware incontinence. In these situations, incontinence can be related to stress maneuvers with repeated small volume urine loss; similarly, older patients may no longer have the sensation of urgency that accompanies bladder overactivity. The Medical, Epidemiologic, and Social Aspects of Aging, or MESA, questionnaire can be used to help quantify symptoms and to determine if the patient is suffering from both stress and urge incontinence, called mixed urinary incontinence (See Fig. 13.1).

One way of identifying SUI severity is to quantify the number of sanitary pads the patient uses daily, but the number and type of pad alone can be misleading. Thus, a

MESA URINARY INCONTINENCE QUESTIONNAIRE (UIQ)

NAME :_____   DATE :_____
            LAST,   FIRST   MI

Please check (√) the appropriate box.

1. Over the past 12 months, have you had urine loss beyond your control?
    _____ Yes   _____ No

2. How long ago did your urine loss start? _____ years _____ months _____days

3. When does the urine loss usually occur?

        _____ Day time only

        _____ Night time only

        _____ Both day time and night time

4. Do you use anything for protection against leaked urine?

        _____ Yes (Go to the next question)   _____ No

5. On <u>average,</u> how many of each of these do you use for protection? (Please write the number used
    and check each day or week)
                                                                        <u>Number</u>
                                                                        <u>Used</u>

    Sanitary napkins   _____   ____each day or ____each week
    Pads like those placed on furniture (ex. Blue pads)   _____   ____each day or ____each week
    Adult wetness control garments (ex. Attends, Depends) _____   ____each day or ____each week
    Toilet paper or facial tissues   _____   ____each day or ____each week
    Something else (please list)   _____   ____each day or ____each week

    _____ _____   ____each day or ____each week

    _____ _____   ____each day or ____each week

6. While awake, when you are having urine loss problems, how much urine would you say you lose without
    control EACH TIME?

        _____ A few drops to less than ½ teaspoon
        _____ ½ teaspoon to less than 2 tablespoons
        _____ 2 tablespoons to ½ cup
        _____ ½ cup or more

7. When you lose urine, does it usually:

        _____ Just create some moisture
        _____ Wet your underwear
        _____ Trickle down you thigh
        _____ Wet the floor

8. Generally, how many times do you usually urinate from the time you wake up to the time before you

    go to bed? _____ times.

9. Generally, how many times do you usually urinate after you have gone to sleep at night? _____ times

Fig. 13.1 MESA Urinary Incontinence Questionnaire (Diokno et al. 2002)

Urge Incontinence Questions

1. Some people receive very little warning and suddenly find that they are losing, or about to lose urine beyond their control.
    How often does this happen to your?
    _____Often (3)   _____Sometimes (2)   _____Rarely (1)   _____Never (0)

2. If you can't find a toilet or find a toilet that is occupied and you have an urge to urinate, how often do you end up losing
    urine and wetting yourself?
    _____Often (3)   _____Sometimes (2)   _____Rarely (1)   _____Never (0)

3. Do you lose urine when you suddenly have the feeling that your bladder is full?
    _____Often (3)   _____Sometimes (2)   _____Rarely (1)   _____Never (0)

4. Does washing your hands cause you to lose urine?
    _____Often (3)   _____Sometimes (2)   _____Rarely (1)   _____Never (0)

5. Does cold weather cause you to lose urine?
    _____Often (3)   _____Sometimes (2)   _____Rarely (1)   _____Never (0)

6. Does drinking cold beverages cause you to lose urine?
    _____Often (3)   _____Sometimes (2)   _____Rarely (1)   _____Never (0)   TOTAL SCORE=_____/18

URGE SYMPTOMS INDEX LOOK-UP TABLE				
1/18 = 6%	5/18 = 28%	9/18 = 50%	13/18 = 72%	17/18=94%
2/18 = 11%	6/18 = 33%	10/18 = 56%	14/18 = 78%	18/18 = 100%
3/18 = 17%	7/18 = 39%	11/18 = 61%	15/18 = 83%	
4/18 = 22%	8/18 = 44%	12/18 = 67%	16/18 = 89%	

Stress Incontinence Questions

1. Does coughing gently cause you to lose urine?
    _____Often (3)   _____Sometimes (2)   _____Rarely (1)   _____Never (0)

2. Does coughing hard cause you to lose urine?
    _____Often (3)   _____Sometimes (2)   _____Rarely (1)   _____Never (0)

3. Does sneezing cause you to lose urine?
    _____Often (3)   _____Sometimes (2)   _____Rarely (1)   _____Never (0)

4. Does lifting things cause you to lose urine?
    _____Often (3)   _____Sometimes (2)   _____Rarely (1)   _____Never (0)

5   Does bending over cause you to lose urine?
    _____Often (3)   _____Sometimes (2)   _____Rarely (1)   _____Never (0)

6. Does laughing cause you to lose urine?
    _____Often (3)   _____Sometimes (2)   _____Rarely (1)   _____Never (0)

7. Does walking briskly cause you to lose urine?
    _____Often (3)   _____Sometimes (2)   _____Rarely (1)   _____Never (0)

8. Does straining, if you are constipated, cause you to lose urine?
    _____Often (3)   _____Sometimes (2)   _____Rarely (1)   _____Never (0)

9. Does getting up from a sitting to a standing position cause you to lose urine?
    _____Often (3)   _____Sometimes (2)   _____Rarely (1)   _____Never (0)   TOTAL SCORE=_____/27

STRESS SYMPTOMS INDEX LOOK-UP TABLE						
1/27 = 4%	5/27 = 19%	9/27 = 33%	13/27 = 48%	17/27 = 63%	21/27 = 78%	25/27 = 93%
2/27 = 7%	6/27 = 22%	10/27 = 37%	14/27 = 52%	18/27 = 67%	22/27 – 81%	26/27 = 96%
3/27 = 11%	7/27 = 26%	11/27 = 41%	15/27 = 56%	19/27 = 70%	23/27 = 85%	27/27 = 100%
4/27 = 15%	8/27 = 30%	12/27 = 44%	16/27 = 59%	20/27 = 74%	24/27 = 89%	

Fig. 13.1 (continued)

Table 13.1 Medications that cause transient UI

Medication	Effect on urinary system
Alpha-adrenergic receptor antagonists	Smooth muscle relaxation of the bladder neck and urethral causing SUI (mainly women)
Tricyclic antidepressants Alpha-adrenergic agonists	Anticholinergic effect and alpha-adrenergic receptor agonist effect causing post-void dribbling, straining, and hesitancy in urine flow and even urinary retention
Psychotropics	May decrease afferent input resulting in decrease in bladder contractility. Can accumulate in the elderly causing confusion resulting in functional incontinence
Cholinesterase inhibitors	Increase bladder contractility and may cause incontinence
Narcotic analgesics, opioids	Decrease bladder contractility, decrease afferent input. Depress the central nervous system causing sedation, confusion, and immobility, leading to urinary retention and UI
Calcium channel blockers	Impair bladder contractility, causing UI
Diuretics	Overwhelm the bladder with rapidly produced urine for up to 6 h after ingestion
Methylxanthines	Polyuria, bladder irritation

Adapted from Ouslander (2004)

clinician should ascertain not only whether the patient is using a thin liner versus a full diaper but also how wet they are when she changes them. Some patients change their pads after only a few drops of leakage, whereas others only change their pads when they are fully soaked. Additionally, one should inquire about a patient's overall voiding habits to evaluate for any concomitant voiding or bowel dysfunction. Does she also have daytime frequency and urgency, nighttime frequency or leakage while sleeping (nocturnal enuresis), any history of hematuria or dysuria, straining to void, or post-void micturition (dribbles of urine leaking out after she finishes urinating)? Constipation can frequently cause urinary leakage, so ensuring that a patient with leakage is having soft, formed bowel movements is very important. Hematuria or dysuria in a smoker could be an indication of a transitional cell cancer of the bladder or ureter and merit a full hematuria workup. A voiding diary can be helpful in the woman with frequency and nocturia, which can also provide insight on fluid intake, as polydipsia can exacerbate any type of urinary incontinence.

Incontinence can often accompany pelvic organ prolapse (POP), and the history should also include if the patient reports a sensation of a bulge coming out of her vagina. As laxity in the structural supports of the pelvis can cause UH, prolapse can occur in more severe cases. In a woman with a concomitant cystocele or rectocele, she may note the need to "splint," where she places a finger in the vagina to assist with emptying of the bladder and/or bowels. It is imperative to know that women with advanced POP often do not have SUI, as this can be "masked" by the bulge kinking off the urethra. In such cases, women may report having SUI in the past that spontaneously resolved, likely once their prolapse worsened.

Other pertinent aspects of the history include a complete medical history, with prior surgeries and current medications noted. Some medications can worsen SUI in patients, such as alpha-adrenergic antagonists, such as doxazosin (see Table 13.1). Current or prior tobacco use can lead to chronic cough, as can pulmonary conditions such as asthma or COPD. Chronic cough as a side effect of angiotensin-converting inhibitors is rare, but it should be noted in the patient's medication history. Obesity can also be a source of SUI, and weight loss of 10 % can often correct the incontinence. Treatment of chronic cough can in and of itself relieve SUI and should be pursued either before or concomitantly with any treatments for SUI, as successful treatment is less likely if this symptom is not addressed adequately. Lastly, a full gynecologic history, including gravida/parity status, vaginal versus caesarean section deliveries, and any complications of pregnancies, should be noted. Menopausal status and the use of any type of hormone replacement are also important, although hormonal replacement therapy may only marginally help the woman with SUI.

Diagnostic Evaluation

Physical Exam

The goal of a proper physical examination is to reproduce the leakage that the patient reports while identifying anatomic abnormalities that could account for the incontinence. Examination with a full bladder is paramount in the evaluation of SUI. However, some patients may leak with an empty bladder evaluated with a supine empty bladder stress test (SEBST) – leakage from the urethral meatus during cough or Valsalva maneuver at the time of the pelvic examination. In 2010 Nager et al. reported that patients with a positive SEBST had increased pad weight and number of leaks per day compared to patients with a negative SEBST, that is, a positive supine empty bladder stress test is highly indicative of severe stress incontinence. Urethral hypermobility on exam is indicated by brisk, upward movement of the urethra of at least 30° with an increase in abdominal pressure. One method of measuring the degree of urethral mobility is via the "q-tip test," in which a soft lubricated applicator is passed through the urethra to the level of the bladder neck. The woman is asked to cough and/or Valsalva and the degree of rotation is measured, with >30° considered hypermobile. However, this test is not used as often clinically due to urethral discomfort.

A "stress test" is considered positive if one demonstrates urinary leakage; however, absence of urinary leakage does not mean the patient doesn't have SUI. 34 % of women with SUI have a negative stress test, which could be positional or due to inadequate filling of the bladder (Nager et al. 2010). If negative, reassess with the patient standing. Absence of urethral mobility, i.e., a "fixed" urethra, in the presence of stress leak is important since the most commonly used surgery for SUI, the midurethral sling, has a higher failure rate in these patients. This finding is more common in the elderly female, who may also have a finding of atrophic vaginitis.

Other findings to note on exam are whether there are signs of a urethral diverticulum, which can be identified as a fluid-filled sac along the urethra that expresses fluid through the meatus on palpation. These can also be quite tender, particularly if they are actively infected. Patients with a urethral diverticulum will often report the symptom of post-void dribbling, stress incontinence, or even continuous incontinence. The examination of the patient's pelvic floor while asking her to perform a

Kegel maneuver – squeeze down around your finger and evaluate the strength of her pelvic floor musculature – can be very helpful. A woman with a weak pelvic floor and incontinence may significantly benefit from pelvic floor physical therapy.

A pelvic exam must also identify the presence of pelvic organ prolapse and its severity. This is especially important in a patient who reports previously having stress incontinence that spontaneously resolved as her vaginal bulge worsened. Some patients have such a large cystocele that it ultimately kinks off the urethra.

A rare cause of incontinence, particularly in the young nulliparous female, is the presence of an ectopic ureter, which can drain directly into the vagina. Usually, this is associated with a symptom of continuous, rather than activity-related, incontinence. Lastly, one should perform a general neurologic examination, evaluating for intact sensation and any deficits.

Diagnostic Tests

It is clinically indicated to obtain a urinalysis in every patient with SUI, looking for microscopic hematuria, which should prompt a workup according to the American Urological Association guidelines, or a urinary tract infection, which should be treated prior to additional workup.

Measuring post-void residual is also part of the basic evaluation for SUI, especially if there is planned surgical intervention. Incomplete emptying or urinary retention, the definition of which can vary but is generally accepted as a PVR >150 mL, identifies those who may have an issue with bladder emptying after surgery. An elevated PVR could be related to a neurologic deficit or a large cystocele that may need to be repaired simultaneously. These patients merit further workup, particularly in the absence of advanced-grade pelvic organ prolapse.

Urodynamic testing (UDT) is a routine outpatient diagnostic test designed to reproduce symptoms while assessing for other functional abnormalities of the lower urinary tract. In the woman with SUI alone, UDT is not routinely indicated. The Value of Urodynamic Evaluation, or VaLUE, study was a randomized trial comparing office evaluation only versus office evaluation and urodynamics prior to SUI surgery (Nager et al. 2012). This large multicenter study showed that in 97 % of patients, urodynamics merely confirm the office evaluation; that is, in the vast majority of patients, urodynamic testing is not necessary to make a proper diagnosis. At 1-year follow-up, these patients had similar outcomes. The uncomplicated index patients included in the VaLUE study were defined as a woman with stress-predominant incontinence, a post-void residual of less than 150 mL, negative urinalysis or urine culture, and urethral hypermobility with a positive stress test on examination.

Which patients should undergo urodynamic testing?

1. Any patient who reports SUI and in whom one cannot demonstrate it on exam with a full bladder in the standing position, prior to any surgical intervention.
2. Any patient with concern for, or a proven neurologic disease – leakage in this patient may be due to altered bladder compliance and neurogenic detrusor overactivity. Consider video urodynamics to look for vesicoureteral reflux at

higher detrusor pressures – this can ultimately lead to deterioration of the upper tracts (kidneys).
3. Any patient who has previously undergone an anti-incontinence procedure and has persistent or recurrent incontinence. UDT can help evaluate if the prior surgery is causing urethral obstruction.
4. Patients with high-grade pelvic organ prolapse without stress incontinence may have occult stress incontinence, which can be "unmasked" during UDT.
5. Mixed incontinence patients who have both SUI and urgency, frequency, and urge urinary incontinence should undergo UDT to help the clinician decide which treatments should be initiated first.

The AUA and the Society for Urodynamics, Female Pelvic Medicine, and Urogenital Reconstruction (SUFU) published a set of guidelines in 2012 to assist clinicians in determining which patients may benefit from further urodynamic testing (Winters et al. 2012). For straightforward stress urinary incontinence, no routine imaging studies are indicated.

Management

Because SUI is a quality-of-life disease, the treatment is contingent upon the patient's bother. Remember, some patients are not severely bothered by what you may perceive as a severe symptomatology and choose not to pursue any treatment. Conservative first-line treatment consists of pelvic floor physical therapy and behavioral changes (see Table 13.2). Teaching a client Kegel exercises (see Table 13.3) can be done in the office or with referral to physical therapist (PT) who specializes in pelvic floor therapy. When referring a patient to pelvic floor PT, the physical therapists use a number of modalities to target the levator muscle group, including intravaginal muscle strengthening exercises, biofeedback, and electrical stimulation. Behavioral therapy is helpful in patients who report excessive fluid intake (>100 oz. total daily) or who have incontinence due to delayed voiding, where leakage occurs due to overfilling. Addressing any causes of chronic cough or straining can resolve SUI in many women. Cough is a known side effect of angiotensin-converting enzyme (ACE) inhibitors, such as lisinopril, in some individuals. Appropriate referrals to otolaryngology for chronic cough or even discussion with their primary physician to adjust medications can be helpful.

Table 13.2 Behaviors to reduce stress incontinence

Behavior	Intervention
Fluid intake	Fluid intake should be 6–8 8 oz glasses of fluid per day
Bowel function	Regulate bowel function to avoid straining and constipation
Smoking	Quit to relieve chronic cough associated with smoking
Obesity	Lose weight to decrease pressure on sphincter

Table 13.3 Kegel exercises

Kegel exercise instructions
1. Identify pelvic floor muscles
2. Squeeze and hold up to 10 s
3. Relax for 10 s after each contraction (relaxing is just as important as contracting)
4. Do not use the stomach, buttocks, or thighs
5. Do ten sets daily in each position, sitting, standing, and laying
6. Doing too many exercises can fatigue your muscles

For those patients with situational incontinence only (i.e., only occurring during certain sporting activities), one can use a urethral insert to "plug" the outlet and reduce leakage. The FemSoft is a soft, plastic insert that can be left in the urethra temporarily. Alternatively, a vaginal tampon has been reported to reduce leakage in younger women. In the most severe cases of sphincteric damage, or in the frail elderly individuals, catheter placement can be offered as a short- or even long-term option, but carries several risks, including urethral damage, hematuria, and urinary tract infections.

For patients who are not interested in or not candidates for physical therapy, or in those with incomplete symptom resolution after PT, the next option is surgery, as there are no Food and Drug Administration-approved pharmaceuticals for SUI. The most common procedure for SUI currently is the mid-urethral sling (MUS). The concept of an MUS, initially described as a tension-free vaginal tape, was first described by Ulmsten in 1996 (Ulmsten et al. 1996). A 17-year follow-up of 90 women published in 2013 reported an objective cure rate of over 90 % (Nilsson et al. 2013). The surgical approach involves a small vaginal incision to permit passage of a thin strip of synthetic mesh using a trocar, or a thin metal carrier, through the obturator canal and exiting via the groin (the transobturator sling) or behind the pubic bone exiting via the suprapubic area (the retropubic sling). Once healed in position, the mesh rests underneath the middle of the urethra and, during any increase in intra-abdominal pressure, permits coaptation of the urethra to prevent urinary leakage.

The Trial of Mid-Urethral Slings (TOMUS) study evaluated for a difference in outcomes between the retropubic and the transobturator approach. At 24-month follow-up, both groups were found to have similarly high rates of satisfaction. The retropubic slings were found to have slightly better objective success rates, but also had higher rates of voiding dysfunction requiring surgery (3 % vs. 0 %, $p = 0.002$) and urinary tract infections (Nilsson et al. 2013). The transobturator slings, because they pass through the obturator fossa, can cause damage to the obturator nerve; thus, these patients had a higher rate of neurologic symptoms.

The most common complications of MUS include urinary obstruction, bladder or urethral injury, injury to bowel or vascular structures, and mesh erosion. Urinary obstruction may be reported by the patient and should be promptly managed within the first several weeks postoperatively. Many patients report a slower stream; however, any patient who is unable to void or requires catheterization needs prompt evaluation by the operating surgeon. Immediately after surgery, the mesh has not undergone maximal tissue ingrowth, and it is possible to perform a sling release, either in the operating room or the office. The vaginal incision is opened and the sling is grasped and pulled down to loosen. After about 3 weeks, the surrounding pelvic tissues have begun to grow into the mesh, and the patient may require a sling incision, where the sling must be cut in the operating room. If obstruction is not addressed, the bladder can be damaged due to high voiding pressures, which can ultimately cause myogenic failure (inability to contract normally) and/or bladder wall thickening, which can adversely affect bladder filling.

Bladder and urethral injuries are typically diagnosed via intraoperative cystoure-throscopy. Bladder perforation by a trocar has been reported in 3.5–6.6 % of cases; management includes removal of the offending trocar and repassage as well as temporary catheterization, the duration of which is at the performing surgeon's discretion. In cases where the trocar has only passed through the bladder a single time, some surgeons feel comfortable leaving no catheter; in other cases, with multiple passages (as occasionally occurs in a patient with difficult anatomy), the catheter must remain in place for 1 to 7 days. If mesh erosion into the urethra or the bladder occurs as a late complication, the patient can present with gross hematuria, lower tract symptoms such as frequency or urgency, or recurrent urinary tract infections. Mesh that is eroded into the urinary tract must be removed completely. The choice to perform another sling at that time versus as a delayed approach is up to the surgeon's discretion, but the use of mesh in these revision cases may not be prudent.

Mesh erosion or exposure is a rare occurrence after MUS, but this condition can present as vaginal discharge or bleeding, especially after intercourse or partner discomfort. The patient herself may feel palpable mesh or other material in the vagina, but this is most often seen by the clinician during pelvic exam. If the exposure is minimal or the patient is asymptomatic, the erosion can be observed and the patient can use a topical estrogen cream. This is most commonly done in a woman who is not sexually active. If the patient is having symptoms, there are several management options, including excising the exposed portion, reapproximating vaginal epithelium over the exposure, or even removal of the entire mesh sling. Complete removal can lead to recurrence of the patient's incontinence. It should be noted that full-thickness exposure is not necessary for the sling to cause discomfort, and the finding of point tenderness over a portion of the sling that was not present preoperatively may warrant partial or total sling removal in select cases.

Bowel injuries are exceedingly rare but occur with passage of the trocar through the space of Retzius during retropubic sling placement. This occurs more commonly in women with a history of prior abdominal of pelvic surgery or with an abdominal hernia. Bowel injuries manifest after retropubic MUS with peritoneal signs – severe or persistent abdominal pain, guarding, rigidity, fever, or feculent drainage from the abdominal incision sites. Diagnosis may be solidified by a CT scan with oral contrast. This is a surgical emergency and requires prompt treatment.

A second procedure which dates to the early twentieth century but is still commonly used is the pubovaginal fascial sling. This procedure differs from the mid-urethral sling in several important ways. First, the anatomic location is more proximal than the MUS – the sling itself is placed at the bladder neck. These slings are historically intended to be at least partially obstructing and can be used in patients with intrinsic sphincter deficiency or in patients who have failed previous MUS. Instead of a piece of mesh, tissue is used – typically autologous tissue, taken from the patient's fascia lata on the thigh or from the rectus fascia on the abdominal wall. A vaginal incision is made, just like in the MUS, but the bladder neck is exposed and lateral dissection performed to enter the retropubic space. Next, an abdominal incision is made, typically a Pfannenstiel incision, and if using rectus fascia, this is harvested. The piece of tissue required to perform this procedure is typically 6–10 cm in length and 1–2 cm in width. Permanent suture is used to anchor the fascia on each end to tension it to the abdominal fascia. A ligature passer is passed on either side of the urethra down from the abdominal to the vaginal incision under fingertip guidance. The suture is grasped and brought up so that the fascia is lying flat against the urethra and then tensioned under direct visualization and palpation. This procedure takes longer, may have more blood loss, and typically requires an overnight stay, versus the MUS which permits same-day discharge. The complications are similar to those of the MUS and include injury to bowel, bladder, urethra, or vascular structures or urinary obstruction, but because the patient has no mesh placed and the tissue is her own, the exposure rate is quite low. However, because the fascial sling is much more obstructing than the MUS, many patients develop new-onset urgency, voiding dysfunction, and the need for catheterization. If the fascial sling is overly tensioned, it can be loosened, but this is always done in the operating room (not the office) and is more extensive than loosening a mesh sling.

The Burch colposuspension, which differs from slings as this procedure is performed via an abdominal incision, anchors the anterior vaginal wall at the level of the bladder neck to the iliopectineal line (Cooper's ligament) using 2–4 permanent sutures. This procedure is most commonly performed at the same time as an abdominal hysterectomy. In the Stress Incontinence Surgical Treatment Efficacy Trial, or SISTEr, the Burch colposuspension was compared to the previously discussed bladder neck sling (Albo 2007). With 24-month follow-up, this multicenter trial showed that the fascial sling had higher overall success rates than the Burch procedure and that more patients who had undergone the Burch procedure needed a second surgery to correct their SUI. However, the success of the fascial sling was offset by its higher rate of complications, including UTI, urge incontinence, and the need for surgical treatment to permit voiding.

In patients with a fixed urethra, a fascial sling can be effective, but a less invasive, less obstructive approach is to use a bulking agent, such as calcium hydroxyapatite (Coaptite) or silicon elastomer (Macroplastique). Cross-linked collagen was commonly used in the past, but is no longer available on the market. Bulking agent injection is performed using a cystoscope through the wall of the mid-urethra to "bulk up" the urethral sphincter and allow the walls of the urethra to coapt together, reducing stress incontinence. Patients should be counseled that "cure" of the leakage with this technique is uncommon, but one can expect significant improvement with 1–2 injections. Risks are low and can include transient retention (1–3 days), urinary infection, and urethritis and dysuria in rare cases.

There is currently ongoing research regarding the use of autologous muscle cells injected into the urethra to "regenerate" the urethral sphincter. Muscle cells are harvested via biopsy of the thigh muscles, for example, and grown in an outside laboratory for several weeks before reinjection. Early studies are promising, but this treatment shows promise and may be commercially available in the near future.

Conclusion

SUI is a very correctable problem, and its management has evolved to a less invasive approach, with good long-term follow-up and several well-designed studies demonstrating efficacy of the MUS. Obtaining a thorough and appropriate history, performing a directed physical examination, and assessing urine and voiding function are critical to develop a therapeutic plan for each patient. Carefully assessing the patient's expectations and then providing appropriate counseling on nonsurgical and surgical options are requisites to ensure that each patient receives the outcome that she desires.

Resources for the Nurse Practitioner

http://www.auanet.org/education/guidelines/incontinence.cfm
Diane Newman and Alan Wein Urinary Incontinence 2nd edition Health Professionals Press 2009

Resources for the Patient

http://www.urologyhealth.org//Documents/Product%20Store/Surgical-VaginalMesh-treat-SUI-PatientFactSheet.pdf
http://www.niddk.nih.gov/health-information/health-topics/urologic-disease/urinary-incontinence-women/Pages/facts.aspx

References

Albo ME, Richter HE, Brubaker L et al (2007) Burch colposuspension versus fascial sling to reduce urinary stress incontinence. N Engl J Med 356(21):2143–2155

DeLancey JO (1994) Structural support of the urethra as it relates to stress urinary incontinence: the hammock hypothesis. Am J Obstet Gynecol 170(6):1713–1720; discussion 1720–1713

Diokno AC, Catipay JR, Steinert BW (2002) Office assessment of patient outcome of pharmacologic therapy for urge incontinence. Int Urogynecol J Pelvic Floor Dysfunct 13(5):334–338

Hu TW, Wagner TH, Bentkover JD, Leblanc K, Zhou SZ, Hunt T (2004) Costs of urinary incontinence and overactive bladder in the United States: a comparative study. Urology 63(3):461–465

Nager CW, Kraus SR, Kenton K et al (2010) Urodynamics, the supine empty bladder stress test, and incontinence severity. Neurourol Urodyn 29(7):1306–1311

Nager CW, Brubaker L, Litman HJ et al (2012) A randomized trial of urodynamic testing before stress-incontinence surgery. N Engl J Med 366(21):1987–1997

Nilsson CG, Palva K, Aarnio R, Morcos E, Falconer C (2013) Seventeen years' follow-up of the tension-free vaginal tape procedure for female stress urinary incontinence. Int Urogynecol J 24(8):1265–1269

Ouslander JG (2004) Management of overactive bladder. New Engl J Med 350:786–799

Ulmsten U, Henriksson L, Johnson P, Varhos G (1996) An ambulatory surgical procedure under local anesthesia for treatment of female urinary incontinence. Int Urogynecol J Pelvic Floor Dysfunct 7(2):81–85; discussion 85–86

Winters JC, Dmochowski RR, Goldman HB et al (2012) Urodynamic studies in adults: AUA/SUFU guideline. J Urol 188(6 Suppl):2464–2472

Overactive Bladder

14

Leslie Saltzstein Wooldridge

Contents

Objectives
1. Discuss diagnosis, incidence, and assessment of overactive bladder.
2. Delineate treatments for OAB.
3. Describe the impact on quality of life for patients with overactive bladder.

L.S. Wooldridge, GNP-BC, CUNP, BCIA-PMD
Mercy Health Bladder Clinic, Muskegon, MI, USA
e-mail: dnclswis@me.com

© Springer International Publishing Switzerland 2016 251
M. Lajiness, S. Quallich (eds.), *The Nurse Practitioner in Urology*,
DOI 10.1007/978-3-319-28743-0_14

This chapter on overactive bladder (OAB) is intended to guide the nurse practitioner in his/her practice through the proper linear treatment of patients. In doing so, the incidence and prevalence of OAB in North America will be stated. A review of pertinent history and a physical to determine the diagnosis of OAB will also be presented. Finally, treatment and therapies identified by the American Urologic Association (AUA) and Society for Urodynamics and Female Urology (SUFU) guidelines for treatment of OAB (Gormley 2012–2015) will be discussed.

Definitions (Abrams et al. 2002, 2006)

All definitions are determined by the International Continence Society (ICS) (Haylen 2009).

Overactive bladder (OAB) is defined as the presence of urinary urgency, usually accompanied by frequency and nocturia, with or without urgency urinary incontinence, in the absence of UTI or other obvious pathology.

Frequency is voiding more than eight times in a 24-h period.

Nocturia is the complaint of interruption of sleep one or more times because of the need to void.

Urgency is the complaint of a sudden, compelling desire to pass urine that is difficult to defer

Urge urinary incontinence is the involuntary leakage of urine, associated with a sudden compelling desire to void.

OAB "wet" is OAB with urge urinary incontinence.

OAB "dry" is OAB without urge urinary incontinence.

Warning time is the time from the first sensation of the urgency to void.

Refractory OAB is present in the patient who has failed appropriate behavioral therapy of sufficient length and a trial of at least one antimuscarinic medication administered for 6–12 weeks (*JUrol* 2012: 188:2455–2463).

Incidence and Epidemiology

In the United States it is estimated that 42 million men and women have OAB symptoms. Of that number, approximately 23 million never seek treatment. Of the 19 million that seek treatment, 12 million receive drug therapy. Two million are successful while 10 million people need more and are eligible for third-line therapy. Only 75,000 of those people receive third-line therapy. OAB is a chronic condition and should be treated as such with ongoing therapies. It is estimated that 33 million people are untreated or undertreated for OAB symptomology.

Prevalence of OAB increases with age. Urgency is more common overall in females until the seventh decade when men catch up. OAB symptom prevalence and severity tend to increase with age (Irwin 2006). About a third of the patients with OAB can remit during a given year, but the majority of patients have symptoms for years. There is no specific racial or ethnic information available (Miller et al. 2009).

Risk Factors

Overactive bladder can be idiopathic and develop over years. Obese people with a BMI greater than 30 can predispose someone to OAB (Wing et al. 2010). Atrophic vaginitis and benign prostatic hypertrophy and changes in aging that can predispose women and men if not treated (Kraus et al. 2010). Heavy ingestion of bladder irritants can be a self-imposed OAB (Newman and Wein 2009).

Guidelines for Treatment

The guidelines for treatment of OAB were designed and published (Gormley et al. 2012, 2015) to provide direction for all types of providers who evaluate and treat OAB. This project was conducted as part of the Agency for Healthcare Research and Quality (AHRQ) Evidence Report, Treatment of OAB in Women (2009). A literature search was conducted from 1966 to 2008 and 2008 to 2011. The first guidelines were initially presented May 2012 at the AUA annual meeting and continue to be updated as new information becomes available.

First-line therapy	Second-line therapy	Third-line therapy	Additional treatments
Behavioral management Fluid management Pelvic floor therapy Toileting schedules If partially effective, consider adding medications	Medications Anticholinergics Antimuscarinics Beta 3 adrenergic agents If patient goals are not met consider further treatment	Neuromodulation Percutaneous tibial nerve stimulation (PTNS) Sacral nerve stimulation (SNS) OnabotulinumtoxinA (Botox)	Indwelling catheters Surgery: Augmentation cystoplasty Urinary diversion

History and Physical Examination

The history is one of the most important components of diagnosing OAB. Knowing the onset, duration, characteristics of complaints, and any previous pelvic surgery is very helpful. Included in the history is the patient's amount of urgency, frequency, and urge incontinence. Did any particular event start the bladder problem? (Abrams 2010)

The most objective form of documentation is the use of a bladder record (see Fig. 14.14.1 This document should tell you when and how often the patient voids and was there an urge and what was the severity of that urge. It is also

Before you begin, please read these instructions carefully.

Keep a record for 3 days in a row, using a new form for each 24-hour period

Write down every time you urinate or lose urine, whether it was planned or accidental.

Measure urine. Or estimate total voiding amount.

Other points to remember:

- Use the column on the far left, which is not numbered, to mark the time that you get out of bed in the morning and the time you get into bed at night.
- **Column 1:** Each time you urinate on purpose, record the amount on the line that corresponds with the approximate time. If you go to the bathroom more than once an hour, write both amounts in the space, with a slash: 400/100 cc. or M/S
- **Column 2:** Anytime you have accidental urine loss, make a check mark on the line that corresponds with the approximate time. If it happens twice in an hour, make 2 check marks.
- **Column 3:** Each time you make a check mark in column 2, estimate the amount of urine loss in column 3. Since you won't be able to measure urine leakage, use the number (1-4) that best describes what happened.
- **Column 4:** To provide more details about accidental urine loss, use the letter "S", "U", or "B" to describe the episode
- **Column 5:** Write YES if the episode was bothersome to you, NO if it wasn't
- **Column 6:** Each time you drink fluids, enter the amount and the type of fluid-8oz (or 1 cup) of juice, coffee, or water, for example

Bring the 3 voiding diaries to your next visit-and remember not to empty your bladder just before you see the doctor.

In and Out of bed	Time	Column 1 Intentional urination (quantity) S-M-L or Measured	Column 2 Accidental urine Loss (check)	Column 3 Quantity of urine loss S-M-L	Column 4 Activity at the time of urine loss	Column 5 Bothersome? YES/NO	Column 6 Type and amount of fluids
	Midnight						
	1 am						
	2 am						
	3 am						
	4 am						
	5 am						
	6 am						
	7 am						
	8 am						
	9 am						
	10 am						
	11 am						
	Noon						
	1 pm						
	2 pm						
	3 pm						
	4 pm						
	5 pm						
	6 pm						
	7pm						
	8 pm						
	9 pm						
	10 pm						
	11 pm						
Totals							

Fig. 14.1 Voiding Diary (Adapted from the University of Michigan 2012)

important to note their perception of the need to void. Do they know when their bladder is full? Do they leak immediately after awareness? Do they leak 1–2 min after awareness? If there was a leaking episode, the time and activity at the time of the leak should also be noted. How many pads did they change in a 24 h period? Also include everything the patient had to drink that day, time, type of fluid, and amount. All of these parameters can be correlated when developing a plan of care. At a minimum all patients should be providing 3 days of bladder records. Four days is optimal (Bright et al. 2012).

Rule out all transient causes of OAB including:

- Urinary tract infection.
- Atrophic vaginitis.
- Benign prostatic hypertrophy.
- Excessive flow (CHF, diabetes, diuretics).
- Restricted mobility.
- Medication review: determine any possible causes of OAB from new or current medications.
- Bladder cancer.

Other valuable components of the history include any previous treatment of OAB and the response to those treatments. Identify the comorbidities associated with OAB including diabetes, congestive heart failure, Parkinson's Disease (Sammour 2009), prostate surgery/benign prostatic hypertrophy (Glazener et al. 2011), atrophic vaginitis, stroke (Thomas et al. 2009), multiple sclerosis (Williams 2012; Fowler 2009), bladder cancer, pelvic radiation cystitis, spinal cord injury (Gray and Moore 2009), etc. These problems most often have OAB components inherent in their physiology. It is also imperative to inquire about environmental considerations. Distance to the bathroom, mobility, and lifestyle contributions are all aspects that can exacerbate OAB.

Review all current medications, prescribed and over the counter. Look for medications that might contain alcohol or caffeine. Certain medications used to treat hypertension or peripheral edema including diuretics that are associated with polyuria can cause urgency, frequency, and incontinence.

A focused physical exam is important to rule out any physical abnormality and gives the clinician the opportunity to teach the patient Kegel exercises.

Female Examination

- Vaginal exam including inspection of the perineum, labia, vaginal tissues, urethra, and presence of prolapse. Also check for vaginal spasm, pain, or tenderness in the vagina and note the position. This is the time to teach proper technique for Kegel exercises and determine the strength of the pelvic floor. Rule out hypermobility of the bladder neck by doing the pad stress test or Q-tip test. Normal is <30° pelvic floor descent with valsalva (Hashim and Abrams 2012).
- Rectal exam to rule out constipation, blood, or prolapse.

Male Examination

- Inspection of the genitals to rule out any abnormalities that may cause pain or urgency, condition of the foreskin, presence of urethral discharge, size of scrotum/testes, abnormal lesions, or masses.
- Rectal exam to identify any abnormalities of the prostate, presence or absence of pain or inflammation, constipation or blood or fissures, hemorrhoids, or stool.
- Teach Kegel exercises. Document strength of contraction and note rising of the tip of the penis, which indicates proper technique with that contraction.

All Patients

- Urinalysis: rule out UTI, hematuria, glycosuria. Treat UTI only if symptomatic.
- Check post-void residual to rule out overflow incontinence (>300 ml).
- Functional status: does the patient need assistance with walking that may inhibit their ability to get to the toilet? Wheelchair, walker, or cane? Can they manipulate their own clothing?
- Pain issues that may limit their desire to toilet.
- Note cognition: is the patient alert, oriented? Can he/she identify a toilet and/or urge to void, follow instructions?
- Check lower extremity nerve conduction. Use a tuning fork on the bony prominences of lower extremities to determine intact nerve pathways.
- Is there lower extremity edema that may increase nocturia?
- Perineal sensation (anal wink or bulbocavernosus reflex).
- Note abnormal lab values: elevated blood glucose or calcium.

Diagnostic Testing

Upon admission to the clinic, patients should have their post-void residuals (PVR) checked. A residual of 150 ml or greater can indicate incomplete bladder emptying and can cause constant urgency. Post-void residuals should be done within 10 min of voiding. Any perceived abnormal PVR requires confirmation before being considered significant.

Urodynamic testing can also determine the absence or presence of OAB in the form of detrusor overactivity, but cannot determine frequency. This test is not necessary for everyone but is helpful when the diagnosis is unclear because of a patient having difficulty expressing them with how they are leaking or the physical exam is inconclusive differentiating between the presences of urge versus stress urinary incontinence. Urodynamics is not required to make the diagnosis of OAB and should not be used in the initial screening process (see Chap. 11).

Treatment for OAB: AUA Guidelines (Gormley 2012)

First-Line Therapy: Behavioral Management

Elimination of bladder irritants is the first and foremost treatment for OAB. Common irritants are caffeine, artificial sweeteners, alcohol, grapefruit juice, tomatoes and spices, citrus, and excessive milk. When determining the amount of bladder irritants a patient can have, help them gradually decrease their intake to a minimum. You can also have them drink water simultaneously with their coffee or other drink or alternate their drink of preference with water to help dilute the irritant. Teach your patients to know their own body's tolerance for bladder irritants. Decrease the amount they eat or drink until their urgency, frequency, and incontinence are under control. Patients sometimes need to make choices between their coffee, tea, pop, or alcoholic drink or OAB (Wyman 2009).

Fluid management can be a key issue in the presence or absence of OAB (Wyman 2009). Patients need to know that drinking 6–8 glasses of fluid is normal intake. Half of total intake should be water. Water intake should be increased by at least a cup for every 30 min of strenuous exercise that is done. Intake should be creatively spaced throughout the day. Sip, do not gulp drinks. Patients should stop drinking fluids 3 h prior to bedtime. If they become thirsty, sucking on one ice cube at a time can help. Caffeine should be eliminated after midafternoon to help with a good night's sleep.

Pelvic floor therapy is done several ways. Simple Kegel exercises, biofeedback, or pelvic floor stimulation are components of pelvic floor therapy.

Proper technique when performing Kegel exercises is to isolate the pelvic floor muscle, specifically the levator ani muscle. This is the muscle that helps control urinary leakage. Most women find this exercise difficult to master. However with proper instruction and practice it can be a good way to control detrusor contractions, increase pressure in the urethra, and control urinary leakage. Proper technique is very important in order to achieve positive results. Instruction is easily done with a vaginal exam when placing finger into the vagina, have the patient squeeze and pull the finger into her vagina without moving the rest of her body.

Kegel exercise instructions
1. Identify pelvic floor muscles
2. Squeeze and hold up to 10 s
3. Relax for 10 s after each contraction (relaxing is just as important as contracting)
4. Do not use stomach, buttocks, or thighs
5. Do ten sets daily in each position, sitting, standing, and laying
6. Doing too many exercises can fatigue your muscles

The pelvic floor muscles are a group of striated and skeletal muscle groups. There are two different types of muscle fibers in the pelvic floor: slow-twitch (Type 1) and fast-twitch (Type II) fibers. These fibers control strength and endurance. The levator ani is made up of mostly slow-twitch fibers that work to maintain normal resting and help with endurance. The fast-twitch muscle fibers (type II) aid in strong and forceful contractions. They can fatigue much quicker and faster. To improve these muscle fibers, doing a set of five quick flicks and resting 10 s in between can help strengthen these muscles and aid in recruitment of these muscles with a strong urge to urinate. Doing quick flicks can help reduce the urge to urinate. These too should be done daily, in sets of 2–3 in each position, sitting, standing, and laying.

In order to properly perform pelvic floor exercises, the patient should be cognitively intact. For those who are not, you can use a 6″ ball placed between the knees, while in a seated position with toes pointed inward and squeeze the ball, hold for 10 s and relax (Hulme 1998)

Biofeedback is a teaching technique with which you are taught to improve your pelvic floor muscle strength and learn to see these muscles work properly to help control urination, urgency, or relaxation. Special sensors or electrodes are placed near the pelvic muscles that help in controlling urination. There are two ways to provide "sensors". A vaginal probe, somewhat like a tampon, or a rectal probe can be used. Another method is the use of surface electrodes. Two electrodes are placed around the anus. Another electrode is placed on your thigh and yet another electrode is placed on your abdomen. These electrodes all have wires that are connected to a computer. The activity performed by these muscles can be seen on the computer in the form of lines. The information the patient receives from the signal can then be used to make adjustments in muscle activity. The job of the biofeedback therapist is to interpret the activity and coach the patient into improving the strength and endurance of the pelvic floor muscle. This is done through a variety of exercises that are performed, in the office, in front of the computer to see differences and changes. Practicing these exercises at home is essential in order to make progress and see changes in urinary leakage patterns, urgency, or relaxation. Through practice, patients become more aware of their pelvic muscles and eventually learn to use the muscles without having to depend on biofeedback.

Biofeedback is used in the treatments of stress or urge urinary incontinence. It can also be used for other pelvic floor disorders, bladder control problems, or before and after surgery. There are no side effects or pain to this therapy. It is generally used in conjunction with behavioral therapies and sometimes medication. Treatment sessions vary but usually begin weekly. As symptoms improve, time in between sessions increases. There are computer programs available for biofeedback with programs specific to stress or urge incontinence or techniques in relaxation.

Electrical stimulation is the third type of pelvic floor therapy. It is a controlled delivery via the vagina or rectum of small amounts of stimulation to the nerves and muscles of the pelvic floor and bladder. Stimulation is generated through a vaginal or rectal probe that is placed in the vagina or rectum or surface electrodes. The purpose of this treatment is to relax the bladder muscle and reduce unwanted bladder contractions. The numbers of treatments that are needed are individualized to each patient and their problem.

Urge reduction techniques are ways in which to use your pelvic floor muscles to inhibit detrusor contractions to avoid leaking.

Urge reduction techniques
1. With the strong urge to urinate, stop what you are doing
2. Take a deep breath and do a couple of quick Kegel exercises
3. Distract yourself
4. If the urge goes away, slowly move toward the bathroom
5. Should the urge return, repeat the above
6. The key to controlling the urge is NOT to respond by rushing to the bathroom   This will almost always result in leaking urine

Toileting programs are highly effective with a motivated patient and/or caregiver.

Habit training	Bladder retraining	Prompted voiding
Voiding according to one's schedule Use bladder records as a guideline Can also be helpful for those with little or no sensation to void Prevention technique for those who forget to void Goal is to keep bladder pressure low and prevent leakage	Use of Kegel exercises, urge reduction techniques, and timing to "teach" your bladder how to gradually hold more urine Purpose is to resist the urge to void Gradually lengthen time in between voiding by using relaxation and urge reduction techniques Try to hold an additional 15 min to gradually increase voiding intervals Successful outcomes can take up to 6–8 weeks to accomplish	Caregiver dependent Specific behavioral protocol with opportunity to toilet at regular intervals Timing is based on results of bladder diaries Check the patient at designated times to prevent incontinence Opportunity (prompt) to toilet every 2 h Toileting assistance if requested If the patient is wet, change clothing and/or pads as needed and ask if the patient needs to use the toilet Social interaction and verbal feedback involved *DO NOT SCOLD THE PATIENT!* Assist the patient as necessary Patience is key to success When approaching the patient be positive

Managing nocturia is important to help patients get a good night's sleep. Five uninterrupted hours of sleep is normal for the elderly. Waking once to void at night is also normal for the elderly. However, these strategies can help with leakage:

- No fluids after supper. Suck on ice cubes if thirsty.
- Take evening medications no later than 7 pm unless sleep aids. May take sips of water with medications.
- Elevate legs 45° f (higher than waist or 45–60 min in later afternoon. A simple strategy is to lay on the couch and elevate legs on 2–3 pillows.
- Alter time of diuretic administration to midafternoon (no later than 3 pm).
- Stay up as late as possible in order to sleep longer.
- Bedside commode/urinal for safety if necessary.

Management of constipation with fluids, exercise, increasing natural fiber (artificial fiber can cause excess flatus) or medication is important to keep the bowels regular. A full colon has a tendency to push on the bladder causing urgency and/or leaking.

Pessaries are indicated for pelvic organ prolapse. Fitting a patient with a pessary may help with urgency caused by the pressure on the bladder from the prolapse. Pessaries should be fitted and cared for by a trained professional with experience with pessaries. There are multiple different types and sizes, each used for a unique problem.

When using *incontinent products* for urine containment, make sure they fit and the patient is using pads with appropriate levels of absorption for his/her problem. DO NOT use menstrual pads for urine containment. These products have coarse fibers that may cause irritation and skin breakdown. Also, do not use Kleenex, toilet paper, or paper towels for control of leakage as this too can cause skin breakdown. Only use incontinent products that are marketed as such.

Other strategies for decreasing bladder urgencies
1. Weight loss: obesity is associated with the risk of onset of OAB symptoms
2. Use diuretics judiciously and not before bedtime
3. Make toilet easier to get to: bedside commode and urinals. Condom catheters at bedtime
4. Think of the environment: cold and running water are triggers to void
5. Smoking cessation: nicotine is a bladder irritant

Second-Line Therapy: Medications

Currently there are two major classifications of drugs used for the treatment of OAB: antimuscarinics and beta 3 agonist. The antimuscarinics include oxybutynin, tolterodine, solifenacin, darifenacin, fesoterodine, and trospium. Their actions are similar. These drugs act during the filling/storage phases of the micturition cycle by inhibiting afferent (sensory) input from the bladder, as well as directly on the smooth muscle to decrease contractility (see the chart for detailed information regarding these drugs). These drugs are contraindicated in patients with slow gastric motility, narrow angled glaucoma, and severe renal or hepatic impairment. Major side effects include constipation, dry mouth, and blurred vision. These drugs are to be used with caution with the elderly (Shamliyan 2012a,b).

The second major drug for treating OAB is mirabegron. It is an agonist of the human beta-3 adrenergic receptor. It relaxes the detrusor smooth muscle during the storage phase of the urinary bladder fill-void cycle by activation of beta-3 adrenergic receptor, which increases bladder capacity.

Vaginal estrogen cream has also been studied to have some effect on bladder urgency in postmenopausal women (Robinson and Cardozo 2011). Estrogenation of the vaginal tissues is most commonly achieved by administering 1 g of estradiol or estriol per vagina for 7–14 days at bedtime. For ongoing care and healthy tissues, the dosage recommendation is usually 1 g 2–3 times per week in the vagina by fingertip application or measured applicator.

General Comments Regarding Medications

- Do not administer these drugs to residents with controlled narrow angled glaucoma, significant bladder outflow obstruction, GI obstructive disorders, or renal or hepatic dysfunction.
- All information provided is from package inserts or advertised company literature.
- Effectiveness similar in all drugs.
- None of these drugs should be chewed, divided, or crushed.
- Treatment discontinuation due to adverse effects of drugs is common.
- It is overall recommended for all drugs with anticholinergic properties that they be avoided in the elderly. Behavioral interventions should always be tried first (Beers Criteria 2012; Kerdraon et al. 2014).

Third-Line Therapy: Neuromodulation and Botox

Third-line therapies are indicated for patients with refractory OAB defined as the patient who has failed a trial of symptom-appropriate behavioral therapy of sufficient length to evaluate potential efficacy and who has failed a trial of at least one antimuscarinic medication administered for 6–12 weeks (AUA/SUFU guidelines 2013). See comparison list of third-line therapies (attached).

Percutaneous tibial nerve stimulation (PTNS) is a minimally invasive therapy delivered in the office setting for 30 min. This is a treatment that can be delivered by a NP, PA, or RN under the direction of a physician. PTNS is a series of 12 treatments, typically once a week. It is a nonsurgical, nondrug therapy. This therapy has been approved for treatment of patients with urgency, frequency, and urge incontinence who do not want drugs, cannot tolerate drugs, failed conservative therapy including two OAB medications. PTNS is delivered through a device called Urgent PC along with a lead wire to the stimulator and a surface electrode. Stimulation occurs through a 34-gauge needle electrode inserted approximately 2 in. above the medial malleolus and one finger-width toward the back of the leg at a 60° angle. The patient is tested for proper response of the stimulation from the heel, foot, or toe vibration or flexion of the toes. Any or all of these responses are appropriate to note proper placement. The impulse travels up the tibial nerve to the sacral nerve plexus. This treatment is designed to alter aberrant bladder signals. There are minimal side effects (Staskin et al. 2012). Urgent PC is not to be used in patients who have a pacemaker, internal defibrillator, or those pregnant or planning on pregnancy and those with peripheral neuropathies. Patient response is generally seen after 5–6 treatments and sustained after the 12th treatment and ongoing maintenance therapy (MacDiarmid et al. 2010).

Sacral nerve stimulation (SNS) is an implantable system that stimulates the sacral nerves modulating the neural reflexes that influence the bladder, sphincter, and pelvic floor. SNS is indicated for treatment of urinary retention, fecal incontinence, and the symptoms of OAB including urgency, frequency, and urge incontinence after failure of first and second-line therapy with moderate to severe symptoms. SNS is also approved for fecal incontinence and urinary retention.

The theory of mechanism behind SNS is that the modulation enables more normal detrusor muscle behavior and helps reduce detrusor and pelvic floor muscle spasticity. It is a two-staged procedure. Test stimulation period allows informed choice for the patient and the doctor to proceed with implanting internal device based on effectiveness. Patients undergoing SNS must be cognitively intact in order to use the remote device to maximize treatment. Patients must also be aware that diagnostic MRI's are contraindicated (head is okay). It is also contraindicated in patients with pacemaker, internal defibrillator, or pregnancy.

Intravesical Onobotulinumtoxin-A is an acetylcholine release inhibitor and a neuromuscular blocking agent. It is FDA approved for treatment of urinary incontinence due to detrusor overactivity associated a neurologic condition, e.g., spinal cord injury or multiple sclerosis as well as treatment of idiopathic overactive bladder with symptoms of urge urinary incontinence, urgency, and frequency in patients who have failed first- and second-line therapy. The dosage is 100 units as 0.5 ml (5 units) injections across 20 sites into the detrusor muscle. Detrusor overactivity associated with a neurologic condition should not exceed 200 units. Treatments can be repeated after 12 weeks. Mean repeat time for OAB is 24 weeks, for neurogenic bladder, mean repeat time is 42–48 weeks. Adverse reactions include urinary tract infection, urinary retention, dysuria, and hematuria. (See comparison chart of all three treatments.)

When all third-line therapies fail, Dr. Sandip Vasavada advocates OnabotulinumtoxinA (BOTOX) as most studies were done with patients who have moderate to severe urge incontinence. Dr. Steven Siegel advocated for sacral neuromodulation after failed Botox after a 6–9 month waiting period after the last Botox injection to prevent false positive/negative testing. Dr. Kenneth Peters went one step further to advocate the pudendal route. At this publication time, this route is not FDA approved. In Dr. Peters' experience, he feels the location of the leads in a slightly different position can affect better outcomes as in his 10-year data, "80 % of patients felt their success was greater with PNM compared to SNM." Dr. Stephen Krauss feels the data support a >75 % durable success for augmentation/diversion. However, these procedures are not often done due to their invasive nature (Freilich 2015).

Clinical Pearls
- First-line treatments for OAB have no risk and should be offered to all patients.
- Patient's goals for treatment outcomes should be realistic. OAB is a chronic syndrome and can be difficult to treat.
- Treating the cognitively impaired patient:
  - Treat all medical conditions or transient contributors to OAB.
  - Avoid change in environment.
  - Identify the bathroom.
  - PATIENCE!!! Avoid blaming/scolding. It can trigger disruptive behavior.
  - Watch for nonverbal cues that a person needs to toilet.
  - Prompt to void. Use positive statements vs questions: "Come with me. I will take you to the bathroom" is better than, "Do you have to go to the bathroom?" or, "Do you want to go to the bathroom?"

- Treating the patient with impaired mobility:
  - Pain control may be necessary in order for the patient to get to the bathroom on time. Think scheduled and break through pain management.
  - Safety first: make sure the patient is using assistive devices as needed.
  - Toileting assistive devices may be helpful, i.e., commodes, urinals, or condom catheters.
- Treating the geriatric patient:
  - Awareness of normal aging changes that affect the bladder and pelvic floor including the presence of:
    - Decreased bladder contractility.
    - Uninhibited contractions are present.
    - Decreased bladder capacity.
    - Increased nighttime production of urine.
    - Atrophic vaginitis.
    - Benign prostatic hypertrophy.
- Realization that OAB is a chronic syndrome without an ideal treatment and no treatment will "cure" the condition in most patients.
- Be prepared to manage the transitions between treatment levels appropriately.
- It is appropriate for patients to choose no treatment at all.
- Weigh benefit versus risk with all treatments.
  - Duration of potential adverse reactions.
  - Reversibility of adverse reactions.
- OAB may compromise quality of life but it does not affect survival.

Resources for the Nurse Practitioner
International Continence Society (ICS)
www.ICS.org
American Urogynecologic Society
www.AUGS.org
American Urologic Association: OAB guidelines
http://www.auanet.org/education/auaguidelines.cfm
Society of Urologic Nurses and Associates (SUNA)
www.suna.org
OAB screening tools
www.PfizerPatientReportedOutcomes.com
NIH Bladder Diary

Resources for the Patient
National Association for Continence (NAFC)
www.nafc.org
Patient Pictures
www.patientpictures.com
Simon Foundation
www.simonfoundation.org
Patient Education Fact Sheets:
www.SUNA.org

Third line of therapy options for overactive bladder

	PTNS	Botox	InterStim
Primary location of service	Clinic	Clinic or hospital	Clinic and hospital
Provider	Nurse	Physician	Nurse and physician
Indication	Urinary urgency, frequency, and urge incontinence	Urinary incontinence due to overactivity of bladder as well as urinary urgency and frequency in patients not responding to meds	Urinary urgency, frequency, urge incontinence, nonobstructive urinary retention, or urge fecal incontinence
Contraindications	Patients with defibrillators, pacemakers, pregnant or considering pregnancy, and bilateral lower extremity nerve damage	Urinary tract obstruction, history of frequent urinary tract infections Allergy to Botox	MRI, diathermy, implantable devices (pacemaker, defibrillator), pregnancy
Technique	Twelve treatments, 30 min each No anesthesia	Local anesthesia to bladder and urethra. Sedative 45–60 prior to procedure Twenty injections in the bladder wall through a cystoscope Treatments can be repeated after 12 weeks, generally repeats every 6–8 months	First-stage testing in office ~30 min procedure, local anesthesia, single wire stimulation through lower back Implant procedure in operating room under anesthesia
Complications	Rare, bleeding at site, painful sensation during stimulation that did not interfere with treatment	Urinary tract infection, inability to urinate, or empty bladder (need to catheterize self), bloody urine	Infection, pain at implantation site, lead movement, urinary and bowel problems, electric shock, need for revision
Posttreatment	No restrictions	The patient should void prior to leaving the clinic or hospital	Activity restricted 3–6 weeks post-op Battery change every 5–7 years based on usage
Improvement and cure rates	59–88 %	50–70 %	37–79 %
References	MacDiarmid (2010, 2015)	Allergen Inc (2014)	Medtronic (2013)

Medications for overactive bladder

Medication antimuscarinics	Dosages	Adverse events (>5 %)	Drug/drug interactions	Half-life	Comments
Detrol LA (tolterodine)	2 or 4 mg daily Immediate release Also available, given BID	Dry mouth 23 % Headache 6 % Constipation 6 %	NONE	8 h	No dosage adjustments needed for elderly residents Research available on elderly (Zinner 2002) for safety, efficacy, and adverse events
Ditropan XL (Oxybutynin)	5, 10 or 15 mg daily Available in tablet or syrup 5 mg/5 ml Available generic, immediate release (AE increased and given TID)	Dry mouth 29 % Diarrhea 7 % Constipation 7 % Headache 6 %	Studies not conducted	12 h	Likely to cross blood brain barrier (Kay 2005) May have significant cognitive effects
Enablex b (darifenacin)	7.5 or 15 mg daily	Constipation 20.9 % Dry mouth 18.7 % Headache 6.7 %	Digoxin, ketoconazole, itraconazole, ritonavir, nelfinavir, clarithromycin, and nefazodone (see package insert for details)	13–19 h	Highest % of constipation of all drugs in the class. Think of your patients with concomitant fecal incontinenceData suggest safety in the elderly
Gelnique	10 % sachet 3 % pump	Dry mouth 7 % UTI 7 %	Studies not conducted		Do not take a bath, swim, shower, exercise, or get the application site wet for 1 hour after you apply your dose
Oxytrol (Oxybutynin)	3.9 mg patch Change twice weekly (q3–4 days)	Site pruritis 14 % Site erythema 8.3 %	Studies not conducted	7–8 h	Geriatric effectiveness no different than younger people 49 % of patients in original study were >65 years old Likely to cross blood-brain barrier More convenient mode of delivery. Much fewer GI side effects

Medication antimuscarinics	Dosages	Adverse events (>5 %)	Drug/drug interactions	Half-life	Comments
Sanctura (trospium chloride)	20 mg. BID 60 mg XR daily	Dry mouth 20.1 % Constipation 9.6 %	NONE	20 h	Needs to be taken on an empty stomach or 1 h before meals In residents >75 years, dosage may need to be decreased to 20 mg. QD based on tolerability
Toviaz (fesoterodine fumarate)	4 and 8 mg extended release	Dry mouth 17 % (4 mg) and 35 % (8 mg) Constipation 4 % (4 mg) and 6 % (8 mg)	Doses >4 mg not recommended in patients taking potent CYP3A4 inhibitors	7 h	Hot environment caution Better choice than trospium for patients with >2–3 episodes UI daily
Vesicare (solifenacin)	5 or 10 mg daily	Dry mouth 10.9 % (5 mg) and 27.6 % (10 mg) Constipation 5.4 % (5 mg) and 13.4 % (10 mg)	NONE	45–68 h	No CNS side effects Favorable tolerability profile Better choice than trospium for patients with >2–3 episodes UI daily
Beta-3 adrenergic receptor agonist Myrbetriq (Mirabegron)	25–50 mg daily	Hypertension, nasopharyngitis, UTI and headache <2 % and>placebo	Monitoring needed with drugs metabolized by CYP2D6 (metoprolol and desipramine) and warfarin Digoxin: start at lowest dose of digoxin and monitor serum levels	50 h	Trial of 8 weeks is recommended to determine effectiveness No adjustment of dosage necessary for the elderly

General comments

  Do not administer these drugs to residents with controlled narrow angled glaucoma, significant bladder outflow obstruction, GI obstructive disorders, or renal or hepatic dysfunction

  All information provided is from package inserts or advertised company literature

  Effectiveness similar in all drugs

  None of these drugs should be chewed, divided, or crushed

  Treatment discontinuation due to adverse effects of drugs is common

  It is overall recommended for all drugs with anticholinergic properties that they be avoided in the elderly. Behavioral interventions should always be tried first (Beers Criteria 2012)

References

Abrams P, Cardozo L, Fall M, Griffiths D, Rosier P, Ulmsten U, vanKerrebroeck P (2002) The standardization of terminology of lower urinary tract function report from the standardization sub-committee of the International Continence Society. Neurol Urodyn 21:167–178

Abrams P, Artibani W, Gajewski JB, Hussain I (2006) Assessment of treatment outcomes in patients with overactive bladder: importance of objective and subjective measures. Urology 68(2 Suppl):17–28. Review

Abrams P, Anderson K, Birder L, Brubaker L, Cardozo L, Chapple C, Cottenden A (2010) Fourth international consultation on incontinence recommendations of the international scientific committee: evaluation and treatment of urinary incontinence, pelvic organ prolapse, and fecal incont. Neurourol Urodyn 29:213–240

American Geriatrics Society (2012) Beers Criteria Update Expert Panel. American Geriatrics Society updated Beers Criteria for potentially inappropriate medication use in older adults. J Am Geriatr Soc. 60(4):616–31. doi: 10.1111/j.1532-5415.2012.03923.x. Epub 2012 Feb 29

BOTOX® Best practices for the treatment of overactive bladder patients (2014). Allergan, Inc., Irvine

Bright E, Cotterill N, Drake M, Abrams P (2012) Developing a validated urinary diary: phase 1. Neurol Urodyn 31(5):625–633

Fowler CJ, Panicker JN, Drake M, Harris C, Harrison SC, Kirby M, Lucas M, Macleod N, Mangnall J, North A, Porter B, Reid S, Russell N, Watkiss K, Wells M (2009) UK consensus on the management of the bladder in multiple sclerosis. Postgrad Med J 85(1008):552–9. doi: 10.1136/jnnp.2008.159178. Review

Freilich D (2015) Panel: management of refractory overactive bladder: what to do when third line therapies fail – session highlights. Taken from www.UroToday.com

Fundamentals of SNM resource book: academia medical education (2013). MN Medtronic, Minneapolis

Glazener C, Boachie C, Buckley B, Cochran C, Dorey G, Grant A, Hagen S (2011) Urinary incontinence in men after formal one-to-one pelvic-floor muscle training following radical prostatectomy or transurethral resection of the prostate (MAPS): two parallel randomized control trial. Lancet 378:328–337

Gormley EA, Lightner DJ, Burgio KL, Chai TC, Clemens JQ, Culkin DJ, Das AK, Foster HE Jr, Scarpero HM, Tessier CD, Vasavada SP (2012) American Urological Association; Society of Urodynamics, Female Pelvic Medicine & Urogenital Reconstruction. Diagnosis and treatment of overactive bladder (non-neurogenic) in adults: AUA/SUFU guideline. J Urol 188(6 Suppl): 2455–63. doi: 10.1016/j.juro.2012.09.079. Epub 2012 Oct 24

Gormley EA, Lightner DJ, Faraday M, Vasavada SP (2015) American Urological Association; Society of Urodynamics, Female Pelvic Medicine. Diagnosis and treatment of overactive bladder (non-neurogenic) in adults: AUA/SUFU guideline amendment. J Urol 193(5):1572–80. doi: 10.1016/j.juro.2015.01.087. Epub 2015 Jan 23. Review

Gray M, Moore KN (2009) Urologic disorders adult and pediatric care. Elsevier, St. Louis

Hashim H, Abrams P (2012) Overactive bladder syndrome and urinary incontinence, 1st edn. Oxford University Press, Oxford

Haylen BT, de Ridder D, Freeman RM, Swift SE, Berghmans B, Lee J, Monga A (2009) An International Urogynecological Association (IUGA)/International Continence Society (ICS) Joint Report on the Terminology for Female Pelvic Floor Dysfunction. Neurol Urodyn 29:4–20

Hulme JA (1998) Beyond Kegels Book II: a clinician's guide to treatment algorithms and special populations. Phoenix Publishing, Missoula

Irwin DE, Milsom I, Hunskaar S et al (2006) Population-based survey of urinary incontinence, overactive bladder, and other lower urinary tract symptoms in five countries: results of the IPIC study. Eur Urol 50(6):1306–1315

Kay GG, Granville LJ (2005) Antimuscarinic agents: implications and concerns in the management of overactive bladder in the elderly. Clin Ther 27(1):127–38; quiz 139–40. Review

Kerdraon J, Robain G, Jeandel C, Mongiat AP, Game X, Fatton B, Scheiber-Nogueira MC, Vetel JM, Mares P, Petit AC, Amareno G (2014) Impact on cognitive function of anticholinergic drugs used for the treatment of overactive bladder in the elderly-Abstract. Prog Urol 24(11):672–681. Taken from www.UroToday.com

Kraus SR, Bavendam T, Brake T, Griebling TL (2010) Vulnerable elderly patients and overactive bladder syndrome. Drugs Aging 27(9):697–713

MacDiarmid S (2015) PTNS for overactive bladder: patient selection and technique. Urol Times. Feb 1, 2015. Available at http://urologytimes.modernmedicine.com/urology-times/news/ptns-overactive-bladder-patient-selection-and-technique

MacDiarmid SA, Peters KM, Shobeiri SA, Wooldridge LS, Rovner ES, Leong FC et al (2010) Long-term durability of percutaneous tibial nerve stimulation for the treatment of overactive bladder. J Urol 183(1):234–240

Miller DC, Saigal CS, Litwin MS (2009) The demographic burden of urologic diseases in America. Urol Clin North Am 36:11–27

Newman DK, Wein AJ (2009) Managing and treating urinary incontinence, 2nd edn. Health Professions Press, Baltimore

Robinson D, Cardozo L (2011) Estrogens and the lower urinary tract. Neurourol Urodyn 30(5):754–757

Sammour ZM, Gomes CM, Barbosa ER, Lopes RI, Sallem FS, Trigo-Rocha FE, Bruschini H, Srougi M. (2009) Voiding dysfunction in patients with Parkinson's disease: impact of neurological impairment and clinical parameters. Neurourol Urodyn 28(6):510–5. doi: 10.1002/nau.20681

Shamliyan J, Wyman J, Kane R (2012a) Nonsurgical treatments for urinary incontinence in adult women: diagnosis and comparative effectiveness. Agency for Healthcare Research and Quality. Retrieved 26 Oct 2012, from www.effectivehealthcare.ahrq.gov/reports/final.cfm

Shamliyan T, Wyman JF, Ramakrishnan R, Sainfort F, Kane RL (2012b) Benefits and harms of pharmacologic treatment for urinary incontinence in women. Ann Intern Med 156(12):861–874

Staskin DR, Peters KM, MacDiarmid S, Shore N, deGroat WC (2012) Percutaneous tibial nerve stimulation: a clinically an cost effective addition to the overactive bladder algorithm of care. Curr Urol Rep 13(5):327–334

McAninch JW, Lue TF (2013) Smith's general urology, 18th edn. McGraw-Hill, New York

Thomas LH, Cross S, Barrett J, French B, Leathley M, Sutton CJ, Watkins C (2009) Treatment of urinary incontinence after stroke in adults (Review). www.thecochranelibrary.com. Retrieved 4 Nov 2012, from CINAHL (www.thecochranelibrary.com)

University of Michigan, A (2012) Voiding diary: what it's for, how to fill it out. J Fam Pract 61(9):547–548

Williams D (2012) Management of bladder dysfunction in patients with multiple sclerosis. Nurs Stand 26(25):39–46

Wing RR, Creasman JM, West DS, Richter HE, Myers D, Burgio KL, Franklin F (2010) Improving urinary incontinence in overweight and obese women through modest weight loss. Obstet Gynecol 116(2):284–292

Wyman JF, Burgio KL, Newman DK (2009) Practical aspects of lifestyle modifications and behavioral interventions in the treatment of overactive bladder and urgency urinary incontinence. Int J Clin Pract 63(8):1177–1191

Zinner NR, Mattiasson A, Stanton SL (2002) Efficacy, safety, and tolerability of extended-release once-daily tolterodine treatment for overactive bladder in older versus younger patients. J Am Geriatr Soc 50(5):799–807

Problems in Female Urology: Interstitial Cystitis/Bladder Pain Syndrome, Pelvic Floor Disorders, and Pelvic Organ Prolapse

15

Lindsey Cox

Contents

L. Cox, MD
Medical University of South Carolina,
96 Jonathan Lucas St. MSC 620, CSB 644T, Charleston, SC, USA
e-mail: coxli@musc.edu

© Springer International Publishing Switzerland 2016
M. Lajiness, S. Quallich (eds.), *The Nurse Practitioner in Urology*,
DOI 10.1007/978-3-319-28743-0_15

Objectives
1. Provide a resource for nurse practitioners caring for female urology patients to aid in diagnosis and management of complex pelvic pain, including interstitial cystitis/bladder pain syndrome (IC/BPS).
2. Review other female pelvic floor disorders (PFD) including pelvic organ prolapse (POP).
3. Differentiate among a broad range of differential diagnoses to exclude other causes of pelvic pain.
4. Recognize and manage IC/BPS according to the American Urological Association guidelines.
5. Outline the steps of evaluation and nonoperative as well as surgical management of pelvic floor disorders, e.g., pelvic organ prolapse.

Overview

The specialty of urologic surgery has traditionally had a strong focus on disorders of the male genitourinary tract. Urologists dedicated to treating disorders in women or "female urology" have recently joined with urogynecologists in the formation of a new medical specialty called female pelvic medicine and reconstructive surgery or FPMRS. Urologists trained in FPMRS treat a wide range of benign conditions in women and men, including urinary incontinence, overactive bladder, neurogenic bladder, as well as the topics of this chapter, chronic pelvic pain or IC/BPS and pelvic floor disorders. These topics are interrelated as patient presentation and symptoms can overlap, but each deserves discrete attention as management and therapy are distinctly different, and will be covered separately.

This chapter does describe experimental and off-label uses of medications and devices for IC/BPS; the author urges providers to follow all governmental and manufacturer protocols, precautions, warnings, indications, and contraindications.

IC/BPS

Definitions

Interstitial cystitis/bladder pain syndrome (IC/BPS) is a chronic condition that can be challenging both to diagnose and to treat. Various terms have been used to describe this condition, including painful bladder syndrome (PBS), chronic pelvic pain syndrome (CPPS), and interstitial cystitis alone. This chapter will use IC/BPS for consistency with the American Urological Association (AUA) guidelines (Hanno et al. 2011). The hallmark symptom of IC/BPS is chronic pain in the pelvis, pelvic floor, and/or genitalia; this pain is often accompanied by lower urinary tract symptoms. The condition is noninfectious, non-malignant, and chronic in nature, with research definitions ranging from 6 weeks to 6 months of symptoms meeting case definitions. Symptoms may fluctuate over time but rarely resolve completely.

There is no well-defined pathologic etiology or specific definitive diagnostic testing for IC/BPS, despite much research on the topic; even epidemiologic studies with the goals of defining cases of IC/PBS for study were unable to find a single definition that was both sensitive and specific (Berry et al. 2010). The diagnosis of IC/BPS relies primarily on patient-reported symptoms and careful exclusion of other possible causes of pelvic pain. The National Institute of Diabetes and Digestive and Kidney Diseases (NIDDK) of the US National Institutes of Health (NIH) is funding the Multidisciplinary Approach to the Study of Chronic Pelvic Pain (MAPP) research network to study the spectrum of pelvic pain disorders including IC/PBS (Clemens et al. 2014).

In addition to diagnostic challenges, therapies for IC/BPS are not universally effective, and there are no curative medical therapies. Some studies have shown that patients with characteristic Hunner's ulcers on cystoscopy have slightly different symptoms and responses to therapy when compared to non-ulcerative patients (Chennamsetty et al. 2015).

The AUA guidelines for IC/BPS represent the current best practices for the diagnosis and treatment of patients with IC/BPS. The algorithm presented allows for the provider to work from initial diagnosis through the care of patients with severe and refractory symptoms who have failed multiple treatment approaches.

A recent update (Hanno et al. 2015) to the original guidelines reported the newly published data on epidemiology and the impact of IC/BPS on quality of life. The update also reviews the evidence for changing manual pelvic floor physical therapy from a *Clinical Principle* to a *Standard* and moving injection of botulinum toxin into the bladder from a fifth- to a fourth-line treatment, among other updates based on new scientific studies. These treatments will be discussed in detail under the section entitled *Management*. Patients may benefit from handouts that include the AUA algorithm to help explain the evidence-based approach to escalating therapy.

Epidemiology

A recent epidemiologic study estimated that there are 3.3–7.9 million United States women 18 years old or older with IC/BPS, but only 9.7 % of women surveyed who met criteria had been diagnosed (Berry et al. 2011). Prior studies have shown a ratio of five females for every one male with IC/BPS, but recent evidence suggests that there may also be significant numbers of men who meet epidemiologic definitions but are not diagnosed (Suskind et al. 2012).

Studies have revealed associations between IC/BPS and other non-bladder chronic conditions, including fibromyalgia, chronic fatigue syndrome, irritable bowel syndrome, allergy, asthma, migraine, anxiety, depression, vulvodynia, and back pain (Warren et al. 2011). More research is needed to characterize these relationships. IC/BPS patients with associated conditions (specifically fibromyalgia, chronic fatigue syndrome, irritable bowel syndrome) have lower health-related quality of life scores than those without (Suskind et al. 2013).

Anatomy and Physiology

The external anatomy of the female perineum is pertinent to the diagnosis and management of IC/BPS, as vulvar pain is also common in this population. The normal female external genitalia consist of the labia majora, labia minora, the clitoral hood and clitoral body, the vaginal vestibule, as well as bilateral Skene's glands and ducts (lateral to the urethra) and Bartholin's glands and ducts (posterior and lateral to the vaginal opening). The examiner should be familiar with recognizing the hymenal ring, which is a landmark for grading the level of descent of pelvic organs in POP.

The female pelvic floor is an interrelated group of muscles and their attachments which support the pelvic organs. The openings in the pelvic floor accommodate voiding, childbirth, and defecation. The pelvic floor muscles include the coccygeus and the levator ani group (pubococcygeus, iliococcygeus, puborectalis). These muscles are palpable on vaginal examination, increased tone or tenderness can be targets for intervention with pelvic floor physical therapy.

Normal voiding physiology requires several coordinated steps in order to have comfortable and socially appropriate storage of urine, with voluntary voiding that is complete and efficient. The bladder muscle has multiple neurologic inputs and outputs that must be coordinated by higher centers. In the resting state, the bladder performs its storage function; signals to relax the detrusor muscle of the bladder are relayed through the autonomic nervous system. Both lack of parasympathetic input and sympathetic activity serve to relax the detrusor muscle of the bladder as the bladder fills. The urinary sphincters are contracted or closed during storage. When voluntary voiding is determined to be appropriate, the nervous system signals the pelvic floor and urethral sphincter to relax, the bladder neck opens, and the detrusor muscle contracts. This physiology can be altered in IC/BPS at several levels, including sensitivity to filling, overactivity during storage (possibly with involuntary bladder contractions that cause incontinence of urine), pain or difficulty with voiding, and inefficient emptying. The cause (or causes) of these alterations in IC/BPS is not yet understood.

History

Commonly, patients with IC/BPS present with a chief complaint of pain. They can often describe an inciting event or an event preceding the onset of symptoms. This event may be an episode of acute bacterial cystitis or time when they were forced to hold urine for a prolonged period of time. Some patients describe no inciting event but rather an insidious and gradual worsening of symptoms over the course of the condition, and it is typical for patients to describe flares and remissions of symptoms.

Important considerations for history taking include a thorough medical history with comprehensive history of other chronic pain conditions; neurologic, autoimmune, or rheumatologic and endocrine conditions; as well as general medical conditions. Thorough gynecologic and obstetrical history include menstrual status, detailed history of pregnancies and outcomes, history of sexually transmitted infections, history of sexual function including sexual abuse or assault, history of any abnormal Pap smears and the treatments, history of any gynecologic or urologic disorders including urolithiasis, presence of any urologic or gynecologic cancers including treatments (surgery, chemotherapy, radiation), and current status of these conditions. A frequency-volume chart, or voiding diary, is also recommended (Hanno et al. 2011). A description of the patient's bowel habits can provide an intervention point for adjunctive treatment of dysfunctional elimination or constipation.

Patients may have characteristics or a diagnosis of other pain and non-pain syndromes including fibromyalgia, endometriosis, vulvodynia/vestibulodynia, migraines, chronic back pain, irritable bowel syndrome, chronic fatigue syndrome, depression, or anxiety. The visit to a urologic care provider is often not the first visit for pelvic pain or for other pain-related complaints. Some studies have shown that the complexity of the presentation and the overlap with other syndromes likely results in a delay in diagnosis for patients with IC/BPS (Chrysanthopoulou and Doumouchtsis 2013). It is imperative to detail prior evaluation, treatments and their effects, and the patient level of insight into their pain conditions. Listening to patients at this stage can help develop a broad differential diagnosis, avoid repeating prior testing and treatments, and allow the provider to gain a sense of the patient psychosocial situation which can impact future shared decision-making. This is especially important if patients already have a diagnosis of IC/BPS, so as not to overlook potentially treatable conditions that could be present either concurrently with IC/BPS or alone.

In generating a differential diagnosis, some "red flags" for other conditions can be elicited on history. Patients with neurologic symptoms may need further questioning or workup to rule out multiple sclerosis, pudendal neuralgia, or spinal pathology such as cauda equina syndrome. Musculoskeletal symptoms could be the result of trauma or inflammation; gynecologic symptoms (vulvar pain, vaginal discharge, dysmenorrhea) may point to infectious causes or endometriosis. Urologic symptoms such as hematuria, colicky flank or groin pain can prompt investigations into conditions such as eosinophilic cystitis, lupus cystitis, urothelial carcinoma in situ, atypical infections, or urolithiasis.

Thorough characterization of pain is important to understand the aspects of the condition that are most bothersome and limiting to the patient, as well as to have insight into other (potentially undiagnosed) conditions. Symptom questionnaires for urinary symptoms as well as for pain should be administered at baseline and at subsequent visits to assess for response to treatment (Hanno et al. 2011).

In characterizing pain, it is important to elicit:

(a) Pain location: frequently pain can originate in the suprapubic area; however for some patients, the origin of pain is reported as urethral or vaginal. Pain can radiate throughout the pelvis, including the lower abdomen, flanks, and lower back, and/or pain can radiate toward the vagina or rectum. Patients will often describe a bothersome constant awareness of the bladder. Some patients use terms such as "pressure" or "discomfort" and will actually deny overt "pain."

(b) Timing of pain: patients with IC/BPS may report pain is worse daytime or nighttime, some patients can describe a correlation with pain flares and the menstrual cycle, and frequently pain flares can be correlated with times of psychosocial stress.

(c) Relationship of pain to urinary symptoms: often patients will report that pain is increased with filling and relieved by voiding, some patients will also report dysuria as a characteristic of pain flares, and for a small number this is the initial symptom of IC/BPS.

(d) Exacerbating and ameliorating factors: frequently patients recognize dietary triggers that can worsen pain due to IC/BPS, classically acidic or spicy foods. Patient position can have an effect on pelvic pain caused by pudendal neuralgia, which is often worse with prolonged sitting and improved by standing or by sitting on a toilet seat.

Risk Factors

As discussed, patients with other non-bladder syndromes are more likely to have IC/BPS than patients without these conditions; however there are many unanswered questions as to how these conditions are related. There is also a possible familial component, although this also is an area where further research is needed (Warren et al. 2011).

Physical Exam

Specific Maneuvers

The evaluation begins with a general examination noting patients' appearance and affect. Neurologic exam, extremity exam, abdominal exam, flank exam for CVA tenderness, and a detailed pelvic exam are also recommended. Patients may have had severe pain with pelvic examination and/or negative experiences with examination, therefore it is important to emphasize to patients that the exam will be fully explained to them and completed at their pace. Having a chaperone available that can facilitate the provider's ability to perform the exam expeditiously and at the same time provide support to the patient while the exam is being completed is also helpful.

Abnormal Findings

A limited neurologic examination should include any abnormalities in mental status, gait and balance, sensation and muscle tone of the perineum and pelvic floor. Musculoskeletal and/or abdominal exam may reveal tender points, and a useful eponymous test is performing an evaluation for Carnett's sign. The patient is asked to raise the head and shoulders or to raise both legs with straight knees. The examiner will find a positive Carnett's sign if the abdominal pain worsens with tensing the abdominal wall, indicating that the source of the pain is less likely originating from an intra-abdominal source. Positive Carnett's sign could indicate possible nerve entrapment in the abdominal wall (especially from prior surgery), myofascial pain, or trigger points.

The pelvic exam begins with inspection for skin abnormalities including skin lesions consistent with herpes simplex or other infections, including yeast. The examiner should also be familiar with other chronic vulvar skin conditions like lichen sclerosus and lichen planus. The vulva and vaginal vestibule can be examined with a cotton-tipped swab to map light touch sensation, numbness, or areas of tenderness. The vaginal vestibule and introitus should be examined carefully and notation made of the quality of the vaginal epithelium – signs of atrophy, signs of yeast, signs of contact dermatitis, friable tissue, inflammation, as well as vaginal discharge. Abnormalities such as Bartholin's and Skene's gland/duct cysts should also be noted.

Examining the urethra begins with the urethral meatus. Note should be made of urethral meatal stenosis, urethral prolapse, urethral caruncle, or signs of urethral diverticulum, including any mass along the anterior vaginal wall. Any surgical scars should be noted, and the presence of any visible or palpable mesh or sutures should be reported. Tenderness, spasm, or increased tone of the pelvic floor muscles should be assessed, and voluntary control of both the ability to perform contraction and relaxation of the pelvic floor should be evaluated.

A speculum/halved speculum should be used to visualize the cervix or vaginal cuff scar; the vaginal epithelium should be interrogated for signs of fistula, granulation tissue, or other lesions; and cervical tenderness should also be assessed. Bimanual examination may reveal vaginal wall masses, adnexal tenderness or mass, abnormal uterine size or lie, or one of the common findings for patients with IC/BPS, bladder tenderness to palpation both transvaginally and suprapubically. Attempts to correlate findings on exam to the patient's pain description are extremely helpful.

Pelvic organ prolapse should also be reported and patients should be examined at full valsalva to determine if prolapse is present. Full evaluation of pelvic organ prolapse will be discussed later in the chapter. If the bladder is relatively full, the examiner can also assess for stress urinary incontinence on cough and valsalva. If the patient has complaints of feeling of incomplete emptying, weak stream, or straining to void, the examiner may elect to perform straight catheterization to determine post-void residual or to document sterile urine if infectious causes have not been thoroughly ruled by obtaining a catheterized urine sample to send for further testing.

Diagnostic Tests

Laboratory Evaluation

The initial laboratory evaluation should include a urinalysis and urine culture. These should be evaluated to rule out infection and to screen for other abnormalities. Urinalysis with microscopy should be ordered as a follow-up for any abnormalities on urinalysis, and guidelines for microscopic hematuria workup should be followed. The less common finding of sterile pyuria should be worked up as well in the standard fashion. Urine can also be sent for special testing for atypical organisms that can cause urethritis, namely, ureaplasma urealyticum and ureaplasma parvum as well as mycoplasma species.

If the patient reports associated vulvar and vaginal symptoms or if the examination is concerning for a yeast infection, it is reasonable to send a swab for yeast culture, as there are strains of yeast that are resistant to commonly used over-the-counter and prescription treatments. Other sexually transmitted infections (gonorrhea, chlamydia, and trichomonas) as well as bacterial vaginosis should be ruled out in the setting of vaginal discharge. Urinary biomarkers have been extensively studied as adjuncts to the diagnosis of IC/BPS; these are not typically used outside of the research setting, and there are no clinically available tests for urine markers that are recommended in the AUA guidelines for IC/BPS.

Imaging Studies
There are no imaging studies that are recommended as part of the basic diagnostic algorithm for IC/BPS. Imaging studies may be considered if other conditions are suspected. A CT urogram should be ordered for confirmed microscopic hematuria and gross hematuria or concern for congenital abnormalities such as an ectopic ureter. History of urolithiasis, colicky pain, especially that which radiates to the groin or flank can also prompt CT evaluation for a distal ureteral stone.

Pelvic ultrasound is useful for evaluating findings on abnormal pelvic exam, especially adnexal mass. Transvaginal ultrasound can show the presence and location of mesh in patients with prior pelvic surgery, although it is not required. Concern for urethral diverticulum or unclear examination findings on the anterior vaginal wall can prompt a pelvic MRI.

Procedures
Testing for post-void residual volume by ultrasound or catheterization is recommended for all patients as part of the basic evaluation (Hanno et al. 2011). If catheterization is undertaken and suspicion for IC/BPS is high, a one-time bladder instillation of 40 cc of 2 % lidocaine at the time of examination can help determine if instillation therapy is a viable treatment option for future management.

Urodynamic studies can also be considered, including a simple uroflowmetry to screen for functional or structural obstruction or detrusor underactivity. More sophisticated cystometrogram and pressure flow studies to evaluate complex incontinence or voiding dysfunction.

Cystoscopy is performed when there is concern for bladder cancer or urothelial carcinoma in situ, as well as congenital abnormalities such as an ectopic ureter or iatrogenic concerns such as prior surgery with or without mesh. Vaginoscopy can be added to evaluate for vaginal scarring, septa, fistula, or other unexplained findings on physical examination.

Management

Behavioral, Conservative, Complementary, and Alternative Medicine
The AUA guidelines recommend that all patients should be educated on behavioral modifications, fluid management, dietary changes, exercise, and stress reduction that can help them cope with their IC/PBS diagnosis and symptoms. Specific dietary educational materials on excluding bladder irritants using the elimination diet are

available for patients on the Interstitial Cystitis Association website (http://www. ichelp.org). For patients who are particularly diet sensitive, the supplement Prelief (calcium glycerophosphate; AkPharma) can be used prior to situations when trigger foods cannot be avoided. Dietary changes, fiber supplements, and stool softeners can help avoid constipation, which may be an exacerbating factor for IC/BPS patients. For patients who are interested in therapy that is directed at the bladder but wish to avoid pharmaceuticals, CystoProtek (chondroitin sulfate, quercetin, rutin, glucosamine sulfate, hyaluronate sodium; CystoProtek), aloe vera, or phenazopyridine may be helpful. Providers should not underestimate the contribution of education, self-care, and behavioral modification in the therapy of IC/BPS.

Patients with IC/PBS may benefit from additional multidisciplinary referrals. Patients who have pain outside of the pelvis or pain that is difficult to manage can be referred to an anesthesiologist or physical medicine and rehabilitation provider who specializes in pain management. If patients feel they have a significant psychological impact of their pain/symptoms, they can be offered a referral counseling with a pain psychologist. Patients with impact on sexual function can be referred for sexual health counseling. Referral to gastroenterology for refractory bowel symptoms, including constipation is often warranted, and referral to gynecology for a discussion of treatment of endometriosis, dysmenorrhea, or oral contraceptives/hormonal manipulation for patients with hormone sensitive IC/BPS symptoms can also be worthwhile.

Pelvic floor physical therapy (PFPT) is an important tool for the treatment of patients with pelvic floor muscle tenderness and IC/BPS. PFPT is a second-line therapy for IC/BPS based on strong evidence (Hanno et al. 2015). A recent randomized clinical trial showed that ten sessions of 60 min of myofascial physical therapy resulted in significantly more patients (59 %) reporting they were moderately or markedly improved compared to those undergoing therapeutic massage (26 %) (Fitzgerald et al. 2012).

Medical

Oral IC/BPS Medications
Several oral medications are options for second-line treatment per the AUA guidelines. They are listed here in alphabetical order, as they are listed in the guideline:

1. Amitriptyline is a tricyclic antidepressant that is used off label for chronic pain conditions. Amitriptyline has a high rate of side effects, most commonly sedation/drowsiness and nausea; the sedation can be taken advantage of for patients who have difficulty with sleep due to symptoms; and the anticholinergic effects can help relax the bladder. It is typically started at 25 mg daily and increased to 100 mg daily; lower doses can be used to start the titration if the medication is not tolerated due to side effects. The medication can be titrated up over a period of weeks; studies have shown that patients who reach the 50 mg daily dose show significant improvement in symptom scores or global response to symptom improvement compared to placebo

(Van Ophoven et al. 2004; Foster et al. 2010). These doses are lower than those typically used for antidepressant effects.

2. Cimetidine is an histamine H2-receptor blocker that is not FDA approved for IC/BPS but has been shown to be effective with few side effects in small studies. The dosage used in studies varies from 200 mg three times daily and 300 mg twice daily to 400 mg twice daily (Hanno et al. 2011).

3. Hydroxyzine (pamoate or hydrochloride salt) is a first-generation antihistamine that is also used in certain conditions for its anxiolytic effects. Side effects are typically limited and include sedation with initial use. Doses used in studies range from 10 mg titrated to 50 mg daily-25 mg titrated to 75 mg daily over a period of weeks. The evidence for general use in IC/BPS is unclear; however experts postulate that hydroxyzine may be beneficial for the subset of IC/BPS patients with systemic allergies (Sant et al. 2003).

4. Pentosan polysulfate is the only oral medication that is FDA approved for use in IC/BPS. The polysaccharide drug is proposed to improve the glycosaminoglycan layer that protects the lining of the bladder. There have been conflicting reports on the performance of the pentosan polysulfate in randomized, placebo-controlled trials, but a pooled analysis (Dimitrakov et al. 2007) shows that it likely has a modest benefit for patient-reported symptom improvement, and the expert consensus of the AUA guideline panel recommends pentosan polysulfate as a second-line treatment. The most common adverse effects are diarrhea, abdominal pain, and rectal bleeding.

Oral immunomodulation with cyclosporine A is a fifth-line treatment in the AUA algorithm. Several studies demonstrate efficacy in small groups of patients with refractory IC/BPS symptoms. It appears that cyclosporine A may be most effective in patients with ulcerative IC/BPS. The most common adverse events are rising serum creatinine and hypertension, and therefore patients must be monitored very closely (Hanno et al. 2011; Hanno et al. 2015; Forrest et al. 2012).

Oral medications previously used as anticonvulsants that are widely used as treatments for neuropathic pain (pregabalin and gabapentin) have been used in small trials and case reports for both chronic prostatitis and pelvic pain in men and in women with IC/BPS (Vas et al. 2014; Pontari et al. 2010), but the effectiveness of these medications is unclear.

Lower urinary tract symptoms (LUTS) can also be treated per usual pathways, with the caveat that patients may not experience the responses expected in patients with LUTS without IC/PBS. Patients with significant hesitancy can be trialed on alpha-blockers; those with frequency and urgency can be trialed on antimuscarinics and or mirabegron.

The AUA guidelines specifically recommend against long-term oral antibiotic use as well as systemic glucocorticoid use (Hanno et al. 2011).

Topical ointments containing various drugs can be useful for patients with concomitant vulvar pain or vulvodynia; the most commonly used is lidocaine 5 % ointment. These ointments are variable in the vehicle base, as well as in active ingredient concentration and combination; many compounding pharmacies can add neuropathic agents, tricyclic antidepressants, antispasmodics, as well as other anesthetics (Haefner et al. 2005). Patients with pelvic floor muscle involvement, although the evidence for its use is sparse and contradictory, can also be given a trial of vaginal valium, either 5 or 10 mg tablets or compounded as a suppository (Carrico and Peters 2011; Crisp et al. 2013).

Intravesical Instillations

Using a urethral catheter to directly instill medications into the bladder in a retrograde fashion is a commonly used treatment for patients with IC/BPS and is usually referred to as bladder instillation or intravesical instillation therapy. Patients can be somewhat reluctant to undergo catheterization due to concerns of the catheterization itself being painful; counseling and a knowledgeable nursing staff familiar with IC/BPS patients can help facilitate treatments. A review of the evidence for the various instillations medications summarizes them well (Colaco 2013). A Cochrane review also exists that predates the AUA guidelines, which essentially had no conclusive evidence for any therapy other than resiniferatoxin, which was not shown to be effective (Dawson and Jamison 2007). The intravesical treatments are recommended as second-line treatments by the AUA and are again listed in alphabetical order:

1. Dimethyl sulfoxide (DMSO) is an organosulfur compound that has been used as an intravesical treatment for IC/BPS for decades, with two randomized crossover trials showing efficacy. There is some variability in the amount, dwell time, and interval of instillations; however the guideline reports protocols of successful trials of DMSO alone as using 50 cc of 50 % DMSO for a dwell time of 15 min in weekly or every 2-week intervals for a course of four to six treatments (Hanno et al. 2011). Notably, DMSO is absorbed by the bladder and can be painful if left to dwell too long. Adverse events are noted to be variable, including garlic odor, bladder irritation, and headache, but overall are not serious.
2. Heparin is well known for its use as an anticoagulant; however, structurally it is a glycosaminoglycan, and because of the theory that the glycosaminoglycan layer is inadequate or disrupted in IC/BPS, it has also been widely used as an intravesical treatment for IC/BPS. It is used in preparations ranging from 10,000 to 40,000 IU in 3–10 cc of sterile or distilled water, given one to three times per week with dwell times up to 1 h. Heparin's efficacy has been shown in observational studies, and in more recent studies, it has been combined with alkalinized lidocaine (to take advantage of the shorter-term effectiveness of lidocaine) with good results (Hanno et al. 2011).
3. Lidocaine is a local anesthetic that has been shown to have short-term efficacy in reducing symptoms of IC/BPS in several studies, which are mostly observational (Hanno et al. 2011). In the study protocols, 8–20 cc of 1–2 % lidocaine is often mixed with bicarbonate to alkalinize and potentially increase penetration of the medication, with a dwell time of up to 1 h for daily to weekly instillations. A pretzel-shaped intravesical device that releases lidocaine into the bladder continuously called LiRIS (Lidocaine Releasing Intravesical System) is being tested in clinical trials (Nickel et al. 2012).

The use of other medications in combination with the above or alone has been described in the literature. In clinical practice, various compounds are added to "cocktails" that are provider specific, including bupivacaine, gentamicin, pentosan polysulfate, other glycosaminoglycans (hyaluronic acid and chondroitin sulfate), and various glucocorticoids (triamcinolone or hydrocortisone). Because DMSO is absorbed by the bladder and may affect the absorption of other agents, caution is advised when using DMSO as part of a cocktail. The AUA recommends *against* using intravesical BCG, a commonly used treatment for bladder cancer.

After a patient is determined to have a significant response to bladder instillations, the provider can continue to arrange for office visits for the administration of the treatments, or the patient and family can be taught self-catheterization and prescribed medications and supplies to perform instillations at home. This strategy demands a motivated patient, as well as advanced coordination of care to overcome hurdles with insurance coverage, prescriptions that may require a compounding pharmacy, and the lack of shelf-stable cocktails, but can help patients be independent in their symptom management.

Neuromodulation

Sacral neuromodulation (SNM) is considered a fourth-line treatment for IC/BPS, although it is not FDA approved for this use. SNM is approved for use in patients with urinary frequency and urgency, which often overlap with IC/BPS symptoms. Patients are given a trial of neurostimulation which begins with implantation of a sacral stimulator lead, and then an implanted device is surgically inserted if the patient reports successful alleviation of symptoms and/or improvement on voiding diary. A similar technique that targets the pudendal nerve for stimulation has also been studied in a small cohort and found to be effective for pain and voiding symptom relief (Peters et al. 2007). Patients with implanted neurostimulators should be aware of battery life limitations (around 5 years) and restrictions on undergoing spinal MRI with the device in place.

Percutaneous tibial nerve stimulation (PTNS) is another type of neuromodulation that is approved for use for relief of urinary symptoms secondary to overactive bladder syndrome. In this treatment, a fine needle, the size of those used in acupuncture, is placed along the course of the tibial nerve on the medial aspect of the ankle. The needle is then attached to a device that provides electrical stimulation temporarily, with no permanent implants. Very small studies in patients with IC/BPS have shown decrease in pain intensity with PTNS, although larger- and longer-term studies are needed (Gokyildiz et al. 2012).

Intradetrusor Botulinum Toxin

Cystoscopy with injection of botulinum toxin into the bladder detrusor muscle is an FDA-approved therapy for neurogenic (200U) and non-neurogenic (100U) detrusor overactivity. It has been studied in refractory IC/BPS since 2004. The AUA guidelines initially recommended its use as a fifth-line treatment, partly due to adverse events and the potential for the need to catheterize if unable to void after injection at the 200U dose. The guideline amendment moved botulinum toxin injection to a fourth-line treatment (Hanno et al. 2015). The guideline panel notes that most of the evidence, even the newer studies, is observational, not placebo controlled, and has arms that combine botulinum toxin with hydrodistention, making the overall effect of botulinum toxin injection in IC/BPS difficult to pinpoint. A recent review of the evidence for botulinum toxin use in IC/BPS showed a trend toward using the 100U dose and repeat injection protocols (Jhang et al. 2014). Patients have to be willing to catheterize if botulinum toxin injection causes the inability to empty the bladder well; those who are unable to tolerate catheterization are not candidates for this treatment.

Other Pain Injections
Some providers who treat complex pelvic pain also provide trigger point injections and/or pudendal nerve blocks based on clinical evaluations. Caudal epidural injections and other more sophisticated locoregional pain procedures can be performed as part of multidisciplinary teams that include pain management specialists.

Hyperbaric Oxygen
Hyperbaric oxygen therapy is another investigational treatment that has been shown in very small studies to have a potential role in treating IC/BPS due to its use in other forms of cystitis, but it is not currently an approved or commonly used therapy (Tanaka et al. 2011; Van Ophoven et al. 2006).

Surgical
The most common surgical procedures for IC/BPS are cystoscopy with hydrodistention of the bladder and cystoscopy with treatment for Hunner's ulcers (biopsy, fulguration, triamcinolone injection).

Criteria for Surgery
Patients who have failed conservative management can choose to undergo cystoscopy and hydrodistention as a diagnostic aid as well as for therapeutic benefit. This is a third-line treatment in the AUA algorithm. If characteristic findings are present (petechiae, glomerulations, Hunner's ulcer), these can add to the evidence for a diagnosis of IC/BPS and provide an avenue for treatment (Hunner's ulcer), and determination of anesthetized bladder capacity can identify patients with severe forms of IC/BPS. Some patients will not have these findings but will still have the characteristic flare of symptoms followed by weeks to months of symptom improvement. This pattern of response to hydrodistention also helps firm up a diagnosis of IC/BPS if symptoms are unclear. The long-term efficacy for symptom relief varies but typically declines over a period of months in observational studies. There are no sham-/placebo-controlled studies to determine how effective hydrodistention will be and no category of patients that are particularly likely to have benefit from the treatment.

Very few patients will meet criteria for major surgical intervention for IC/BPS. Patients with intractable pain and very small, contracted bladder have been treated with open surgical techniques, including augmentation cystoplasty, substitution cystoplasty, and continent and incontinent urinary diversion with and without simple cystectomy. The patients must be counseled that these are major surgeries which are irreversible, have significant morbidity, and are not guaranteed to alleviate all pain (Andersen et al. 2012; Rössberger et al. 2007; Peters et al. 2013).

Preoperative Considerations and Additional Tests That May Be Appropriate Prior to Surgery

Preoperative considerations would be similar to any minor endoscopic procedure; guidelines for workup of any patient undergoing general anesthesia should be followed, with inclusion of a urine culture with treatment to sterilize the urine prior to instrumentation.

Medications

Typically the procedure is done with general anesthesia, but because of the high levels of existing preoperative pain, patients are also medicated intraoperatively with urethral 2 % lidocaine jelly and an instillation of 40 ml of 2 % lidocaine at the conclusion of the hydrodistention. While anesthetized, a belladonna and opium suppository can also be administered to prevent bladder spasms in the postoperative period, and patients are given prescriptions to manage the pain flare that typically occurs after the procedure. Triamcinolone, a corticosteroid, is injected into Hunner's ulcers as needed, with the guideline specifying 10 ml of triamcinolone acetonide, 40 mg/ml, injected in 0.5 ml aliquots into the submucosal space of the center and periphery of ulcers using an endoscopic needle, with 60 mg maximum dose (Hanno et al. 2011).

Teaching Points

Reports from cystoscopy and hydrodistention will typically characterize the bladder capacity under anesthesia, as well as the appearance of the bladder mucosa both before and after filling the bladder to capacity. Hydrodistention can cause findings consistent with IC/BPS including terminal hematuria on draining the bladder, petechiae, or glomerulations. There may be no abnormal findings, and a normal cystoscopy does not rule out IC/BPS. Hunner's ulcers are typically erythematous ulcers that can appear anywhere on the bladder mucosa and are present even before hydrodistentions. Suspicious lesions should be biopsied prior to any treatment of the lesion with fulguration or injection.

Postoperative Management and Short-Term Complications

Patients should be counseled that the first few days to week after their hydrodistention, their IC/BPS symptoms may actually flare before they improve. They should be given pain medications, including narcotics, if needed, and phenazopyridine, and advised that they may have dysuria and difficulty voiding. Patients should receive instructions to help identify signs and symptoms of urinary retention and urinary tract infection and should notify their provider if these occur.

An extremely rare but serious intraoperative complication of any cystoscopic procedure, including hydrodistention, with or without treatment of ulcers, is bladder perforation. The bladder can tear or crack during bladder stretching, which may require prolonged catheterization, or in extreme circumstances, intraoperative open surgical repair. The AUA guidelines state that high-pressure, long-duration hydro-distention should not be offered.

Long-Term Complications

Long-term complications from hydrodistention are also unusual. Repeated fulgurations could lead to scarring of bladder and decreased capacity, but only if extensive.

Pelvic Organ Prolapse and Pelvic Floor Disorders

Definitions

Pelvic organ prolapse is a term that describes the overall condition of female pelvic organs descending from their normal position into or through the vagina. The International Urogynecological Association/International Continence Society (IUGA/ICS) terminology committee defines POP as "The descent of one or more of the anterior vaginal wall, posterior vaginal wall, the uterus (cervix), or the apex of the vagina (vaginal vault or cuff scar after hysterectomy)." (Haylen et al. 2010) The description of pelvic organ prolapse has also been standardized and is described by the portion of the vagina that is observed to be prolapsing (Winters et al. 2012). The term "cystocele" is often applied to an observed anterior vaginal wall prolapse, as a bulge in the anterior vaginal wall most commonly occurs with bladder protrusion into the vagina, but may also contain small bowel (enterocele) or the uterus, making the term "anterior vaginal wall prolapse" more appropriate. Uterine or cervical pro-lapse occurs when the uterus or cervix descends into the vaginal canal. Enterocele can occur in the anterior vaginal wall, posterior vaginal wall, or at the vaginal apex. Vaginal vault or vaginal cuff prolapse describes the prolapse of the upper vagina after hysterectomy, uterine prolapse and vaginal vault prolapse also be described as apical compartment prolapse.

A bulge in the posterior vaginal wall that most commonly contains the rectum, is termed a "rectocele." The term "rectal prolapse" is reserved for prolapse of the rec-tal mucosa through the anal opening. A perineocele is a term that describes a bulge caused by a defect in the support of perineal body causing perineal descent.

Epidemiology

There is an 11 % risk of undergoing an operation for POP or urinary incontinence by the age of 80 (Fialkow et al. 2008), and it is projected that there will be as many as 9.2 million women in the United States with POP by 2050 (Wu et al. 2009). Pelvic organ prolapse is known to have a significant impact on women's quality of life, sexual health, and body image (Lowder et al. 2011).

Anatomy and Physiology

The structure and function of the female pelvis are described above. The pelvic floor must support the genitourinary and gastrointestinal organs and at the same time, allow them to perform the functions of voiding, childbirth, and defecation. The normal support of the pelvic organs itself is complex, and dysfunction of the muscles, "ligaments," and "fascia" that keep these organs within the pelvis are not fully understood. Advanced computer modeling is currently being employed to understand the dynamic forces involved in the development of POP (Chen et al. 2013; Jing et al. 2012).

History

Frequently, patients present with a chief complaint of a bothersome vaginal bulge. The patient can describe this as pain but also as "pulling" or "heaviness" in the pelvis or vagina (Haylen et al. 2010). Patients will often describe the sensation that they are sitting on a small ball or other object.

It may be that the patient arrives at the appointment with a history of being told by another provider that they have prolapse, a cystocele, or that one of their pelvic organs has "dropped." It is especially important to reassure these patients that prolapse itself is not a dangerous or life-threatening condition, that it is perfectly acceptable to manage non-bothersome prolapse conservatively, and that sexual activity will not cause them harm.

Similar history-taking considerations exist for female patients with pelvic floor dysfunction as with IC/BPS, including a detailed sexual, gynecologic, and obstetric history, including complications and details of delivery. A thorough evaluation of symptoms of prolapse as well as bowel and bladder function should be reported and assessed with validated questionnaires. Specific questioning should elicit if stress incontinence symptoms were present prior to developing prolapse, which may have improved after prolapse developed. Because prolapse can make it difficult to void, patients should be questioned about hesitancy, feeling of incomplete bladder emptying, position-dependent voiding, and straining. Patients may report using their hand to reduce the prolapse in the vagina or on the perineum, or "splinting," in order to facilitate bladder emptying or defecation. Fecal incontinence, flatal incontinence, straining to defecate, feeling of incomplete defecation, constipation, and other associated symptoms of anorectal dysfunction should be investigated. Symptoms of sexual dysfunction include pain during intercourse (dyspareunia), obstructed intercourse, and vaginal laxity (Haylen et al. 2010).

The examiner should also elicit a detailed surgical history, with review of records if possible. It can be difficult for patients to recall remote surgeries or concomitant procedures performed at the time of hysterectomy. It is useful to determine if a patient has had oophorectomy, and some patients may not know this information, and efforts should be made to confirm the status. Additionally, if pelvic surgeries were performed in recent years, it is also helpful to know what materials were used for any anti-incontinence or reconstructive surgeries in the event that reoperation is necessary.

A wide range of risk factors for POP have been proposed based on epidemiologic studies, but because of our limited understanding on the pathophysiologic causes of POP, modifying patient risks to prevent POP is not a common strategy. Vaginal childbirth and levator ani muscle defects likely have a significant impact on a woman's risk for developing POP (DeLancey et al. 2007; Morgan et al. 2011) and should be evaluated; however current management of prolapse does not differ for patients with and without these risk factors.

Physical Exam

Specific Maneuvers
Prior to the pelvic examination, it is useful to get an idea of the size of the prolapse by asking the patient how the bulge looks/feels when it is at its largest. This will help the examiner know if they are seeing the full extent of the prolapse during examination. Often patients will require specific instruction to achieve the full extent of prolapse. One helpful maneuver is to ask the patient to take a deep breath and hold it and, while not allowing exhale, to bear down, causing a full valsalva. When the prolapse reaches its full extent, the vaginal rugae will smooth out. The patient should be able to demonstrate the control of the pelvic floor and the force of a pelvic floor contraction should be noted.

The pelvic organ prolapse quantification scale, or POP-Q, is a system of measurements that describe pelvic organ prolapse based on a fixed point of reference (the hymenal remnant.) This system was developed to help both researchers and clinicians to standardize the description of prolapse in individual patients which allows for staging of prolapse with comparison of patients. The POP-Q is well described in the literature (Haylen et al. 2010) and is best learned from an experienced practitioner.

The position of the anus should be evaluated, and a rectal exam should be undertaken in the evaluation of bowel symptoms, noting the sphincter tone, ability to contract and to attempt to expel an examining digit, and a rectovaginal exam that can reveal the quality of the tissues and the extent of rectocele, and hard stool in the rectal vault can indicate functional bowel problems.

Abnormal Findings
As described above, thorough pelvic examination should be undertaken with notation of the tissue quality, any skin abnormalities, and any areas of tenderness or pain. Other abnormalities on pelvic exam that may be associated with previous surgeries should be well documented. These would include the presence of mesh or sutures and the presence of scars or banding.

Additionally, patients with prior surgery, medical conditions that would make one prone to fistulas, or complicated childbirth should incite a high index of suspicion for vesicovaginal, rectovaginal, urethrovaginal, peritoneovaginal, or ureterovaginal fistulas. The anus should be examined for asymmetry, indicating muscle injury or weakness. Rectal prolapse should be described and any concerns for fistulas or chronic or poorly healed obstetrical lacerations should be noted.

Diagnostic Tests

Laboratory Evaluation
Urinalysis and culture should document the absence of infection for patients with urinary complaints or who are planned for surgical intervention with urinary tract instrumentation.

Imaging Studies
Dynamic magnetic resonance imaging, 3D ultrasound, and other complex imaging modalities are often used for research in POP but are not recommended as part of the standard evaluation. Imaging can be indicated for abnormal findings on pelvic exam, such as concern for fistula or urethral diverticulum or for dysfunction of the urinary tract (fluorourodynamics) or the gastrointestinal tract (defecography).

Procedures

A post-void residual urine volume can be obtained by ultrasound bladder scan or by catheterization. A full bladder stress test where the patient is examined with a full bladder (either by natural filling or by retrograde bladder filling with a catheter) can be useful to document the presence or absence of stress incontinence. If the patient is considering prolapse repair, the full bladder stress test can also be performed with the prolapse reduced, either with a pessary or a speculum in the vagina, to demonstrate stress incontinence that may occur with the prolapse reduced (occult stress urinary incontinence). More complex voiding dysfunction can be evaluated with a simple cystometric examination or with urodynamics. Defecatory dysfunction can be evaluated with defecography or anorectal manometry.

Management

Behavioral, Conservative, Complementary, and Alternative Medicine
Patients should be counseled regarding concerns about safety, sexual functioning, and body image (Lowder et al. 2011). For many patients, conservative management along with education about their condition and reassurance that POP is not dangerous is a reasonable treatment option.

One physical intervention that is often recommended for patients with prolapse is pelvic floor physical therapy. In contrast to focus on muscle relaxation and muscle control in patients with interstitial cystitis, pelvic floor physical therapy for patients with POP is focused on muscle training and strengthening. Individualized one-on-one pelvic floor physical therapy has been shown in a randomized controlled trial to improve patient-reported symptoms of POP (Hagen et al. 2014). This type of therapy can be offered to patients as a low-risk intervention (Hagen and Stark 2011).

Vaginal pessaries have been used as a mechanical intervention for pelvic organ prolapse for centuries. Contemporary vaginal pessaries are devices made of medical-grade silicone of various shapes and sizes that are designed to treat any size or type of prolapse. Pessary fitting entails choosing the right size and shape of pessary to comfortably reduce a women's prolapse, and a trial of valsalva and voiding in the office at the time of the fitting is typical. Pessary treatment is described as having a moderate dropout rate, but a review of the evidence shows that studies report 50–80 % continuation at 1 year, with a high patient satisfaction in the medium term (Lamers et al. 2011). Pessary maintenance schedules are variable, and maintenance is performed by the patient and/or the provider to varying degrees depending on the patient's situation. Some patients are completely independent in removing and cleaning pessaries and are simply monitored with a yearly speculum exam to ensure that there is no damage to the vaginal tissues, and some patients require periodic removal and cleaning by a provider due to physical or cognitive limitations. The most common side effects of pessary use are vaginal discharge, odor, bleeding pain, and constipation (Lamers et al. 2011). Retained pessaries after loss to follow-up or neglect can cause serious complications, but these are exceedingly rare.

Medical

There are essentially no pharmacologic treatments for POP. Topical estrogen cream can help improve the vaginal tissues and some of the associated irritative voiding symptoms and dyspareunia associated with atrophy and will possibly make pessary use more comfortable, but will not improve prolapse.

Surgical

Surgical treatment for POP can be divided in to obliterative versus reconstructive approaches. Obliterative surgery consists of colpocleisis, which is performed by closing off the vaginal canal to reduce the prolapsed organs with concomitant perineorrhaphy to decrease the size of the genital hiatus, with our without an anti-incontinence procedure (Abbasy and Kenton 2010). Colpocleisis is performed transvaginally and, when performed without hysterectomy, is a safe and fairly low-morbidity operation. Patients must be counseled on the loss of the ability to have vaginal intercourse and should not have colpocleisis performed if they wish to preserve this ability. Patient satisfaction and anatomic success are very high in the literature, with a recent large case series of one type of colpocleisis describing over 92 % satisfaction in 310 elderly women, with 15.2 % complication rate and 1.3 % mortality rate (Zebede et al. 2013).

Reconstructive surgery can consist of a single or multiple procedures designed to restore the anatomy and function of the prolapsed organs. These procedures are typically described by the compartment that they address and the route by which the procedures are performed.

Uterine prolapse, apical compartment prolapse, and vaginal vault prolapse can be repaired transabdominally or transvaginally; both approaches resuspend the vagina by attaching it to a structure within the pelvis for support. Abdominal sacrocolpopexy involves attaching the vaginal apex via a reinforcing graft (often synthetic polypropylene mesh) to the sacral anterior longitudinal ligament (Nygaard et al. 2013). Sacrocolpopexy can be performed as an open, laparoscopic or robotic surgery either post-hysterectomy or at the same time as total or supracervical hysterectomy. Transvaginal native tissue repairs for apical prolapse include a vaginal hysterectomy and suspension of the vaginal apex by attaching it with sutures to the sacrospinous ligament or to the uterosacral ligaments. Vaginal mesh repairs for apical prolapse would include using mesh placed transvaginally to resuspend the vaginal apex, typically by attachment to the sacrospinous ligament. Choice of apical prolapse repair is often surgeon dependent, and the risks and benefits of the planned repair should be discussed on an individualized basis.

Reconstructive surgery for anterior vaginal wall defects, often called "anterior colporraphy" or "anterior repair" can be colloquially described by patients as "bladder lift," "bladder sling," or "bladder suspension," making it imperative to obtain operative reports in patients who have had prior surgery. Anterior compartment repairs are most often transvaginal surgeries and consist of native tissue repairs where the cystocele is reduced using plicating sutures (anterior colporraphy) or transvaginal mesh repairs where polypropylene mesh is used as a graft to reinforce the vaginal wall. Controversy over transvaginal mesh and warnings from the FDA about complications of transvaginal mesh use (Menchen et al. 2012) have lead to a number of lawsuits involving these devices. Nonabsorbable anterior wall mesh grafts do seem to result in a more durable repair (Altman et al. 2011; Maher et al. 2008; Gomelsky et al. 2011); however this must be balanced with the risks of mesh use, and the provider must ensure that these risks are thoroughly understood by the patient prior to proceeding with an augmented repair.

Surgical repairs for posterior wall defects include rectocele repair ("posterior colporraphy" or "posterior repair") and perineorrhaphy. These are most typically completed transvaginally without any graft material as there is no current evidence that grafting of any type improves outcomes in the posterior compartment (Gomelsky et al. 2011).

Criteria for Surgery

The most important preoperative consideration for patients considering prolapse repair is that POP repairs are elective surgeries. Patients should be counseled extensively on the risks and benefits, the durability and the success rates of the procedures, as well as the alternatives to surgery. This counseling has been shown to play an important role as patient's preparedness for surgery is associated with their satisfaction with the outcome of the procedure (Kenton et al. 2007). Patients must meet criteria for general anesthesia, with the exception of colpocleisis, which can be performed under spinal anesthetic.

Preoperative Considerations and Additional Tests That May Be Appropriate Prior to Surgery

Patients with POP are frequently middle aged or older and may have significant comorbidities. Guidelines should be followed for preoperative workup for any patient undergoing general anesthesia. Patients should also have preoperative urine cultures if there is concern for UTI, or the urinary tract is going to be extensively instrumented.

Medications

Medications used during surgery include vasopressin or local anesthetic with epinephrine for hydrodissection, as well as phenazopyridine, methylene blue, or indigo carmine to aid in confirmation of ureteral efflux during cystoscopy. Providers vary in the use of vaginal packing with or without medications. Guidelines for perioperative surgical prophylactic antibiotics should also be followed.

Teaching Points

Prolapse repair is a dynamic field of surgery and an active area of research in the specialty of FPMRS. Anatomic success is not the only factor that is important when judging the success of an operation for prolapse, as the absence of symptoms (vaginal bulge) is strongly related to how much overall improvement patients subjectively report after surgery (Barber et al. 2009). Failure rates determined by varying definitions of success show a wide range in the literature; however most studies show that there is a reasonable chance that a patient may undergo a second surgical prolapse repair, which makes complex reoperative surgery not uncommon for the pelvic surgeon, and patients must be counseled on risks for repeat surgical repair.

Intraoperatively, the surgeon must recognize that patients under anesthesia have relaxation of the pelvic floor musculature and that these muscles will regain normal tone. Surgical planning should take into account the patient preoperative exam, symptoms, personalized goals, and examination under anesthesia.

Postoperative Management

Postoperatively, patients undergoing most major POP repairs will be observed for a 23 h stay. Patients will be catheterized during surgery and will undergo void trial typically on postoperative day #1. If a vaginal pack is placed, the packing will need to be removed prior to trial of voiding. If patients are unable to void, often they can be taught intermittent catheterization to be performed post-void to facilitate transition back to normal voiding, which is typically on the order of days to a few weeks. If the patient is unable to self-catheterize, she can be sent home for a short time with an indwelling Foley catheter. Pain control is often achieved with oral narcotics and anti-inflammatories, and bowel regimen to prevent straining and constipation is imperative.

Short-Term Complications

Short-term complications include all of the usual considerations that go along with any major surgical intervention. Because of the need for lithotomy positioning, nerve injury at several sites has been described and careful intraoperative position-ing is critical. Small risks of abdominal wound infections, port site complications, or complications from vascular, genitourinary, or gastrointestinal injuries during minimally invasive or open intra-abdominal surgery exist. A meta-analysis of sacro-colpopexy complication rates showed a rate of wound infection of 2.4 % and a rate of cystotomy of 2.8 % (Hudson et al. 2014).

Transvaginal surgery also carries a risk of postoperative bleeding, in vaginal, paravaginal, and intra-abdominal spaces, and special consideration should be given to bleeding into the retroperitoneum after sacrospinous ligament suspension suture placement. Intra-abdominal bleeding or bowel complications can occur (obstruc-tion or injury) during vaginal hysterectomy or enterocele repair where the perito-neum is entered, or with passage of mesh kit trocars. A series of 438 consecutive transvaginal native tissue repairs also showed a very low rate of complications, with a cystotomy rate of 0.2 % and a reoperation rate for hemorrhage of 0.9 %, without differences in serious complications for patients undergoing sacrospinous ligament suspension or hysterectomy (Mothes et al. 2014). There are risks of blad-der or ureteral injury during hysterectomy regardless of route, as well as in anterior and apical prolapse repairs and passage of mesh kit trocars, and a high index of suspicion is warranted and routine cystoscopy is recommended. Wound complica-tions for vaginal wounds rarely include infection. However, vaginal wounds can require management in the immediate postoperative period due to bleeding or dehiscence, and in the short term, granulation tissue can form within the vagina at the site of vaginal incisions, which can often be treated in the office, or as a short outpatient procedure. Urinary tract infection can occur regardless of type of sur-gery, and patients should be counseled on the signs and symptoms of this relatively common occurrence.

Long-Term Complications

Long-term complications of prolapse repair can include small bowel obstruction (if peritoneum is entered), dyspareunia, lower urinary tract dysfunction, mesh complications (exposure, erosion, pain), and failure of the repair or recurrent pro-lapse. Following prolapse surgery, around 12 % of women develop de novo urinary frequency and urgency, and 9 % develop voiding dysfunction (Maher et al. 2013). Follow-up of mesh grafts used in prolapse shows an exposure rate around 7.3–18 % for transvaginal mesh (Gomelsky et al. 2011; Maher et al. 2013), and a long-term study of abdominal sacrocolpopexy showed that 10.5 % of patients would be expected to have a mesh or suture erosion at 7 years of follow-up (Nygaard et al. 2013), keeping in mind that in all studies, mesh exposures in the vagina were often managed conservatively.

Resources for the Nurse Practitioner

(i) AUA Guideline: Diagnosis and Treatment of Interstitial Cystitis/Bladder Pain Syndrome.   http://www.auanet.org/education/guidelines/ic-bladder-pain-syndrome.cfm

(ii) American Urogynecologic Society. www.augs.org

(iii) Interactive POP-Q http://www.bardmedical.com/products/pelvic-health/pop-q/

Resources for the Patient
  (i) Urology Care Foundation Patient Information http://www.urologyhealth.org/urology/index.cfm?article=67
 (ii) Interstitial Cystitis Association http://www.ichelp.org
(iii) American Urogynecologic Society. www.augs.org
(iv) Voices for Pelvic Floor Dysfunction http://www.voicesforpfd.org/p/cm/ld/fid=5

Clinical Pearls
- Be mindful of cultural/religious considerations, relative to members of the opposite sex performing these examinations and procedures.
- Management of constipation is key to management of both prolapse and IC/BPS.
- Current guidelines recommend against long-term antibiotic and systemic glucocorticoid use for IC/BPS.
- Patients who are unwilling to perform ISC, or lack the manual dexterity for ISC, are not candidates for botulinum toxin bladder injections.
- Education, self-care, and behavioral modifications are keys to successful management of IC/BPS.
- Always consider preoperative urine cultures in this population, if the GU tract will be extensively instrumented.

References

Abbasy S, Kenton K (2010) Obliterative procedures for pelvic organ prolapse. Clin Obstet Gynecol 53(1):86–98. doi:10.1097/GRF.0b013e3181cd4252

Altman D, Väyrynen T, Engh ME, Axelsen S, Falconer C (2011) Anterior colporrhaphy versus transvaginal mesh for pelvic-organ prolapse. N Engl J Med 364(19):1826–1836. doi:10.1056/NEJMoa1009521

Andersen AV, Granlund P, Schultz A, Talseth T, Hedlund H, Frich L (2012) Long-term experience with surgical treatment of selected patients with bladder pain syndrome/interstitial cystitis. Scand J Urol Nephrol 46:284–289. doi:10.3109/00365599.2012.669789

Barber MD, Brubaker L, Nygaard I et al (2009) Defining success after surgery for pelvic organ prolapse. Obs Gynecol 114(3):600–609. doi:10.1097/AOG.0b013e3181b2b1ae

Berry SH, Bogart LM, Pham C et al (2010) Development, validation and testing of an epidemiological case definition of interstitial cystitis/painful bladder syndrome. J Urol 183(5):1848–1852. doi:10.1016/j.juro.2009.12.103

Berry SH, Elliott MN, Suttorp M et al (2011) Prevalence of symptoms of bladder pain syndrome/interstitial cystitis among adult females in the United States. J Urol 186(2):540–544. doi:10.1016/j.juro.2011.03.132

Carrico DJ, Peters KM (2011) Vaginal diazepam use with urogenital pain/pelvic floor dysfunction: serum diazepam levels and efficacy data. Urol Nurs 31(5):279–284, 299, http://www.ncbi.nlm.nih.gov/pubmed/22073898

Chen L, Ramanah R, Hsu Y, Ashton-Miller JA, Delancey JOL (2013) Cardinal and deep uterosacral ligament lines of action: MRI based 3D technique development and preliminary findings in normal women. Int Urogynecol J Pelvic Floor Dysfunct 24:37–45. doi:10.1007/s00192-012-1801-4

Chennamsetty A, Ehlert MJ, Peters KM, Killinger KA (2015) Advances in diagnosis and treatment of interstitial cystitis/painful bladder syndrome. Curr Infect Dis Rep 17(1):454. doi:10.1007/s11908-014-0454-5

Chrysanthopoulou EL, Doumouchtsis SK (2013) Challenges and current evidence on the management of bladder pain syndrome. Neurourol Urodyn 30(February 2013):169–173. doi:10.1002/nau.22475

Clemens JQ, Mullins C, Kusek JW et al (2014) The MAPP research network: a novel study of urologic chronic pelvic pain syndromes. BMC Urol 14:57. doi:10.1186/1471-2490-14-57

Colaco MA, Evans RJ (2013) Current recommendations for bladder instillation therapy in the treatment of interstitial cystitis/bladder pain syndrome. Curr Urol Rep 14(5):442–447. doi:10.1007/s11934-013-0369-y

Crisp CC, Vaccaro CM, Estanol MV et al (2013) Intra-vaginal diazepam for high-tone pelvic floor dysfunction: a randomized placebo-controlled trial. Int Urogynecol J Pelvic Floor Dysfunct 24:1915–1923. doi:10.1007/s00192-013-2108-9

Dawson TE, Jamison J (2007) Intravesical treatments for painful bladder syndrome/interstitial cystitis. Cochrane Database Syst Rev (4):2007–2009. doi:10.1002/14651858.CD006113.pub2

DeLancey JOL, Morgan DM, Fenner DE et al (2007) Comparison of levator ani muscle defects and function in women with and without pelvic organ prolapse. Obstet Gynecol 109:295–302. doi:10.1097/01.AOG.0000250901.57095.ba

Dimitrakov J, Kroenke K, Steers WD et al (2007) Pharmacologic management of painful bladder syndrome/interstitial cystitis: a systematic review. Arch Intern Med 167(18):1922–1929. doi:10.1001/archinte.167.22.2452

Fialkow MF, Newton KM, Lentz GM, Weiss NS (2008) Lifetime risk of surgical management for pelvic organ prolapse or urinary incontinence. Int Urogynecol J Pelvic Floor Dysfunct 19:437–440. doi:10.1007/s00192-007-0459-9

Fitzgerald MP, Payne CK, Lukacz ES et al (2012) Randomized multicenter clinical trial of myofascial physical therapy in women with interstitial cystitis/painful bladder syndrome and pelvic floor tenderness. J Urol 187(6):2113–2118. doi:10.1016/j.juro.2012.01.123

Forrest JB, Payne CK, Erickson DR (2012) Cyclosporine a for refractory interstitial cystitis/bladder pain syndrome: experience of 3 tertiary centers. J Urol 188(October):1186–1191. doi:10.1016/j.juro.2012.06.023

Foster HE, Hanno PM, Nickel JC et al (2010) Effect of amitriptyline on symptoms in treatment naïve patients with interstitial cystitis/painful bladder syndrome. J Urol 183(5):1853–1858. doi:10.1016/j.juro.2009.12.106

Gokyildiz S, Kizilkaya Beji N, Yalcin O, Istek A (2012) Effects of percutaneous tibial nerve stimulation therapy on chronic pelvic pain. Gynecol Obstet Invest 73:99–105. doi:10.1159/000328447

Gomelsky A, Penson DF, Dmochowski RR (2011) Pelvic organ prolapse (POP) surgery: the evidence for the repairs. Br J Urol 107(11):1704–1719. doi:10.1111/j.1464-410X.2011.10123.x

Haefner HK, Collins ME, Davis GD et al (2005) The vulvodynia guideline. J Low Genit Tract Dis 9:40–51. doi:10.1097/00128360-200501000-00009

Hagen S, Stark D (2011) Conservative prevention and management of pelvic organ prolapse in women. Cochrane Database Syst Rev (12):CD003882. doi:10.1002/14651858.CD003882.pub4. Copyright

Hagen S, Stark D, Glazener C et al (2014) Individualised pelvic floor muscle training in women with pelvic organ prolapse (POPPY): a multicentre randomised controlled trial. Lancet 383:796–806. doi:10.1016/S0140-6736(13)61977-7

Hanno PM, Burks DA, Clemens JQ et al (2011) AUA guideline for the diagnosis and treatment of interstitial cystitis/bladder pain syndrome. J Urol 185(6):2162–2170. doi:10.1016/j.juro.2011.03.064

Hanno PM, Erickson D, Moldwin R, Faraday MM (2015) Diagnosis and treatment of interstitial cystitis/bladder pain syndrome: AUA guideline amendment. J Urol 193(5):1545–1553. doi:10.1016/j.juro.2015.01.086

Haylen BT, De Ridder D, Freeman RM et al (2010) An International Urogynecological Association (IUGA)/International Continence Society (ICS) joint report on the terminology for female pelvic floor dysfunction. Neurourol Urodyn 29:4–20. doi:10.1002/nau.20798

Hudson CO, Northington Gina M, Lyles RH, Karp DR (2014) Outcomes of robotic sacrocolpopexy: a systematic review and meta-analysis. Female Pelvic Med Reconstr 20:252–260, http://journals. lww.com/jpelvicsurgery/Abstract/2011/11000/Bladder_Pain_Syndrome__A_Review.4.aspx

Jhang J-F, Jiang Y-H, Kuo H-C (2014) Potential therapeutic effect of intravesical botulinum toxin type A on bladder pain syndrome/interstitial cystitis. Int J Urol 21(Suppl 1):49–55. doi:10.1111/iju.12317

Jing D, Ashton-Miller JA, DeLancey JOL (2012) A subject-specific anisotropic visco-hyperelastic finite element model of female pelvic floor stress and strain during the second stage of labor. J Biomech 45:455–460. doi:10.1016/j.jbiomech.2011.12.002

Kenton K, Pham T, Mueller E, Brubaker L (2007) Patient preparedness: an important predictor of surgical outcome. Am J Obstet Gynecol 197(May 2005):654.e1–e6. doi:10.1016/j.ajog.2007.08.059

Lamers BHC, Broekman BMW, Milani AL (2011) Pessary treatment for pelvic organ prolapse and health-related quality of life: a review. Int Urogynecol J 22:637–644. doi:10.1007/s00192-011-1390-7

Lowder JL, Ghetti C, Nikolajski C, Oliphant SS, Zyczynski HM (2011) Body image perceptions in women with pelvic organ prolapse: a qualitative study. Am J Obstet Gynecol 204(5):441. e1–e5. doi:10.1016/j.ajog.2010.12.024

Maher C, Baessler K, Glazener CMA, Adams EJ, Hagen S (2008) Surgical management of pelvic organ prolapse in women: a short version Cochrane review. Neurourol Urodyn 27(1):3–12. doi:10.1002/nau.20542

Maher C, Feiner B, Baessler K, Schmid C (2013) Surgical management of pelvic organ prolapse in women. Cochrane database Syst Rev (4):CD004014. doi:10.1002/14651858.CD004014.pub5

Menchen LC, Wein AJ, Smith AL (2012) An appraisal of the food and drug administration warning on urogynecologic surgical mesh. Curr Urol Rep. doi:10.1007/s11934-012-0244-2

Morgan DM, Larson K, Lewicky-Gaupp C, Fenner DE, DeLancey JOL (2011) Vaginal support as determined by levator ani defect status 6 weeks after primary surgery for pelvic organ prolapse. Int J Gynaecol Obstet 114(2):141–144. doi:10.1016/j.ijgo.2011.02.020

Mothes AR, Mothes HK, Radosa MP, Runnebaum IB (2014) Systematic assessment of surgical complications in 438 cases of vaginal native tissue repair for pelvic organ prolapse adopting Clavien – Dindo classification. Arch Gynecol Obstet 291(6):1297–1301. doi:10.1007/s00404-014-3549-1

Nickel JC, Jain P, Shore N et al (2012) Continuous Intravesical lidocaine treatment for interstitial cystitis/bladder pain syndrome: safety and efficacy of a new drug delivery device. Sci Transl Med 4:143ra100-ra143ra100. doi:10.1126/scitranslmed.3003804

Nygaard I, Brubaker L, Zyczynski HM et al (2013) Long-term outcomes following abdominal sacro-colpopexy for pelvic organ prolapse. JAMA 309(19):2016–2024. doi:10.1001/jama.2013.4919

Peters KM, Feber KM, Bennett RC (2007) A prospective, single-blind, randomized crossover trial of sacral vs pudendal nerve stimulation for interstitial cystitis. BJU Int 100:835–839. doi:10.1111/j.1464-410X.2007.07082.x

Peters KM, Jaeger C, Killinger KA, Rosenberg B, Boura JA (2013) Cystectomy for ulcerative interstitial cystitis: Sequelae and patients' perceptions of improvement. Urology 82(4):829–833. doi:10.1016/j.urology.2013.06.043

Pontari MA, Krieger JN, Litwin MS et al (2010) Pregabalin for the treatment of men with chronic prostatitis/chronic pelvic pain syndrome: a randomized controlled trial. Arch Intern Med 170:1586–1593. doi:10.1001/archinternmed.2010.319

Rössberger J, Fall M, Jonsson O, Peeker R (2007) Long-term results of reconstructive surgery in patients with bladder pain syndrome/interstitial cystitis: subtyping is imperative. Urology 70:638–642. doi:10.1016/j.urology.2007.05.028

Sant GR, Propert KJ, Hanno PM et al (2003) A pilot clinical trial of oral pentosan polysulfate and oral hydroxyzine in patients with interstitial cystitis. J Urol 170(3):810–815. doi:10.1097/01.ju.0000083020.06212.3d

Suskind AM, Berry SH, Ewing BA, Elliott MN, Suttorp MJ, Clemens JQ (2012) The prevalence of interstitial cystitis/bladder pain syndrome (Ic/Bps) and chronic prostatitis/chronic pelvic pain syndrome (Cp/Cpps) in Men; results of the rand interstitial cystitis epidemiology (rice) male study. J Urol 187(January):e29–e30. doi:10.1016/j.juro.2012.02.115

Suskind AM, Berry SH, Suttorp MJ et al (2013) Health-related quality of life in patients with interstitial cystitis/bladder pain syndrome and frequently associated comorbidities. Qual Life Res 22:1537–1541. doi:10.1007/s11136-012-0285-5

Tanaka T, Nitta Y, Morimoto K et al (2011) Hyperbaric oxygen therapy for painful bladder syndrome/interstitial cystitis resistant to conventional treatments: long-term results of a case series in Japan. BMC Urol 11(December 2004):11. doi:10.1186/1471-2490-11-11

Van Ophoven A, Pokupic S, Heinecke A, Hertle L (2004) A prospective, randomized, placebo controlled, double-blind study of amitriptyline for the treatment of interstitial cystitis. J Urol 172(2):533–536. doi:10.1097/01.ju.0000132388.54703.4d

Van Ophoven A, Rossbach G, Pajonk F, Hertle L (2006) Safety and efficacy of hyperbaric oxygen therapy for the treatment of interstitial cystitis: a randomized, sham controlled, double-blind trial. J Urol 176:1442–1446. doi:10.1016/j.juro.2006.06.065

Vas L, Pattanik M, Titarmore V (2014) Treatment of interstitial cystitis/painful bladder syndrome as a neuropathic pain condition. Indian J Urol 30(3):350–353. doi:10.4103/0970-1591.128513

Warren JW, Van De Merwe JP, Nickel JC (2011) Interstitial cystitis/bladder pain syndrome and nonbladder syndromes: facts and hypotheses. Urology 78:727–732. doi:10.1016/j.urology.2011.06.014

Winters JC, Togami JM, Chermansky CJ (2012) Vaginal and abdominal reconstructive surgery for pelvic organ prolapse. In: Wein AJ, Kavoussi LR, Novick AC, Partin AW, Peters CA (eds) Campbell-Walsh urology, 10th edn. Elsevier, Philadelphia

Wu JM, Hundley AF, Fulton RG, Myers ER (2009) Forecasting the prevalence of pelvic floor disorders in U.S. Women: 2010 to 2050. Obstet Gynecol 114(6):1278–1283. doi:10.1097/AOG.0b013e3181c2ce96

Zebede S, Smith AL, Plowright LN, Hegde A, Aguilar VC, Davila GW (2013) Obliterative LeFort colpocleisis in a large group of elderly women. Obstet Gynecol 121(2):279–284, doi:http://10.1097/AOG.0b013e31827d8fdb

Diagnosis and Management of Localized Prostate Cancer

Pamela M. Jones and Jason Hafron

Contents

Objectives

1. Discuss the diagnosis and incidence of localized prostate cancer.
2. Review screening and staging of prostate cancer.
3. Discuss treatment options in localized prostate cancer.

P.M. Jones, FNP-C (✉)
Advanced Prostate Cancer Clinic, Michigan Institute of Urology, St Clair Shores, MI, USA
e-mail: JonesP@michiganurology.com

J. Hafron, MD
Department of Urology, Beaumont Health System, Royal Oak, MI, USA

© Springer International Publishing Switzerland 2016
M. Lajiness, S. Quallich (eds.), *The Nurse Practitioner in Urology*,
DOI 10.1007/978-3-319-28743-0_16

Keywords/Definitions

The prostate gland is a small, smooth exocrine gland that surrounds the urethra. It is located inferior to the bladder and anterior to the rectum. The purpose of the prostate is to secrete seminal fluid to protect the sperm from the acidity of the vaginal tract during reproduction.

The prostate-specific antigen (PSA) test is a serum test used for screening for prostate cancer and other prostate abnormalities. PSA is a protein enzyme produced by the prostate gland to liquefy semen. PSA levels are low in men with healthy prostates.

The Gleason score (GS) is the standard grading system for prostate cancer based on pathologic tissue evaluation obtained from a prostate biopsy or prostate surgery. The tissue is graded based on the glandular structure or pattern as it appears under the microscope. The two most common patterns (the predominant one is primary) are added to obtain the Gleason score (sum).

Incidence and Epidemiology

Prostate cancer is the most common noncutaneous cancer in American men (Cooperberg et al. 2013). The American Cancer Society (ACS) projects that 1 out of 7, or 220,000, men will be diagnosed with prostate cancer annually. Second to lung cancer, prostate cancer is the leading cause of death in American men, with more than 26,000 deaths expected in 2016. The prevalence of prostate cancer increases with age. The risk of a prostate cancer diagnosis for men aged 65 and older is about 60 % (ACS 2016). The number of prostate cancer diagnoses far exceeds the mortality rate due to increased screening, diagnosis, and improvements in treatment. The explanation of the improvement in mortality rates is not without controversy, and significant rates of overdiagnosis and overtreatment are present (Cooperberg et al. 2013).

The anatomy of the prostate gland is divided into three distinct zones: peripheral, central, and transition The peripheral zone consists of 70 % of the glandular tissue and is the most common site of prostate cancer. It is palpated during a digital rectal examination (DRE). The central zone contains the ejaculatory ducts and contributes about 25 % of the glandular tissue. It is a rare site for prostate cancer. The transition zone consists of 5 % of the glandular tissue, but about 15 % of prostate cancers originate in this zone. The transition zone of the prostate is mostly known as the area in which benign prostatic hyperplasia (BPH) develops (Kampel 2013). Most prostate cancers are multifocal and involve multiple zones of the prostate.

Prostate cancer develops when the rates of cell division and cell death are no longer equal, leading to uncontrolled tumor growth. Following the initial transformation event, further mutations of a multitude of genes, including the genes for PTEN and p53, can lead to tumor progression and metastasis. Most prostate cancers (95 %) are adenocarcinomas.

History/Presentation

The majority of early prostate cancers are identified in patients who are asymptomatic, as result of the prevalent use of PSA screening and digital rectal exams. Genitourinary symptoms such as frequency, urgency, nocturia, incomplete emptying, and hesitancy are more commonly related to BPH, prostatitis, and other benign conditions; these symptoms are rarely those of prostate cancer due to local growth of the prostate tumor into the urethra or bladder. It is also common for both BPH and prostate cancer to occur simultaneously. Until otherwise proven, for older men who present with urinary symptoms, prostate cancer remains in the differential for diagnosis.

PSA screening was initiated in the 1980s, and its use peaked in the 1990s. The controversy of overdiagnosis and overtreatment remains despite the fact more sensitive tests and techniques are being developed to detect which prostate cancers need to be treated and which diseases will likely remain latent. Although research continues, PSA screening remains a mainstay for the detection of prostate cancer. The controversy regarding the timing of PSA screening continues to vary and evolve among many medical organizations (see Chap. 22).

Risk Factors

The cause of prostate cancer is not clearly understood. However, there are multiple risk factors associated with it. The leading risk factors are age, race, and family history. Dietary, environmental, genetic, and hormones are other factors also reported to increase the risk of prostate cancer, with varying levels of reported evidence. Age is a significant risk factor for development of prostate cancer. Autopsy studies have revealed a high prevalence of premalignant (high-grade prostatic intraepithelial neoplasia [HGPIN]) and malignant disease (mostly low grade) starting in the third and fourth decade of life and increasing steadily thereafter (Sakr and Partin 2001). Prostate adenocarcinoma prevalence significantly increases from the fifth decade onward, with a 1-in-3 chance of carrying incidental cancer in the 60- to 69-year-old age group and with 46 % of 70- to 81-year-old men harboring prostate cancer (Yin et al. 2008).

The prevalence rates of prostate cancer remain significantly higher in African-American men than in white men, while the prevalence in Hispanic men is similar to that of white men. The prevalence in men of Asian origin is lower than that of whites. Although mortality rates are continuing to decline among white and African-American men, mortality rates in African-American men remain more than twice as high as in any other racial group. There are possible etiologies for the noted disparity in prostate cancer mortality. Some data reveals that African-American men tend to present with prostate cancer at a younger age, higher prostate cancer grade and more advanced in stage. Therefore, the higher mortality rate could potentially be due to more advanced disease at the time of diagnosis, i.e., stage migration (Zagars et al. 1998). The explanation for racial stage migration includes disparities in socioeconomic status leading to less access to health care and PSA screening, as well as racial differences in tumor biology, possibly attributable to dissimilarity in dietary, hormonal, or molecular factors leading to more aggressive tumors (Morton 1994; Powell 1998).

A family history of prostate cancer presents as a hereditary risk factor for this disease. Men with a family history of prostate cancer in one or more first-degree relatives have a higher risk of developing prostate cancer and are also likely to present 6–7 years earlier. Genetic studies suggest that a strong familial predisposition may be responsible for as many as 5–10 % of prostate cancer cases. Several reports have suggested a shared familial risk (inherited or environmental) for prostate cancer. BRCA-2 mutations increase the risk for a more aggressive prostate cancer that develops at a younger age (ACS 2016).

Physical Exam

A complete history and physical examination with a digital rectal exam (DRE) are essential in the assessment of a potential prostate cancer patient. When a DRE is performed, the technique used and the comfort of the patient are important for yielding optimal results from the exam.

In preparation of the exam, the patient should be allowed to urinate, and then properly positioned. The patient should be positioned bent over at the waist with elbows/forearms on the examining table, with the feet shoulder-width apart. The lateral decubitus position on the examining table is also a commonly used position for a DRE. The NP should be prepared with a pair of gloves, lubricant, and tissue for cleanup.

DRE Technique

- Lubricate examining index finger of dominant hand.
- Spread the buttocks apart to take a visual inspection of the gluteal folds, anus, and perineum.
- Tell patient to anticipate touch as gentle pressure is applied to opening of anus.
- Slowly advance finger through sphincter into the rectum.
- Begin the palpation of the prostate at the apex toward the base while including the lateral sulci with finger sweeping from side to side to examine the entire prostate.
- Upon removal of examining finger, make note of any blood.

The physical exam reveals the health status and abnormal findings that may indicate a need for further evaluation. Abnormal DRE findings, such as a firm/hard and very enlarged prostate, induration, and nodularity, are possible indications of prostate cancer (Seidel et al. 2003). The findings above, in addition to DRE abnormalities that include pain, tenderness on exam, enlargement, a boggy prostate, or abnormal findings in the rectum, warrant further evaluation (see Chap. 20). Consideration and appropriate referral should also be given to discovery of swelling, enlarged lymph nodes, back pain, palpable bone pain, weakness, fatigue, or decreased appetite during the history or physical exam. These signs and symptoms could also suggest locally advanced prostate cancer or other malignancies.

Diagnostic Testing

Laboratory Studies

The recommendations for a PSA screening test vary among organizations and are somewhat controversial. The decision to order a PSA test should be discussed with the patient and should be a shared decision between the patient and the health-care provider. The AUA provides a shared decision-making tool to help providers fulfill this standard (see Chap. 22). The decision to perform PSA testing in asymptomatic men is encouraged in patients with risk factors such as African-American race or a family history of prostate cancer. A PSA test such as a DRE should be ordered as a diagnostic tool to further evaluate urinary complaints or abnormal clinical findings. While a PSA test is recommended in the case of abnormal clinical findings, a normal PSA result should not negate further evaluation if prostate cancer is suspected. Again, the range of PSA levels is a continuum of risk, and prostate cancer, albeit small, can be present at low or normal PSA levels.

A PSA result of 2.5 ng/ml or less is considered normal. However, younger men tend to have lower PSA levels than older men. The positive predictive value (PPV) of a PSA 4–10 ng/ml is about 20–30 %, and PSA >10 ng/ml has a PPV of 74 % (Cooperberg et al. 2013). When the PSA level is ≥10 ng/ml, the risk of finding prostate cancer is as high as 60 % (Kampel 2013). Essentially, the higher the PSA, the higher the risk for prostate cancer

Imaging Studies

Multiple imaging studies may be utilized to assist in visualizing the prostate and determining the stage of prostate cancer. The information obtained from these studies is useful when determining treatment options. Imaging studies may also be used to determine an extraprostatic spread of cancer and to evaluate clinical symptoms. The specific imaging tests and rationale for their use will be briefly discussed here.

Transrectal Ultrasound (TRUS) A type of ultrasonography commonly used in guiding prostate biopsies. The prostate is easily visualized on the TRUS and can guide placement of the biopsy needle into each region of the prostate. TRUS is also used to determine the size and volume of the prostate gland. If it is able to detect non-palpable lesions, the visualization may be helpful in the staging and diagnosis of prostate cancer.

Computed Tomography (CT) Scan The cross-sectional imaging of a CT scan may be helpful in revealing organ, bone, and soft tissue details of the abdomen and pelvis. More specifically, the CT scan can identify large or bulky diseases of the prostate, involvement of the bladder, or nodal involvement. Unless contraindicated for a specific patient, the CT scan is performed with IV contrast for enhancement of tissues and lesion detection. Typically, in patients with localized prostate cancer, CT imaging is reserved for high-risk cases (PSA >20 and/or Gleason score >8 and/or T3 disease on DRE) to rule out metastatic disease. The CT scan may also be used for treatment planning, if a patient elects to undergo radiation therapy treatment.

Magnetic Resonance Imaging (MRI) The MRI images are produced using a magnetic field with radio frequency. An MRI is superior to a CT scan when imaging soft tissue, the prostate capsule, and the lymph nodes. Traditionally, an MRI is not utilized in early, localized prostate cancer; however, recently a multiparametric MRI with or without an endorectal coil has been shown to visualize prostate cancer within the prostate gland. Additionally, the fusion of MRI images with TRUS images during biopsy are innovative uses for improvement in the detection of prostate cancer. In these settings, an MRI is used to improve staging, characterization, and risk stratification of the disease to help the clinicians guide therapy.

Bone Scan This nuclear medicine imaging is used to identify disease that has spread to the bone. When prostate cancer metastasizes, the most common site of the spread is to the bone (Box 16.1). Typically, in patients with localized prostate cancer, bone scan imaging is reserved for high-risk (PSA >20 and/or Gleason score >8 and/or T3 disease on DRE) or locally advanced prostate cancer to rule out metastatic disease. Bone scans may also be ordered when a patient develops pain unrelated to the prostate gland itself.

Box 16.1 Common Sites of Prostate Cancer Metastasis (Kampel)
Sites of Spread
- Bones
- Lymph nodes
- Lung
- Liver
- CNS (Brain)

Procedures

A prostate needle biopsy is performed with TRUS guidance and a local anesthetic block to the prostate, commonly in an outpatient setting, either in an office or surgery center. Prior to the biopsy, an enema is usually recommended. Recently, urologists have combined magnetic resonance imaging (MRI) of the prostate with ultrasound to perform an MRI fusion biopsy. MRI fusion biopsies allow the surgeon to target, track, and map the prostate biopsies.

Table 16.1 Side effects/complications of a prostate biopsy

Pain or discomfort	UTI, small risk
Hematuria	Rectal bleeding, small risk
Hematospermia	Fainting immediately following procedure (vasovagal reaction)
Urinary retention	Sepsis (rare)
Fever	

In 2012, Gonzalez et al, renewed the complications and risks related to prostate biopsy. It is important to educate patients on the side effects and the potential complications of this procedure (Table 16.1). Patients should discontinue anticoagulant therapy and nonsteroidal anti-inflammatory medications prior to the biopsy. Antibiotic therapy is required before and after the biopsy procedure. AUA recommends a fluoroquinolone or cephalosporin for prophylaxis. However, the protocol of local practices and flora should guide the choice of antibiotic therapy (AUA 2016, 2008). Patients should also be aware of potential complications (Table 16.1).

When the results of the biopsy are positive for prostate cancer, this pathology and histology along with the PSA, DRE, and imaging results are used to determine the grade and stage of the cancer. This information is necessary in identifying the risk of spread/metastasis. As mentioned earlier in this chapter, most prostate cancers are of adenocarcinoma histology, more specifically acinar-type adenocarcinoma.

Prostate cancer is graded by using the Gleason score or sum (GS). It is graded on a system ranging one, meaning well differentiated, up to five, meaning poorly differentiated. The higher the score, the more likely the tumor will spread. The GS correlates well with the prognosis, stage for stage, however the patient is managed (Albala et al. 2011).

The staging for prostate cancer is identified by using the American Joint Committee on Cancer (AJCC) TNM system. The T (primary tumor), N (nodes), and M (metastatic disease) are determined by clinical and/or pathologic findings. Staging helps identify if the cancer localized, locally advanced, or spread to other areas of the body. TNM staging does not include tumor grade or PSA level (Table 16.2).

Management of Localized Prostate Cancer

Multiple management options are available for newly diagnosed patients with localized prostate cancer. Clinical and pathological characteristics at presentation are important prognostic factors that must be considered when deciding management and treatment options. These characteristics are utilized to determine the relative risk of disease progression for an individual patient upon deciding treatment. Multiple risk instruments are used for prostate cancer. For the purpose of this chapter, the D'Amico risk classification groups (1998), commonly used in the management of prostate cancer, will be illustrated here:

Table 16.2 Anatomic stage/prognostic groups

Group	T	N	M	PSA[a]	Gleason
I	T1a-c	N0	M0	PSA <10	Gleason ≤6
	T1a-c	N0	M0	PSA <20	Gleason 7
	T1a-c	N0	M0	PSA ≥10 but <20	Gleason ≤6
IIA	T2a	N0	M0	PSA <10	Gleason ≤6
	T2a	N0	M0	PSA <20	Gleason ≤7
	T2b	N0	M0	PSA <20	Gleason ≤7
	T2c	N0	M0	Any PSA	Any Gleason
IIB	T1-2	N0	M0	PSA ≥20	Any Gleason
	T1-2	N0	M0	Any PSA	Gleason ≥8
III	T3a-b	N0	M0	Any PSA	Any Gleason
IV	T4	N0	M0	Any PSA	Any Gleason
	Any T	N1	M0	Any PSA	Any Gleason
	Any T	Any N	M1	Any PSA	Any Gleason

Source: American Joint Committee on Cancer, *Prostate Cancer Staging* (7th ed.), American Joint Committee on Cancer, Web
[a]If PSA or Gleason is not available, grouping should be determined by T stage and/or either PSA or Gleason, as available

- Low risk: PSA ≤10 ng/ml, Gleason ≤6, and stage T1 or T2a
- Intermediate risk: PSA 10–20 ng/ml, Gleason 7, or clinical stage T2b
- High risk: PSA >20 ng/ml, Gleason 8–10, or clinical stage T2c or T3a

Management options for localized prostate cancer range from conservative to aggressive. The best treatment options should be clearly presented to each prostate cancer patient. This will require consultation with other clinical specialists, including radiation oncologists and medical oncologists. In certain cases, management of prostate cancer may involve multiple modalities of treatment.

Watchful waiting is an option in which the decision is not to forgo definitive prostate cancer treatment at the time of diagnosis. This is the most conservative option. Patients with severe health risks due to comorbidities and/or limited life expectancy are cases when this option is a consideration. This option may be without routine follow-up.

Active surveillance is another option where definitive treatment is not received at the time of diagnosis. This option is usually considered for certain low- and intermediate-risk prostate cancer patients. These patients are "actively" and carefully followed with PSA level tests, DREs, and biopsies according to clinical guidelines and protocols. These patients are treated accordingly when there are signs of progression. Although between 20 and 41 % of the patients on this regimen may require treatment at 3–5 years following the diagnosis, for most patients, treatment at progression appears to be as effective as it would have been if delivered at the time of diagnosis (Cooperberg et al. 2013), although more costly in total.

Radiation therapy (RT) is an outpatient option for definitive treatment for prostate cancer. Like surgery, radiation therapy has multiple techniques and has advanced over the years. Radiotherapy is a commonly used modality for localized prostate cancer. Each radiation modality has a clinical indication for use. Complications and side effects are a result of the toxicity effects from the radiation on normal tissue in the treatment field. These acute (short-term) or late (≥ 3 months after RT is completed) toxicity effects usually occur three weeks into the treatment course but may occur sooner. These are similar to each RT modality, with varying intensity based on dose, treatment field, and modality.

External beam radiotherapy (EBRT) is the least invasive form of radiation for prostate cancer treatment. It is indicated for low-, intermediate-, and high-risk groups (Hansen and Roach, 2007). EBRT is delivered via X-rays using photon and more recently proton energies. Improved treatment planning and imaging involves three-dimensional conformal radiotherapy (3DCRT) and intensity-modulated radiation therapy. These techniques have allowed for improvement in targeting and shaping volumes, which permits higher doses to the prostate, involving less of the surrounding tissue and decreasing acute and late toxicities. Hyperfractionation is delivered in more fractions (treatments) with a lower dose per fraction. Hypofractionation is delivered in fewer fractions with a higher dose per fraction. EBRT usually begins one week after an hour planning session (simulation). It is delivered in daily fractions five days per week up to approximately nine weeks depending on the prescribed dose or whether it is hyperfractionated versus hypofractionated.

Brachytherapy is an interstitial radiation therapy technique where radioactive seeds are implanted directly into the prostate, with TRUS guidance. The radioactive seeds are deposited into the tissues using a robotic device preloaded with tiny catheters/tubes. Patients are not radioactive at completion of brachytherapy treatment. There are low-dose-rate (LDR) and high-dose-rate (HDR) brachytherapy techniques. The HDR technique will be the focus in this section. This is a minimal invasive treatment requiring spinal anesthesia and a potential overnight stay in the hospital. HDR brachytherapy alone (monotherapy) or in combination with EBRT are the two forms of brachytherapy commonly used. HDR alone is indicated for low- and intermediate-risk groups. It can be delivered in two implants a week apart with two fractions/treatments each or as one implant with two fractions. Single-fraction HDR brachytherapy is being studied currently.

Combined HDR/EBRT is indicated for intermediate- and high-risk groups. The HDR dose per fraction is less than in monotherapy. Patients receiving this modality undergo two implants one week apart, each with two HDR treatments, along with a 4–5 week course of EBRT (Table 16.3).

Surgery

Surgery for prostate cancer involves the removal of the entire prostate gland and the seminal vesicles. The pelvic lymph nodes will only be removed if the preoperative risk of lymphatic spread is high enough to warrant surgical resection. Preoperative

Table 16.3 Radiation therapy modalities with acute/late toxicities

Modality	Acute toxicities	Late toxicities
EBRT	Frequency, nocturia, urgency, dysuria, frequency BMs, diarrhea, rectal urgency and irritation, urinary retention (rare), fatigue	Dysuria, frequency, urgency, hematuria d/t RT cystitis, urethral stricture, diarrhea, rectal urgency, rectal bleeding, d/t proctitis, gradual ED (>30 %) at 5 years
Brachytherapy/HDR	Frequency; urgency; dysuria; urinary retention; diarrhea; rectal frequency, urgency, and spasms; perineal hematoma	Urethral stricture, retention, incontinence, cystitis, proctitis, ED (40 %) 5 years
Combined EBRT/HDR	No significant changes as toxicities are similar to those of single modality	No significant changes as toxicities are similar to those of single modality

risk is based on preoperative nomograms or published risk tables. The goals of surgical resection are to remove all of the prostate cancer while preserving the urethral sphincter and the cavernous nerves if the man is potent. The decision for surgery is based on the patient's overall life expectancy, comorbidities, prostate cancer risk, and previous surgical history. Generally, surgery is reserved for men under 70 years of age and in overall good health. The current techniques to remove the prostate include open radical retropubic prostatectomy, laparoscopic radical prostatectomy, robotic-assisted laparoscopic radical prostatectomy, and radical perineal prostatectomy. The decision to utilize any of these techniques is based on the patients' body habitus, surgical history, and the surgeons' experience.

Open radical retropubic prostatectomy is the traditional method for removal of the prostate gland. The procedure is performed through a mid-line infraumbilical incision under general or spinal anesthesia. The procedure commonly takes 3–4 h and requires 1–2 day hospitalization. Patients will have a Foley catheter in their bladders for 7–14 days. Common side effects of the procedure include urinary incontinence, erectile dysfunction, and bleeding.

Robotic-assisted laparoscopic radical prostatectomy is a minimally invasive approach performed through small incisions, with a robotic interface used to perform the procedure. Robotic surgery affords the surgeon outstanding surgical vision and computer-assisted movement. Patients have less abdominal trauma due to smaller incisions and most will have less pain compared with open surgery. Additionally, blood loss is less with robotic surgery. Patients will require general anesthesia and remain in the hospital for one night and require a Foley catheter for seven days. Side effects may include urinary incontinence, erectile dysfunction, and urethral strictures.

Laparoscopic radical prostatectomy is the same approach as a robotic prostatectomy without a robotic interface between the patient and surgeon. The outcomes and side effects are similar to the robotic-assisted laparoscopic radical prostatectomy.

Radical perineal prostatectomy involves removal of the prostate through an incision made through the perineum. The recovery time after this surgery may be shorter than with the open radical retropubic approach. Outcomes and side effects are similar to other approaches, with the exception of preservation of erectile function. The maintenance of erectile function following perineal prostatectomy is limited.

Cryosurgery involves the freezing of the whole prostate gland or focal areas to lethal cell kill temperatures. The procedure is typically performed using small probes that are placed under transrectal ultrasound guidance through the perineum into the prostate. During treatment, the surgeon can monitor the ice ball to ensure it encompasses the entire prostate. Common side effects include urinary symptoms, hematuria, erectile dysfunction, and (rarely) rectal injuries.

Follow-up for all procedures requires scheduled PSA testing generally every six months. Following surgery it is expected for the PSA to return to zero. If the PSA does not return to zero or rises above zero, unresected or recurrent prostate cancer should be suspected. However, following radiation or cryosurgery, the PSA will reach a nadir that is above zero. In these patients, significant rises from the PSA nadir indicate recurrent prostate cancer. Usually the urologist will obtain a bone scan and CT scan and consider a prostate biopsy to determine the location of the recurrent prostate cancer at that point.

Additionally, the patients return of erectile function and continence is closely monitored following any treatment. If a preoperative potent patient underwent a nerve-sparing surgical procedure, penile rehabilitation programs are helpful. Typically, these programs encourage sexual activity with the use of pharmacother apy and therapeutic devices. Frequently, patients will be placed on a scheduled dose of phosphodiesterase inhibitor. Lastly, patients are encouraged to perform Kegel exercises and often are referred for pelvic floor physical therapy if available to help restore urinary continence. Patient support and encouragement are critical especially at the early stages of recovery.

Clinical Pearls
1. The use of an antibiotic prior to removal of a catheter following prostatectomy maybe helpful.
2. Handouts on what to expect during and after the surgery help alleviate anxiety. Include
   (a) Length of surgery
   (b) Length of hospitalization
   (c) Catheter removal date
   (d) Follow-up date
   (e) Medications that will be prescribed routinely post-op (pd5 inhibitors)
   (f) Kegel exercises how and when to do

Resources for the Nurse Practitioner
AUA Guideline for the Management of Clinically Localized Prostate Cancer (2007)
http://www.auanet.org/education/guidelines/prostate-cancer.cfm
http://urologyhealth.org//Documents/Product%20Store/Prostate-Cancer-
Screening-Checklist-Foundation-English.pdf

Resources for the Patient
ustoo.org. A nonprofit organization established in 1990 that serves as a resource of
volunteers, with peer-to-peer support and educational materials to help men and
their families/caregivers make informed decisions about prostate cancer detection, treatment options, and related side effects.
cancer.org. The official website of the American Cancer Society. The website contains information and resources for patients and families with prostate cancer.
http://www.urologyhealth.org/Documents/Product%20Store/Localized-Prostate-
Cancer.pdf
http://www.urologyhealth.org/Documents/Product%20Store/Surgery-for-Prostate-
Cancer-Fact-Sheet.pdf

References

Albala DM, Morey AF, Gomella LG, Stein JP (2011) Oxford American handbook of urology.
Oxford University Press, New York, pp 190–221. Print
American Cancer Society (2016) Cancer facts & figures for prostate cancer. Am Cancer Soc. Web
American Urological Association (2008) Best practice policy statement on urologic surgery anti-
microbial prophylaxis. American Urological Association Education and Research.
American Urological Association (2016) AUA white paper on implementation of shared decision
making into urological practice. American Urological Association Education and Research,
Inc. Web
Cooperberg MR et al (2013) Neoplasms of the prostate gland. In: McAninch JW, Lue TF (eds)
Smith & Tanagho's general urology, 18th edn. McGraw-Hill Co., New York, pp 357–370.
Federle MP, Rosado-de-Christenson ML, Woodward PJ, Abbott GF (2007) Diagnostic and
surgical imaging anatomy. Salt Lake City. Print
D'Amico AV et al (1998) Biochemical outcome after radical prostatectomy, external beam radia-
tion therapy, or interstitial radiation therapy for clinically localized prostate cancer. JAMA
280(1998):969–974. Web
Gonzalez CM et al (2012) AUA/SUNA white paper on the incidence, prevention and treatment of
complications related to prostate needle biopsy. American Urological Association. 2012. Web
Hansen EK, Roach M (2007) Handbook of evidence-based radiation oncology. Springer,
New York, pp 293–311. Print
Kampel LJ (2013) Dx/Rx: prostate cancer, 2nd edn. Jones & Bartlett Learning, Burlington,
pp 3–134. Print
Morton RA (1994) Racial differences in adenocarcinoma of the prostate in North American men.
Urology 44:637–645. Print
Powell IJ (1998) Prostate cancer in the African American: is this a different disease? Semin Urol
Oncol 16:221–226. Print

Sakr W, Partin AW (2001) Histological markers of risk and the role of high-grade prostatic intraepithelial neoplasia. Urology 57(1):115–120. Print

Seidel HM, Ball JW, Dains JE, Benedict GW (2003) Mosby's guide to physical examination, 5th
edn. Mosby, Inc. St. Louis, pp 675–693. Print

Yin MI, Bastacky S, Chandran U, Becich MJ, Dhir R (2008) Prevalence of incidental prostate
cancer in the general population: a study of healthy organ donors. J Urol 179(3):892–895. Web

Zagars GK, Pollack A, Pettaway CA (1998) Prostate cancer in African-American men: outcome
following radiation therapy with or without adjuvant androgen ablation. Int J Radiat Oncol Biol
Phys 42(5):17–523. Print

Urothelial Carcinoma: Cancer of the Bladder, Ureters, and Urethra

17

Staci Mitchell and Julie Derossett

Contents

S. Mitchell, MSN, FNP-BC (✉)
Department of Urology, University of Michigan Health System, Ann Arbor, MI, USA
e-mail: stacilin@med.umich.edu

J. Derossett, BSN, RN
Division of Cancer Center Urology, Department of Urology,
University of Michigan Health System, Ann Arbor, MI, USA

© Springer International Publishing Switzerland 2016
M. Lajiness, S. Quallich (eds.), *The Nurse Practitioner in Urology*,
DOI 10.1007/978-3-319-28743-0_17

Objectives
1. Explain the diagnosis, assessment, and management of urothelial carcinoma.
2. Identify the incidence, risk factors, and signs and symptoms associated with cancer of the bladder, ureters, and urethra.
3. Discuss the pathology, staging, and diagnostic evaluation of urothelial carcinoma.
4. Review management of urothelial carcinoma.

Overview

Urothelial carcinoma is defined as the abnormal division of cells within the layers of tissue or urothelium of the renal pelvis, bladder, ureters, and urethra. Cancer of the bladder, ureters, and urethra most commonly are misdiagnosed as urinary tract infections or nephrolithiasis. Patients are given multiple courses of antibiotics and/ or pain medication without resolution of their symptoms. Diagnosis and management of the disease is delayed, with risk of disease progression.

Incidence

Bladder Cancer

In 2015, it is estimated that there will be 74,000 new cases of bladder cancer and an estimated 16,000 people will die from this disease (Surveillance, Epidemiology, and End Results [SEER] 2015). Bladder cancer represents 4.5 % of all new cases in the United States. In 2012, there were an estimated 577,403 people living with bladder cancer in the United States. It is the second most common urologic cancer and has the highest recurrence rate of any cancer. With advancing age, bladder cancer is more common in men than women, with a median age at diagnosis of 73. Bladder cancer is most frequently diagnosed among people aged 75–84, with the highest mortality among this group as well.

When comparing race, more Caucasian Americans are diagnosed with bladder cancer than African Americans and more Asian Americans than American Indians and Hispanic Americans. There are a higher percentage of Caucasian men (39.0 %) than African American men (21.4 %) diagnosed with bladder cancer in the United States. There is a higher incidence of bladder cancer in Caucasian women (9.4 %) than in African American women (6.9 %).

Bladder cancer is the ninth leading cause of cancer death in the United States. There are 3.9 % deaths in people ranging in age from 45 to 54, 11.7 % in people 55–64, 20.7 % in people 65–74, 21.1 % in people between the ages of 75–84, and 33.7 % in people over the age of 80 (SEER 2015). The median age at death is 79. The percentage of people diagnosed with bladder cancer surviving 5 years is 77.4 %,

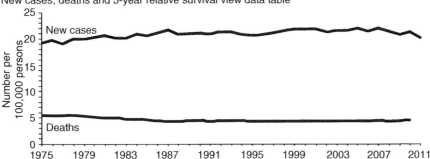

New cases, deaths and 5-year relative survival view data table

Fig. 17.1 Changes over time. Keeping track of the number of new cases, deaths, and survival over time (trends) can help scientists understand whether progress is being made and where additional research is needed to address challenges, such as improving screening or finding better treatments. Using statistical models for analysis, rates for new bladder cancer cases have been falling on average 0.6 % each year over 2002–2011. Death rates have been stable over 2001–2010. 5-year survival trends are shown below the figure. http://seer.cancer.gov/statifacts/html/ur.nb.html

and this 5-year relative survival rate has increased over the last 30 years. In 1975, the percentage of people diagnosed with bladder cancer surviving 5 years was 71.5 % compared to 80.6 % in 2006. The 5-year survival rate also depends upon the cancer stage or extent of disease at the time of diagnosis. The highest 5-year survival rate is those diagnosed with cancer in the originating layer of cells of the bladder or in situ (95.9 %) as compared to localized bladder cancer, confined to the primary site (69.2 %). When bladder cancer spreads outside of the bladder to the regional lymph nodes, the 5-year survival rate decreases to 34.0 % and dramatically decreases to 5.4 % when the cancer is staged at distant or has metastasized to other organs (Fig. 17.1).

Ureteral Cancer

The incidence of cancer within the upper tracts (renal pelvis and ureter) is much lower, is more common in people older than 65, and accounts for about 5 % of all cancers of the kidney and upper urinary tract. According to cancer surveillance reports published from SEER (2014), there were 1333 people diagnosed with ureteral cancer between 1988 and 2001 in the United States, and 808 were male compared to 525 female. There were 1158 Caucasian Americans compared to 42 African Americans diagnosed with ureteral cancer.

The most common type of cancer that originates within the kidney in adults is renal cell carcinoma (RCC) (85 %). Transitional cell carcinoma (TCC) is the most common type of cancer of the renal pelvis and ureter. The prognosis of upper tract cancer is directly related to the stage at diagnosis (Table 17.1). The recurrence of bladder cancer after treatment for renal pelvis or ureteral cancer occurs in 30–50 % of cases (SEER 2014).

Table 17.1 Renal pelvis and ureter cancer

Stage	Survival rate (%)
Localized, low grade, no invasion beyond lamina propria	100
Localized, grades I–III, without subepithelial invasion	80
Localized, high grade with infiltration of pelvic wall	20–30
Regional, extension beyond renal pelvis	5

Adapted from SEER (2014)

Urethral Cancer

Primary urethral cancer is extremely rare, with fewer than 2000 cases reported and less than 1 % of the total incidence of malignancies (Guidos et al. 2014). At the time of diagnosis, the disease is usually advanced, making it difficult to distinguish between primary urethral cancer and locally advanced urothelial carcinoma of the bladder.

African Americans are twice as likely than Caucasians to develop primary urethral carcinoma. The SEER database reports that the majority of primary urethral cancers (55–77.6 %) are urothelial (transitional cell) carcinoma. Other histology types reported include squamous cell carcinoma (11.9–21.5 %), adenocarcinoma (5–16.4 %), and rare cases of melanoma. The incidence of urethral cancer increases with age, with the majority of cases diagnosed at age 75 or older (Swartz et al. 2006).

Anatomy and Physiology

The wall of the bladder has four main layers. The innermost lining is comprised of cells called urothelial or transitional cells, known as urothelium or transitional epithelium. Beneath the urothelium is a thin layer of connective tissue, blood vessels, and nerves, the lamina propria. The next layer is the muscle of the bladder, the muscularis propria. Outside of this muscle is a layer of fatty connective tissue that separates the bladder from other organs.

The types of bladder cancer are identified by the layers, or cells, in which the cancer originates and the depth of invasion. Transitional cell (urothelial) carcinoma (TCC) is the most common type of bladder cancer and originates in the innermost lining of the bladder. TCC has the appearance of urothelial cells that line the inside of the bladder; urothelial cells also line the renal pelvis, ureters, and urethra, meaning TCC can occur at any site along the ureter or renal pelvis. Transitional cell carcinoma is classified further based on depth of invasion and subtype (Table 17.2).

Table 17.2 Classifications of bladder cancer

Type	Description	
Transitional cell (urothelial) carcinoma (TCC)	Most common type of bladder cancer Originates in the innermost lining of bladder. Urothelial cells line the renal pelvis, ureters, and urethra; TCC can also occur in these organs	*Noninvasive*: remained in the inner lining (transitional epithelium) *Invasive*: grown into the lamina propria or into the muscularis propria *Superficial or non-muscle-invasive*: describe noninvasive tumors as well as invasive tumors that have grown into the lamina propria but not the muscularis propria *Papillary carcinoma*: grows in stalk-like formations toward the center of the bladder. Appear to resemble stalks of cauliflower, but do not extend into the deeper layers. Called noninvasive papillary carcinoma *Papillary urothelial neoplasm of low malignant potential (PUNLUMP)*: very low grade and noninvasive; appear at lateral posterior wall of the bladder and ureteric orifices. Rarely associated with invasion or metastasis and have a good prognosis *Flat carcinomas*: do not grow toward the center of bladder and remain in the inner layer. Also called noninvasive flat carcinoma or flat carcinoma in situ (CIS)
Squamous cell carcinoma (SCC)	1–2 % of bladder cancers are squamous cell carcinoma and nearly all are invasive Associated with squamous metaplasia May occur at multiple areas of the bladder, most commonly found at lateral wall and trigone On cystoscopy, the tumor appears nodular and has a plaque-like, irregular surface. Most of the tumors are large, exophytic, and necrotic and bulge into the bladder cavity Having bladder diverticula may increase likelihood of developing SCC	
Adenocarcinoma	Rare Accounts for 0.5–2 % of all bladder cancers Higher rate of extravesical disease as compared to urothelial carcinoma Tumor often appears as a solitary lesion and has a tendency for local invasion, and the symptoms appear late	
Small cell carcinoma	Aggressive, poorly differentiated neuroendocrine neoplasm similar to small cell carcinoma of the lung Rare, accounting for <500 new cases annually Can involve any area of the bladder; most common sites are lateral wall and bladder dome	

(continued)

Table 17.2 (continued)

Type	Description
Sarcoma	Malignant mesenchymal tumor that is rare 50 % of bladder sarcomas are leiomyosarcomas, and ~ 20 % are rhabdomyosarcomas May be present in any region of the bladder, but most commonly identified in the trigone or fundus
Carcinosarcoma and sarcomatoid carcinoma	Rare and highly aggressive Sarcomatoid carcinomas of the bladder are primarily spindle cell tumors with epithelial differentiation, most commonly urothelial
Lymphoepithelioma-like carcinoma	Rare epithelial tumor characterized by lymphoid infiltrate suggestive of lymphoma Typically muscle-invasive at time of diagnosis Appears to have a better prognosis than other primary bladder cancers

Nonurothelial bladder cancers are rare and more aggressive than TCC. Presenting symptoms of nonurothelial bladder cancer appear late and tend to indicate an invasive and more advanced diagnosis, with a poor prognosis. Nonurothelial bladder cancers are further classified as epithelial or nonepithelial. According to Hayes and Gilligan (2014), approximately 90 % of these cancers are epithelial in origin, including squamous cell carcinomas (SCCs), adenocarcinomas, and small cell (neuroendocrine) tumors. Nonepithelial cancers are rare and include sarcomas, carcinosarcomas, sarcomatoid cancers, paragangliomas, pheochromocytomas, primary bladder melanomas, and lymphomas. Melanoma and lymphoma are the most common cancers that metastasize to the bladder. Cancer from the colon, rectum, prostate, or uterus can extend directly into the bladder.

Risk Factors

Urothelial carcinoma is associated with several risk factors: smoking, environmental/chemical exposures, chronic urinary tract infections, and family history of bladder cancer. Smoking is the primary risk factor, and former smokers are twice as likely to develop bladder cancer as those who never smoked, while current smokers are four times more likely (National Institutes of Health [NIH] 2014). Smokers are four times as likely to develop transitional cell kidney and ureter cancer as nonsmokers.

Workplace exposure is associated with an increased risk as well. Industrial chemicals such as aromatic amines, benzidine, and beta-naphthylamine along with rubber, leather, textiles, and paint products have been linked to urothelial carcinoma. Hairdressers, painters, machinists, printers, truck drivers (diesel fumes), and firefighters (chemical/foam fire retardants) are at risk due to exposure to chemicals on the job. Urothelial carcinoma is also commonly identified in populations living near factories, chemical plants, and highly industrialized areas. Chronic overuse of analgesic medications (analgesic nephropathy) has also been associated with upper tract urothelial carcinoma.

Chronic urinary tract irritants such as bacterial infections, foreign bodies (recurrent bladder calculi, catheters), and chronic outlet obstruction have been associated with a higher incidence of developing urothelial carcinoma. The use of chronic indwelling catheters in patients with spinal cord injury has been associated with urothelial malignancies. A population-based retrospective analysis of spinal cord-injured patients conducted by West et al. (1999) concluded that squamous cell carcinoma was more common in spinal cord-injured patients with indwelling urethral catheters and suprapubic catheters (42 %) than those using clean intermittent catheterization, condom catheterization, or spontaneous voiding (19 %).

Additional studies have cited other etiologies specifically identified for cancer of the urethra. Wiener et al. (1992) demonstrated HPV DNA in 4 (29 %) of 14 cases of primary urethral cancer. Kaplan et al. (1967) found that 37 % of males with urethral cancer had some history of venereal disease.

Specific Risk Factors to Assess

- Smoking: Assess type of tobacco used (cigarette, cigar, e cigarettes, chewing tobacco, snuff), number of years smoked, number of packs per day, and date of cessation for former smokers.
- Chemicals in the workplace: Assess for environmental exposures of current and former places of residence; people that live in highly industrialized areas have a higher risk.
- People who have had bladder cancer have a greater risk for getting the disease again.
- People with family members who have had bladder cancer can have a slightly greater chance of getting the disease.
- Bladder cancer is more common in people aged 55 and older.
- Bladder cancer is more common in men than women.
- Lifelong bladder irritation and infections: People who have had multiple bladder infections are at greater risk for bladder cancer. This includes a history of urinary retention requiring an indwelling catheter or the need for intermittent self-catheterization.
- Low fluid intake may add to the risk.
- Arsenic is a poison that raises the risk of bladder cancer. In some parts of the world, arsenic may be found at high levels in drinking water; the chance of exposure in the United States depends on location and whether water is from a well or a sanitation system.

History

A complete and through history is crucial in the diagnosis of urothelial carcinoma. Identifying risk factors and assessment of signs and symptoms will be helpful in guiding diagnostic evaluation and the evaluation of differential diagnosis.

Medical History A complete medical history is necessary to evaluate for prescribing medications, diagnostic testing, and treatment planning. Especially important to note is any previous radiation to the abdomen and pelvis.

Surgical History A history of previous procedures and/or surgeries, especially of the urinary system and to the abdomen and pelvis, will help in treatment planning.

Medication History A thorough medication history is necessary to evaluate for drug interactions and contributes to a differential diagnosis. Note the use of anticoagulation medications, nicotine gum/patch, testosterone replacement in men, and previous antibiotic.

Allergies Especially important is noting allergies to antibiotics and IV contrast.

Social History A complete social history should include alcohol use (amount and type), illicit drug use (amount and type), support system, and home environment. Baseline sexual function is also important to note.

Clinical Presentation The assessment of each symptom should include duration, frequency, severity, intermittent or chronic; and treatments utilized. Urothelial carcinoma can mimic other conditions (Table 17.3).

Physical Examination

A complete head-to-toe physical examination should be performed. Abdominal exam should focus on any potential enlargement of the spleen or liver, masses and tenderness with direct palpation, and/or suprapubic pain. Females need a pelvic and rectal exam to assess for mass and fullness. Males need a complete genitourinary exam including the penis, meatus, scrotum, testis, epididymis, and rectum including prostate to assess for nodules and mass/fullness of rectal wall. Both men and women should have palpation for lateral inguinal lymph nodes and direct palpation of sites of skeletal pain.

Baseline performance status may also be assessed, with a tool such as the Eastern Cooperative Oncology Group (ECOG) performance status measure (Oken et al. 1982). These will help to assess the patient's disease progression, assess how the disease affects the daily living abilities of the patient, and determine appropriate treatment and prognosis.

Table 17.3 Symptom assessment

Signs and symptoms that can be associated with urothelial carcinoma	Signs and symptoms that can be associated with urothelial carcinoma *of the urethra*	Symptoms of advanced (metastatic) disease
Fever, chills, sweats, nausea/vomiting Gross hematuria (visible blood in the urine): most common sign; usually painless and should never be ignored Clots and/or tissue within the urine Microscopic hematuria Lower urinary tract symptoms (LUTS): frequency, urgency, nocturia, and dysuria (pain or burning) Incomplete emptying of the bladder Urinary incontinence Back/flank pain (upper tract carcinoma) Abdominal/pelvic pain Urethral discharge	Diminished stream, straining to void Frequency, nocturia, itching, dysuria (most commonly reported with carcinoma in situ) Urinary retention from progressive urethral stricture disease Hematuria, urethral or vaginal spotting Purulent, foul smelling, or watery discharge Hematospermia Perineal, suprapubic, or urethral pain Dyspareunia Swelling Tenesmus Priapism No symptoms except for findings on physical exam including hard nodule in the perineum, labia, or along the shaft of the penis	Unexplained weight loss Loss of appetite Fatigue New skeletal pain Chest pain/shortness of breath Cachexia

Box 17.1 Clues on Physical Examination

Abnormal physical exam findings that may be associated with bladder cancer and/or metastatic disease

Unintentional weight loss, especially over a short period of time	Palpable pelvic/rectal fullness/mass
Changes of cognition, mood, affect	Palpable urethral mass: men and women
Palpable enlarged cervical, supraclavicular lymph nodes, and/or inguinal lymph nodes	Lower extremity edema: can be an indicator of deep vein thrombosis (DVT). Unilateral edema can be an indicator of metastatic disease
Pain with direct palpation of vertebral bodies, bilateral ribs, pelvis, bilateral hips, and thighs	Declining performance status, especially a rapid decline
Palpable abdominal mass	*Men:* palpable prostatic nodules (possible prostate cancer), scrotal/testis mass

Diagnosis

There are alternative diagnoses that can mimic bladder cancer (Box 17.2). Gross or microscopic hematuria is often treated like a urinary tract infection or nephrolithiasis; multiple courses of antibiotics or pain medications may have been prescribed without a full evaluation for urothelial carcinoma. Never assume hematuria is a urinary tract infection.

Urothelial Carcinoma of the Upper Tracts Transitional cell (TCC) or urothelial carcinoma of the renal pelvis and ureters is the most common type of cancer that affects the upper tracts. Approximately 10 % are squamous cell carcinomas. A primary tumor within the bladder can involve the ureteric orifice and extend into the ureter.

After definitive treatment of carcinoma within the bladder, there is a high recurrence rate of urothelial carcinoma within the upper tracts. Thirty to fifty percent of patients with cancer of the upper tracts have or will have bladder cancer.

Urothelial Carcinoma of the Urethra Urethral carcinoma is characterized by unique anatomic and histologic differences between males and females. The average male urethra is 21 cm and divided into anterior and posterior components. The shorter female urethra is approximately 4 cm with less complex anatomy. In both men and women, the histologic pattern of the urethral mucosa progresses from transitional epithelium to squamous epithelium as it continues distally. The mucosal cells of the urethra are replaced at a rapid rate which can lead to dysplasia and neoplasia; these mucosal cells histologically classify urethral cancer as TCC or adenocarcinoma secondary to metaplasia (Guidos et al. 2014). Inflammation, infection, and irritation may also impede the natural DNA repair mechanisms of the urethral mucosal cells (Guidos et al. 2014).

The most common sites of tumor invasion in females are the labia, vagina, and bladder neck. In males, the most common sites of extension are the vascular spaces of the corpora and periurethral tissues, deep tissues of the perineum, urogenital

---

Box 17.2 Diagnoses That Can Mimic Urothelial Carcinoma

Urinary tract infection (UTI)

Nephrolithiasis

Hemorrhagic cystitis: noninfectious (history of radiation to the pelvis)

Renal cell carcinoma

Overactive bladder

Benign stricture disease (bladder outlet obstruction, overflow incontinence)

Benign prostatic hypertrophy (BPH) in men

Gynecologic causes in women

Urethral trauma

Anticoagulation medication

diaphragm, prostate, and the penile and scrotal skin, where it can cause abscesses and fistula (Guidos et al. 2014). Urethral tumors usually invade locally and extend into adjacent soft tissues. At time of diagnosis, the tumors are often locally advanced and are associated with a poor prognosis.

Staging of Urothelial Carcinoma

Management of urothelial carcinoma is dependent upon the stage and grade of the cancer. Staging is based on the 2010 American Joint Committee on Cancer (AJCC) TNM guidelines. The "T" stage refers to clinical staging only, based on the results of diagnostic testing. The "p" stage is determined by the pathologic examination of the tissues *after* the removal of the bladder, ureter, or urethra. For example, Ta is the clinical stage of noninvasive papillary carcinoma and pTa is the pathologic stage of noninvasive papillary carcinoma.

Diagnostic Testing

Laboratory Evaluation

Comprehensive Blood Panel Assesses for electrolyte imbalances, liver function, and the most important baseline renal function: creatinine, BUN, and glomerular filtration rate (GFR). Evaluating baseline renal function is necessary to determine if it is appropriate for the patient to receive intravenous contrast with imaging. Patients should *not* receive IV contrast with CT scans if creatinine is 2.0 mg/dl or higher.

Complete Blood Count with Platelets and Differential Assesses for an elevated white blood cell count (WBC) to evaluate for possible infection, baseline hemoglobin, and hematocrit.

Coagulation Studies (PT, PTT, INR) Assess the potential for bleeding disorders and baseline INR (especially if on anticoagulation medications).

Urinalysis Always send a urine specimen to the lab for a macroscopic and a microscopic analysis. A macroscopic urinalysis will identify the presence of bacteria and red blood cells (RBC). Never rely on an office urinalysis; this can only give preliminary data on the presence of nitrates and/or blood, while a complete laboratory evaluation is important to evaluate for differential diagnosis.

Urine Culture and Sensitivity Sending the urine for a culture and sensitivity despite the results of the macro- and microscopic urinalysis is a prudent choice, especially if the patient is symptomatic. The culture will identify the type of bacteria present, and sensitivities will identify the appropriate antibiotic to treat the bacteria present in the sample.

Urine Cytology A urine cytology is the most valuable and reliable urine test to detect bladder cancer. A voided urine sample is sent for a laboratory evaluation to determine the presence of cancer cells. The results can be negative, positive, or atypical; atypical urine cytology does not necessarily confirm or deny the presence of cancer cells. Further evaluation based on risk factors and signs and symptoms is recommended. Urine cytology is most helpful in diagnosing high-grade tumors and carcinoma in situ (CIS). Low-grade noninvasive tumors may be missed by routine cytologic analysis. Urine cytology is also used for surveillance after the initial treatment of bladder cancer to detect a recurrence.

FISH (UroVysion Fluorescence In Situ Hybridization) This is a urine-based genetic test for the diagnosis and surveillance of bladder cancer. This method detects genetic alterations of the urothelial cells found in the urine, using fluorescent DNA probes binding to the regions of chromosomes 3, 7, and 17 as well as on the 9p21 (Riesz et al. 2007). A positive test result will identify the amount of positive cells present in the sample.

Diagnostic Studies

Because the presentation of TCC is extremely variable and staging plays a vital part in planning treatment, a wide variety of diagnostics may be used (Table 17.4). An ultrasound post-void residual (PVR) is a noninvasive and time-efficient test that can be completed in the office. Immediately after a voluntary void, the patient's bladder is scanned with a portable ultrasound bladder scanner. The amount of residual urine left in the bladder is measured.

Hydronephrosis or swelling of the kidneys can be identified on CT scan, MRI, or renal US and is an indicator of obstructed urine flow from the kidneys through the ureters to the bladder. This is a significant finding and can indicate tumors within the ureters, at either of the ureteral orifice, excessive tumor burden within the bladder, and/or metastatic disease.

Cystoscopy is the gold standard of care in evaluating the bladder and urethra for cancer. It is typically completed in the outpatient clinic, but can be done in the operating room when bladder biopsies are needed. In the outpatient setting, the patient is prepped using a topical anesthetic, often xylocaine gel. The cystoscope is gently advanced through the urethra into the bladder. Attached to the cystoscope is a port for the administration of normal saline into the bladder to improve visualization of the bladder wall and the bilateral ureteral orifice. This also aids in the collection of urine samples. The lining of the urethra is also visualized and assessed for an area of abnormality. Visualization can be reduced by bleeding, or debris, and flat urothelial lesions such as CIS may be difficult to distinguish from normal bladder tissue. If cystoscopy findings are negative in the setting of a positive urine cytology, further evaluation of the upper tracts is indicated.

Bladder biopsies are tissue samples taken from the bladder lining using the cystoscope. The tissue samples are sent to pathology for examination and are essential for obtaining a tissue diagnosis. These samples provide the histology, grade, and the depth of invasion. After bladder biopsies, the patient may experience gross hematuria, passing clots, dysuria, urgency, and frequency, symptoms that are typically

Table 17.4 Imaging studies to evaluate TCC

Study	Discussion
Ultrasound	Abdominal or renal ultrasound is an appropriate initial test to evaluate abdominal/flank pain, nausea/vomiting, and hematuria
Chest imaging (X-ray and chest CT)	Baseline chest X-ray including anterior, posterior, and lateral views is helpful in evaluating for pulmonary and cardiac disease and nodules or mass Pulmonary nodule protocol chest CT may be considered to further evaluate areas of concern present on X-ray and/or concern for metastatic disease
Computerized tomography (CT) urogram	*Should always be considered in cases of hematuria* Evaluate for any allergies to IV contrast Specialized CT scan that fully evaluates the upper urinary tracts (kidneys and ureters) and the bladder; typically includes abdomen and pelvis Helps to identify tumors present within the urinary system, other organs, and within the abdomen and pelvis Lymphadenopathy (size, location, and number of enlarged lymph nodes) is also assessed Bladder wall thickness can also be identified and measured; this is associated with the presence of a bladder wall tumor
Stone protocol CT scan	Evaluates renal calculi as a potential source of pain/hematuria Usually done without contrast
Intravenous pyelogram (IVP)	X-ray test that provides pictures of the kidneys, bladder, ureters, and urethra Evaluate for any allergies to IV contrast Shows size, shape, and position of the urinary tract and collecting system within the kidneys Intravenous contrast is injected, and a series of x-ray pictures are taken at timed intervals Identifies diseases of the urinary tract, such as kidney stones, tumors, or infection Identifies congenital urinary tract defects
Retrograde pyelogram	Type of X-ray that allows visualization of the bladder, ureters, and renal pelvis A catheter is inserted through the urethra and up into the bladder and/or ureters; contrast is injected through the catheter to opacify the lining of the urinary system Identifies filling defects (e.g., stones or tumors) Option when an intravenous excretory study (IVP or contrast CT scan) cannot be done because of renal disease or allergy to intravenous contrast Relative contraindications include the presence of infected urine, pregnancy, and contrast allergy
MRI (magnetic resonance imaging)	Sensitive test to detect the presence of metastatic disease MRI urogram is similar to a CT urogram: fully evaluates upper tracts and the bladder May not be appropriate for patients with metal implants, pacemakers/defibrillators, and significant claustrophobia
Bone scan (whole body)	Crucial diagnostic test to evaluate for concerns of metastatic disease to the skeletal system
Diuretic renal scan (DRS)	Further evaluates appearance, function, and presence of obstruction (hydronephrosis) of the kidneys Renal function is described by the $T^{1}\!/\!_{2}$ times before and after Lasix administration of each kidney, estimated contribution of each kidney to effective renal plasma flow, and split renal function of each kidney Clarifies degree of obstruction and loss of function for each kidney Also known as a Lasix renal scan or renogram

self-limiting and resolve within 2–3 days. During this time, a short course of phenazopyridine (Pyridium) can help to alleviate the symptoms.

Ureteroscopy with biopsy is an upper tract endoscopy completed in the operating room under anesthesia and is performed by a urologist. A ureteroscope is inserted through the urethra and advanced into the right and/or left ureter. The lining of the ureter and the ureteral orifice are inspected, and biopsies of any visually abnormal areas may be taken.

Urethroscopy A urethroscopy is an endoscopy of the lining of the urethra and is completed at the time of a cystoscopy. If abnormalities are seen on outpatient cystoscopy, then the patient is taken to the operating room for biopsy.

Lymph Node Biopsy A biopsy of enlarged lymph nodes can be completed by either a fine needle aspiration (FNA) or under CT guidance to identify and confirm metastatic disease.

Management of Urothelial Carcinoma

Treatment for urothelial carcinoma can be quite challenging for patients. Review of important behavioral modifications before treatment can improve patient outcomes during and after treatment.

- *Smoking Cessation*: The number one most important task is to quit tobacco use; many patients cannot accept that smoking has a direct correlation to the diagnosis of urothelial carcinoma. Tobacco consultation teams, support groups, cognitive therapy, and medication management programs can be extremely helpful.
- *Chemical and Environmental Exposures*: Reducing exposures to chemicals will minimize risks even further and remind patients to follow all safety guidelines when handling chemicals.
- *Physical Wellness*: Encouraging daily activity such as walking, gentle strengthening exercises (if appropriate for the patient), biking, and swimming before starting treatment will help to improve strength and endurance. This will help facilitate recovery and improve patient outcomes.
- *Nutrition*: Maintaining proper nutrition is essential during and after treatment. Side effects from systemic chemotherapy can alter a patient's appetite and ability to eat. It is common for patients to lose 15–20 lb after a radical surgical resection. Referral for nutrition counseling will help to outline an appropriate meal plan for each patient.
- *Hydration*: Maintaining good hydration will maintain urinary tract health. Dehydration can cause electrolyte imbalance and impair renal function; instruct patients to avoid bladder irritants such as alcohol, caffeine, and soda.
- *Psychosocial Support*: Providing continued support through treatment, recovery, and surveillance will improve patient outcomes and decrease distress. Referral to a Psychology Oncology Program or social work can assist with anxiety and depression, not only for the patient but for the caregiver as well. Social work can

also assist the caregiver and patient with financial concerns, transportation, meals, and household chores.

- *Optimize Medical Comorbidities*: Optimizing medical comorbidities prior to treatment will improve outcomes; well-controlled diabetes, hypertension, and chronic obstructive pulmonary disease (COPD) will maximize recovery. Consultation with primary care providers and specialty providers is necessary coordination of care.

Management of Urothelial Carcinoma of the Bladder

Intravesical Immunotherapy and Chemotherapy

Intravesical therapy is an important treatment modality in the management of non-muscle-invasive (Ta) or minimally invasive bladder cancers. This treats persistent microscopic tumors persistence and prevents tumor re-implantation, new tumor formation, and possible tumor grade and stage progression (Wade et al. 2010). Intravesical therapy is given directly into the bladder through the urethra with a catheter and typically begins 2–4 weeks after a transurethral resection (TURBT). An initial induction course is once per week for 6 consecutive weeks, followed by cystoscopy and/or bladder biopsies in 4–6 weeks. Depending upon response, the patient may go on to maintenance intravesical therapy in the form of immunotherapy or chemotherapy. Immunotherapy is the instillation of agents that work by triggering the body's immune response to destroy cancer cells that may be present in the bladder after a transurethral resection. Intravesical chemotherapy is the instillation of chemotherapeutic agents that inhibit or slow cancer cell production.

Intravesical Immunotherapy
Bacillus Calmette-Guerin (BCG) is a live attenuated strain of *Mycobacterium bovis*, first indicated as a tuberculosis vaccine, and has been used in intravesical immunotherapy since the 1970s. The mechanism of action is a T-helper type I immune response and is considered first-line treatment for non-muscle-invasive bladder cancer.

Interferon is an immunotherapeutic agent that may be used as monotherapy or in combination with BCG. The mechanism of action is lymphocyte activation and potentiates a T-helper type I immune response.

Intravesical Chemotherapy
Mitomycin C (MMC) is the most common intravesical chemotherapeutic agent used for non-muscle-invasive bladder cancer. It is an antibiotic and inhibits DNA synthesis; it can be used for induction and maintenance therapy. MMC can also be used in a perioperative fashion at the time of a transurethral resection (TURBT). The rationale for perioperative dosing is the destruction of residual microscopic tumor at the site of TURBT and of circulating cells, thereby preventing re-implantation at the time of TURBT (Wade et al. 2010).

Gemcitabine is an intravesical chemotherapeutic agent that has been used to treat non-muscle-invasive bladder cancer. This agent may be used in intermediate-risk patients as an alternative to MMC, and in high-risk, BCG refractory patients, and may be active in reducing tumor recurrence.

Thiotepa is one of the earliest agents used for intravesical chemotherapy. It is an alkylating agent that acts to cross-link nucleic acids. Higher doses (>60 mg) can cause myelosuppression. Leukocyte and platelet counts should be obtained before each instillation, and treatment is delayed as necessary (Hall et al. 2007).

Side Effects of Intravesical Therapy Intravesical therapy produces a local reaction to the bladder urothelium which can cause significant symptoms during treatment. The most common side effects are irritative voiding symptoms (dysuria, frequency, urgency), pain in the bladder, gross hematuria, low-grade fever, and malaise. These usually occur in the first 24–48 h after treatment. If symptoms persist, a urine culture should be completed to rule out a bacterial urinary tract infection. If the urine culture is negative, then medications such as anticholinergics, topical antispasmodics (phenazopyridine), analgesics, and NSAIDS can be used to alleviate symptoms.

If the urine culture is positive, intravesical therapy is held, and the patient is treated with the appropriate antibiotic determined by the culture sensitivities. A follow-up urine culture 2–3 days post-antibiotic therapy is completed to confirm resolution of the infection prior to the continuation of treatment. If the patient has difficulty voiding, small frequent voids, and weakening urinary stream, they should be evaluated with an ultrasound prior to resuming treatments.

Side effects can become increasingly severe over time with long-term intravesical therapy, and doses may be half or one-third. In some cases, patients are not able to tolerate subsequent treatments and the therapy is discontinued. In some patients, severe chemical cystitis can occur, especially with MMC or thiotepa, and can be managed with intravesical dimethyl sulfoxide (DMSO includes methylprednisolone, dimethyl sulfoxide, lidocaine HCL 2 %, sodium bicarbonate) given once per week for 6 weeks. Antihistamines, long-acting anticholinergics, and oral prednisone can also be used.

Surgical Management

Transurethral resection of the bladder tumor (TURBT) is both diagnostic and therapeutic and can be used in the initial management of non-muscle-invasive (Ta) disease and recurrent Ta disease. The configuration (flat, sessile, or papillary), location (trigone, base, dome, or lateral walls), size (centimeters), and number of tumors are noted during a TURBT. These characteristics provide critical staging information imperative for treatment recommendations. If there is tumor present at the bladder neck or within the prostatic urethra, biopsy or resection of the prostatic urethra is included at the time of the TURBT. A single dose of MMC given immediately following a TURBT in patients with both low- and high-risk non-muscle-invasive urothelial carcinoma reduces the risk of recurrence. Potential complications include irritative lower urinary tract symptoms, bleeding, bladder perforation, urethral stricturing, and scarring of the ureteral orifices that could potentially lead to renal obstruction.

Radical cystectomy is the standard of care for invasive urothelial carcinoma and is indicated when there is infiltrating muscle-invasive bladder cancer without evidence of metastasis or with low-volume regional metastasis (stages T2–T3b), extensive disease not amenable to cystoscopic resection, invasive prostatic urethral involvement, or low-grade disease that has been refractory to intravesical immunotherapy or chemotherapy. Conditions that can influence cystectomy include bleeding diathesis, evidence of gross, unresectable metastatic disease (unless performed for palliation), and medical comorbidities that preclude operative intervention such as advanced heart disease and poor pulmonary function. Five-year survival rate for radical cystectomy plus pelvic lymph node dissection and negative nodes is 85–100 % for T2a disease but 10–30 % for node-positive disease.

For men, a cystoprostatectomy is performed, involving bilateral lymphadenectomy and removal of the bladder, peritoneal covering, perivesical fat, distal ureters, prostate, seminal vesicles, and vas deferens. Men without tumors at the bladder base or prostate may be considered for a nerve-sparing procedure. For women, an anterior exenteration is completed (bilateral pelvic lymphadenectomy, cystectomy, hysterectomy, salpingo-oophorectomy, partial anterior vaginectomy).

Several types of urinary diversions can be completed with a cystectomy. When considering a urinary diversion, it is crucial to discuss with the patient his/her preference, along with the surgical criteria for each diversion. For an ileal conduit, the patient must be willing to have a stoma that continuously drains urine into an external appliance. With a continent cutaneous urinary diversion, the patient must be willing and able to catheterize the pouch through and external stoma at least every 3 h. With an orthotopic neobladder, the patient must understand that initially it is labor intensive to train the neobladder. He/she must also be willing and physically able to perform intermittent straight catheterization if needed; neobladder patients must also understand that they may experience urinary incontinence or retention.

Management of Urothelial (Transitional Cell) Carcinoma of the Renal Pelvis and Ureter

The treatment for localized upper tract transitional cell carcinoma is surgery and medical management. Nephroureterectomy is the standard of care for upper tract disease and is indicated in patients with renal pelvis TCC, regionally extensive disease, and high-grade or high-stage lesions. A nephroureterectomy can be performed by an open or a laparoscopic approach. The kidney, ureter, and bladder cuff are removed. If the upper tract disease is confined to the distal segment of the ureter, a distal nephrourectomy with re-implantation of the proximal ureter can be completed. The 5-year survival stage after a total nephroureterectomy is 91 % for stages Tis, Ta, and T1 and 0 % for stage N3/M1.

Medical management of upper tract urothelial tumors involves the instillation of chemotherapeutic agents mitomycin C, thiotepa, and immunotherapy BCG. These agents can be administered either percutaneously, through a ureteral catheter (percutaneous nephrostomy tube), or intravesically in patients with vesicoureteral reflux. This approach is most appropriate for patients with multiple superficial disease or carcinoma in situ.

Management of Urothelial Carcinoma of the Urethra

Management of urothelial carcinoma of the urethra varies with stage and location of the lesion. Tumors of the distal urethra are usually discovered earlier and at a lower stage. Tumors of the proximal urethra usually present at a more clinically advanced stage. Surgical management of small superficial tumors includes laser resection, transurethral resection, fulguration, and Mohs surgery. Large tumors or tumors that invade other structures or tissues require a radical resection. Indications for urethrectomy include tumor in the anterior urethra; prostatic stromal invasion that is noncontiguous with the primary site; positive urethral margin during radical cystectomy; or diffuse CIS of the bladder, prostatic ducts, or prostatic urethra.

The management of distal urethral tumors is different for men and women. For superficial tumors in women, treatment may include transurethral resection, electroresection and fulguration, laser surgery, or brachytherapy with or without external beam radiation. For invasive tumors in women, treatment may include an anterior exenteration with or without lymphadenectomy. The management of superficial tumors in men may include transurethral resection, electroresection and fulguration, or laser surgery. Tumors that are located near the tip of the penis may include a partial penectomy with or without lymphadenectomy. For tumors in the distal urethra (but not at the tip of the penis) that are noninvasive, a partial urethrectomy with or without lymphadenectomy may be performed. Invasive urethral tumors in men may require a radical penectomy with or without lymphadenectomy; treatment modalities may include radiation therapy with or without chemotherapy and chemotherapy given together with radiation.

The management of cancer that involves the proximal urethra is also different for men and women. In women with small tumors, radiation therapy and/or surgery (anterior exenteration with lymph node dissection and urinary diversion) may be performed. In men, management may include radiation therapy, or radiation therapy and chemotherapy, followed by surgery (cystoprostatectomy, penectomy, lymph node dissection, and urinary diversion).

Preoperative Education Prior to Surgery for Urothelial Carcinoma

Prior to surgery, the patient will meet with an enterostomal therapist for education and marking for stoma placement. Education will include strategies for living a full life with an ostomy, resources for obtaining ostomy supplies, peristomal skin care, and proper fit of the appliance. Patients may consider a family member or a friend that may be available to assist with ostomy care. The goal for patients is to become confident and independent with care of their stoma and application of their appliance.

Neobladder training will include strategies to promote optimal functional capacity of the neobladder. These include voiding utilizing the Crede's maneuver, timed voiding with gradually increasing the voiding interval, intermittent self-catheterization and irrigation, and pelvic floor therapy.

Patients with a urinary diversion should obtain a medical ID bracelet/necklace to identify the presence and type of their diversion.

Postoperative Management In the immediate postoperative period, there are several complications that can occur after cystectomy. The most common complication that may require readmission to the hospital is failure to thrive. The patient has difficulty recovering at home and is unable to maintain proper nutrition and hydration, resulting in weakness and electrolyte imbalance. Intermittent outpatient IV hydration and monitoring of labs including a comprehensive and a CBC with platelets and differential may be considered. If condition continues to decline, readmission to the hospital is considered for supportive care.

A wound infection and/or dehiscence may also occur after cystectomy. Erythema, redness, drainage, or pain at the abdominal incision may occur. Oral antibiotics, such as Keflex, on an outpatient basis may be considered. If condition progresses to fever, chills, foul odor, and elevated white blood cell count, the patient may require readmission for IV antibiotics and/or a possible surgical wound irrigation and debridement followed by dressing changes. After cystectomy, patients are discharged with an abdominal binder to help support the abdominal incision. A wound with intact underlying fascia may be managed with wet to dry dressing changes on an outpatient basis. This will require patient and caregiver education of wound management and signs/symptoms of infection. If the underlying fascia becomes compromised, then a surgical repair may be considered.

Alteration of the intestinal tract can lead to bowel complications after surgery, including development of a postoperative ileus or hypomotility of the GI tract. Symptoms of an ileus may include moderate, diffuse abdominal discomfort, constipation, abdominal distention, nausea and vomiting, vomiting bile, lack of bowel movement and/or flatulence, and excessive belching. This condition may require readmission for hydration and bowel rest.

A urinary tract infection or pyelonephritis can also occur after surgery. If a UTI is suspected, a urine specimen should be sent for culture and sensitivity. Most uncomplicated UTI can be treated on an outpatient basis with oral antibiotics and increased fluid intake. On occasion, a UTI can progress to pyelonephritis requiring readmission and IV antibiotics and hydration. In severe cases, pyelonephritis can lead to sepsis with aggressive management in the intensive care unit.

Surveillance Recommendations for Urothelial Carcinoma

Non-Muscle-Invasive Urothelial Carcinoma The frequency for local recurrence and the potential for stage progression, especially in those with high-risk disease, require vigilant surveillance lifelong. The clinical follow-up includes an appropriate patient history including voiding symptoms and hematuria, urinalysis, cystoscopy, and urine cytology according to the NCCN (2014) guidelines. This includes cystoscopy at 3–6-month intervals and urine cytology for the first 2 years and at increasing intervals as clinically indicated thereafter. Upper tract imaging should be considered every 1–2 years for high-grade tumors.

Muscle-Invasive Urothelial Carcinoma Following Cystectomy and Urinary diversion The NCCN (version 2.2014) guidelines for surveillance after cystectomy include imaging of the chest, upper tracts, abdomen, and pelvis every 3–6 months for 2 years based on risk of recurrence and then as clinically indicated. A urine cytology and comprehensive blood panel should be completed every 3–6 months for 2 years then as clinically indicated. Also, a vitamin B12 and folic acid should be completed annually. In addition, a urethral wash is recommended every 6–12 months. A urethral wash is completed primarily in male post-cystectomy ileal conduit patients to detect abnormal cells within the urethra.

Resources
The following is a list of resources available for the patient and for the provider.
- American Bladder Cancer Support www.bladdercancersupport.org
- American Cancer Society www.cancer.org
- American Society for Clinical Oncology www.cancer.net
- American Urological Association Foundation www.auafoundation.org
- Bladder Cancer Advocacy Network (BCAN) www.bcan.org
- Bladder Cancer Webcafe www.blcwebcafe.org
- CancerCare www.cancercare.org
- Lance Armstrong Foundation www.livestrong.org
- National Cancer Institute www.cancer.gov
- National Comprehensive Cancer Network (NCCN) www.nccn.org
- United Ostomy Associations of America, Inc. www.uoaa.org
- The Wellness Community www.thewellnesscommunity.org
- The Wound, Ostomy and Continence Nurses Society™ (WOCN®) www.wocn.org

Clinical Pearls

- Tobacco use is the leading risk factor for urothelial carcinoma.
- A complete evaluation of symptoms is essential, as urothelial carcinoma can mimic other conditions such as UTI and renal calculus. Never assume hematuria is a urinary tract infection.
- Always complete an US post-void residual (PVR) to evaluate for urinary retention.
- Never ignore blood in the urine. All hematuria must be further evaluated with urinalysis (microscopic and macroscopic), urine culture and sensitivity, urine cytology, CT urogram, and cystoscopy.
- The presence of hydronephrosis on imaging is a significant finding that must be further evaluated and treated.
- A CT urogram is an essential diagnostic tool to fully evaluate the bladder and upper tracts.
- Side effects from intravesical therapy usually occur within the first 24–48 h after treatment.
- Side effects from intravesical therapy can become increasingly severe with each subsequent treatment.
- An enterostomal therapy consultation and follow-up is essential for patients with an ileal conduit urinary diversion.
- Maintaining good voiding habits is essential in maintaining neobladder health.
- The frequency for local recurrence and the potential for stage progression of patients with urothelial carcinoma require lifelong surveillance.

References

American Joint Committee on Cancer (2010) AJCC cancer staging manual, 7th edn. Springer, New York

Bladder Cancer WebCafe (2015) Internal pouches-continent reservoirs. http://blcwebcafe.org/content/view/126/136/lang,english/

Guidos J, Powell C, Donohoe J et al (2014) Urethral cancer. Medscape. http://emedicine.medscape.com/article/451496-overview

Hall MC, Chang SS, Dalbagni G, Pruthi RS, Schellhammer PF, Seigne JD, Skinner EC, Stuart Wolf J Jr (2007) Guideline for the management of nonmuscle invasive bladder cancer: stages Ta, T1 and Tis: update (2007). The American Urologic Association. J Urol 178(6):2314–2330. http://www.auanet.org/education/guidelines/bladder-cancer.cfi

Hayes J, Gilligan T (2014) Nonurothelial bladder cancer. UpToDate. http://www.uptodate.com/contents/nonurothelial-bladder-cancer

Kaplan GW, Bulkey GJ, Grayhack JT (1967) Carcinoma of the male urethra. J Urol 98(3):365–371 [Medline]

National Comprehensive Cancer Network (2014) NCCN clinical practice guidelines in oncology (NCCN guidelines). Bladder Cancer (Version 2.2014). http://www.tri-kobe.org/nccn/guideline/urological/english/bladder.pdf

National Institutes of Health (2014) Smoking and bladder cancer. http://www.nih.gov/research-matters/august2011/08292011cancer.htm

Oken MM, Creech RH, Tormey DC, Horton J, Davis TE, McFadden ET, Carbone PP (1982) Toxicity and response criteria of the Eastern Cooperative Oncology Group. Am J Clin Oncol 5:649–655, Eastern Cooperative Oncology Group, Robert Comis M.D., Group Chair. The ECOG Performance Status is in the public domain therefore available for public use

Riesz P, Lotz G, Páska C, Szendrôi A, Majoros A, Németh Z, Törzsök P, Szarvas T, Kovalszky I, Schaff Z, Romics I, Kiss A (2007) Detection of bladder cancer from the urine using fluorescence in situ hybridization technique. Pathol Oncol Res 13(3):187–194, Epub 2007 Oct 7

SEER (2014) Training modules, types of kidney and ureter caner. U. S. National Institutes of Health, National Cancer Institute. http://training.seer.cancer.gov/kidney/intro/review.html

SEER (2015) Cancer statistics factsheets: bladder cancer. National Cancer Institute, Bethesda. http://seer.cancer.gov/statfacts/html/urinb.html

Swartz MA, Porter MP, Lin DW, Weiss NS (2006) Incidence of primary urethral carcinoma in the United States. Urology 68(6):1164–1168

Wade JS, Wiegand LR, Correa JJ, Politis C, Dickinson SI, Kang LC (2010) Bladder cancer: a review of non-muscle invasive disease. Cancer Control 17(4):256–268

West DA, Cummings JM, Longo WE, Virgo KS, Johnson FE, Parra RO (1999) Role of chronic catheterization in the development of bladder cancer in patients with spinal cord injury. Urology 53(2):292–297

Wiener JS, Liu ET, Walther PJ (1992) Oncogenic human papillomavirus type 16 is associated with squamous cell cancer of the male urethra. Cancer Res 52(18):5018–5023

Further Reading

Bates AW, Norton AJ, Baithun SI (2000) Malignant lymphoma of the urinary bladder: a clinico-pathological study of 11 cases. J Clin Pathol 53:458

Bessette PL, Abell MR, Herwig KR (1974) A clinicopathologic study of squamous cell carcinoma of the bladder. J Urol 112(1):66–67 [Medline]

Brenner DW, Yore LM, Schellhammer PF (1989) Squamous cell carcinoma of the bladder after successful intravesical therapy with Bacillus Calmette-Guerin. Urology 34:93–95 [PubMed]

Casey RG, Cullen IM, Crotty T, Quinlan D (2009) Intermittent self-catheterization and the risk of squamous cell cancer of the bladder: an emerging clinical entity? Can Urol Assoc J 3(5):E51–E54

Dahm P, Gschwend JE (2003) Malignant non-urothelial neoplasms of the urinary bladder: a review. Eur Urol 44:672

Faysal MH, Freiha FS (1981) Primary neoplasm in vesical diverticula. A report of 12 cases. Br J Urol 53(2):141–143 [Medline]

Feggetter G (1937) Sarcoma of the bladder. Br J Surg 25(98):382–387

Gilligan T (2014) Small cell carcinoma of the bladder. UpToDate. www.uptodate.com

Grossman HB, Natale RB, Tangen CM (2003) Neoadjuvant chemotherapy plus cystectomy compared with cystectomy alone for locally advanced bladder cancer. N Engl J Med 349(9):859–866 [Medline]

Herr HW (1999) The value of a second transurethral resection in evaluating patients with bladder tumors. J Urol 162(1):74–76

Herr HW (2005) Restaging transurethral resection of high risk superficial bladder cancer improves the initial response to Bacillus Calmette Guerin therapy. J Urol 174(6):2134–2137

Herr HW, Donat SM (2006) A re-staging transurethral resection predicts early progression of superficial bladder cancer. BJU Int 97(6):1194–1198

Indrees MT, Cheng L (2013) Pathology of urinary bladder squamous cell carcinoma overview of squamous cell bladder carcinoma. Medscape. http://emedicine.medscape.com/article/1611983-overview#aw2aab6b4

Kempton CL, Kurtin PJ, Inwards DJ et al (1997) Malignant lymphoma of the bladder: evidence from 36 cases that low-grade lymphoma of the MALT-type is the most common primary bladder lymphoma. Am J Surg Pathol 21:1324

Lamm DL, Blumenstein BA, Crissman JD et al (2000) Maintenance Bacillus Calmette-Guérin immunotherapy for recurrent TA, T1 and carcinoma in situ transitional cell carcinoma of the bladder: a randomized Southwest Oncology Group Study. J Urol 163(4):1124–1129

Large M, Eggener S (2015) Radical cystectomy. Medscape. http://emedicine.medscape.com/article/448623-overview#aw2aab6b2b1aa

Locke JR, Hill DE, Walzer Y (1985) Incidence of squamous cell carcinoma in patients with long term catheter drainage. J Urol 133:1034–1035 [PubMed]

Lopez-Beltran A, Pacelli A, Rothenberg HJ et al (1998) Carcinosarcoma and sarcomatoid carcinoma of the bladder: clinicopathological study of 41 cases. J Urol 159:1497

Lynch CF, Cohen MB (1995) Urinary system. Cancer 75:316–329 [PubMed]

Morales A, Eidinger D, Bruce AW (1976) Intracavitary Bacillus Calmette-Guerin in the treatment of superficial bladder tumors. J Urol 116:180

National Cancer Institute (2015) Transitional cell cancer of the renal pelvis and ureter. http://www.cancer.gov/cancertopics/pdq/treatment/transitionalcell

National Cancer Institute (2015) Tumor grade fact sheet. http://www.cancer.gov/cancertopics/factsheet/detection/tumor-grade

National Cancer Institute (2015) Urethral cancer treatment. http://www.cancer.gov/cancertopics/pdq/treatment/urethral/Patient/page5

National Kidney and Urologic Diseases Information Clearinghouse (NKUDIC) (2015) A service of the National Institute of Diabetes and Digestive and Kidney Diseases (NIDDK), National Institutes of Health (NIH). Urinary Diversion. http://kidney.niddk.nih.gov/Kudiseases/pubs/urostomy/index.aspx

Proulx GM, Gibbs JF, Lee RJ et al (1999) Sarcoma of the bladder: a case report review of the literature. Radiol Oncol 33:63–68

Raj GV, Herr H, Serio AM, Donat SM, Bochenr BH, Vickers AJ et al (2007) Treatment paradigm shift may improve survival of patients with high risk superficial bladder cancer. J Urol 177(4):1283–1286

SEER (2015) Survival Monograph: Cancer Survival Among Adults: US SEER Program, 1988–2001, Patient and Tumor Characteristics. SEER Program. NIH Pub. No. 07–6215. National Cancer Institute, Bethesda

Shelley MD, Jones G, Cleves A, Wilt TJ, Mason MD, Kynaston HG (2012) Intravesical gemcitabine therapy for non-muscle invasive bladder cancer (NMIBC): a systematic review. BJU Int 109:496–505. doi:10.1111/j.1464-410X.2011.10880.x

Tainio HM, Kylmala TM, Haapasalo HK (1999) Primary malignant melanoma of the urinary bladder associated with widespread metastasis. Scand J Urol Nephrol 33:406

Understanding Cancer Series: Cancer (2014) U.S. National Institutes of Health, National Cancer Institute. http://www.cancer.gov/cancertopics/understandingcancer/cancer

U.S. national Library of Medicine. NIH National Institutes of Health. http://www.nlm.nih.gov/medicineplus/eney/art.cle1000525.htm

Valerio M, Lhermitte B, Bauer J, Jichlinski P (2011) Metastatic primary adenocarcinoma of the bladder in a twenty-five years old woman. Rare Tumors 3(1):e9

Whalen RK, Althausen AF, Daniels GH (1992) Extra-adrenal pheochromocytoma. J Urol 147:1

Kidney Cancer

18

Luke Edwards and Jason Hafron

Contents

L. Edwards, MD • J. Hafron, MD (✉)
Department of Urology, Beaumont Health System, Royal Oak, MI, USA
e-mail: Jason.Hafron@beaumont.edu

© Springer International Publishing Switzerland 2016
M. Lajiness, S. Quallich (eds.), *The Nurse Practitioner in Urology*,
DOI 10.1007/978-3-319-28743-0_18

Overview

The purpose of this chapter is to provide a basic foundation of knowledge for nurse practitioners specializing in urologic care regarding renal tumors, particularly renal cell carcinoma. Cystic lesions which are a frequent cause for urologic consultation will be discussed as well as some of the more commonly encountered benign renal tumors. This chapter will focus mostly on diagnosis, work up, and the management of malignant renal masses. Management must be tailored to each individual patient based on renal function and comorbidities, as well as characteristics of the mass itself.

Definitions

Clear Cell Carcinoma   The most common type of RCC.

Papillary Carcinoma   The second most common type of RCC, further characterized as type I (less aggressive) and type II (more aggressive).

Chromophobe Carcinoma   The third most common type of RCC, generally less aggressive than other subtypes.

Fuhrman Grade   A grading system to predict tumor behavior based on nuclear characteristics. It is used for clear cell and papillary RCC but not the other less common subtypes.

Percutaneous Renal Biopsy   A needle core biopsy obtained through the skin to obtain renal tissue in order to obtain a histological diagnosis. Performed with either ultrasound or CT guidance.

Paraneoplastic Syndromes   Constellation of both systemic symptoms and laboratory abnormalities which can be associated with RCC and may remit with tumor resection.

Bosniak Criteria   A classification system to risk stratify cystic renal lesions based on CT or MRI characteristics.

Table 18.1 The prevalence
of metastatic disease based
on tumor size

Primary tumor size (cm)	Risk of mets at diagnosis (%)
≤3	<4
3–4	7
4–7	16
7–10	30
>10	43

Incidence

Renal cell carcinoma (RCC) is the most common malignant renal cancer with an incidence of 54–58,000 new cases per year in the United States and accounts for roughly 13,000 cancer deaths per year (Jamel et al. 2010). RCC is most commonly diagnosed in the sixth and seventh decade of life. A male predominance does exist with the disease (Siegel et al. 2011). The incidence of RCC is increasing over the last 30 years and many attribute this to the increased utilization of cross-sectional imaging (Hock et al. 2002).

Anatomy and Pathology

Most RCCs are thought to originate from the epithelium of the proximal convoluted tubules. While beginning in the renal cortex, these masses often grow out bulging into perinephric fat aiding in their visualization on imaging studies. Additionally they demonstrate a propensity to involve the renal vein either by direct invasion or tumor thrombus. Historically nearly 30 % of patients have metastatic disease at presentation, with the most common sites being lung, followed by bone, and regional lymph nodes. Metastases occur via both hematologic and lymphatic spread. The prevalence of metastatic disease correlates with tumor size at presentation in nonlinear sigmoidal relationship (Nguyen and Gill 2009) as demonstrated in Table 18.1.

Not all RCCs behave the same and there is a spectrum of behavior in terms of metastatic risk and recurrence. Grading is based on Fuhrman nuclear grade which takes into account both nuclear size, contour, and nucleoli and ranges from grade I to grade IV. Higher grades connote a higher degree of aggression and portends a worse prognosis.

There are various subtypes of RCC, and a few bear mentioning. The most common type of RCC by far is clear cell RCC, the name given due to the abundance of clear cytoplasm seen on histologic examination of tumor specimen. Clear cell accounts for 70–80 % of all RCC. The second most common subtype is papillary RCC. This is seen more commonly in patients with end-stage renal disease. There are two subtypes of papillary RCC, type I and type II. The distinction is important with regards to prognosis and recurrence as papillary type II has been shown to be more aggressive, whereas type I is considered more indolent. The third most common subtype of RCC is chromophobe, which, like type I papillary, demonstrates less aggressive behavior.

Benign Renal Masses

The two most common benign renal tumors are oncocytoma and angiomyolipomas (AML). An estimated 3–5 % of solid renal masses are oncocytomas (Romis et al. 2004). There is no imaging modality which can reliably differentiate oncocytoma from malignant masses and thus tissue is required for diagnosis, obtained either by percutaneous biopsy or surgical excision.

AMLs are benign tumors that are characterized by three major histologic components: fat cells, smooth muscle, and blood vessels. Unlike oncocytoma, AMLs can be diagnosed reliably with imaging alone. The presence of macroscopic fat on CT imaging is considered diagnostic. While AMLs are benign, they carry the risk of spontaneous life-threatening hemorrhage, and this risk increases with larger tumors. For tumors >4 cm in diameter treatment is preferred given this potentially serious adverse event. Smaller AMLs can be managed with serial imaging on a surveillance protocol.

Cystic Renal Lesions

Often times a patient may be referred to a urology clinic based on renal ultrasound findings which demonstrate a cystic mass. These lesions, with the exception of simple cysts which can be reliably diagnosed by ultrasound, should undergo further imaging usually in the form of CT to better elucidate their nature. A useful classification system for cystic masses has been developed and is commonly used in clinical decision making, namely, Bosniak classification, which is further described in Table 18.2. This classification is particularly helpful in that the different classes have widely varying risks of being malignant (Israel and Bosniak 2005) and thus have important differences in clinical management. Briefly, classes I and II are considered benign and do not require further imaging. Class IIF are lesions that in all likelihood are benign, but consideration should be given to periodic imaging as a form of surveillance. Class III and IV are considered likely malignant and are the only classes characterized by enhancement, which is absent from the others. Accordingly, class III and IV lesions are managed with surgical intervention.

History and Presentation

Flank pain, a palpable mass, and hematuria has historically been described as the classic triad of RCC, however given the increased use of cross-sectional imaging, this triad is rarely seen in today's practice. Additional symptoms with which patients may present include hypertension, hypercalcemia, in addition to constitutional symptoms such as fevers, night sweats, malaise, and weight loss. This constellation of symptoms should prompt body imaging.

RCC is notorious for paraneoplastic syndromes which can occur in the setting of localized disease. These include hypercalcemia, hypertension, anemia or polycythemia, and liver dysfunction which is termed Stauffer's syndrome when seen in the

Table 18.2 Bosniak classification system of renal cysts

Bosniak class	Features	Risk of malignancy	Management
I	Water density, homogenous, no septa, calcifications, or enhancement	None	Reassurance
II	Thin septa, fine calcifications, no enhancement	Negligible	Reassurance
IIF	Hyperdense, multiple thin septa, may have thick calcifications but no enhancement	3–5 %	Periodic surveillance
III	Thickened walls or septa in which enhancement is present	50 %	Surgical excision
IV	Same as III with additional clearly enhancing soft tissue components	75–90 %	Surgical excision

absence of metastatic disease. Paraneoplastic syndromes can be observed in 10–40 % of RCC cases and often remit after the tumor is removed. The persistence of these abnormalities after surgical excision may suggest undetected metastatic disease and portends a worse prognosis (Hanash 1982).

Fortunately many patients seen in practice today are asymptomatic with masses noted on imaging obtained for other reasons, with greater than half of all RCC cases now detected incidentally (Pantuck et al. 2000). Studies suggest that patients with incidentally detected masses as opposed to symptomatic presentation may have improved survival although it is difficult to fully account for lead and length time bias (Gudbjartsson et al. 2005). Review of Surveillance, Epidemiology, and End Results (SEER) data from 2002 to 2008 demonstrates 62 % of patients diagnosed during that time period had localized disease (Hanash 1982) (SEER Database).

Risk Factors

The cause of renal cell carcinoma is unclear and most cases are sporadic. Smoking has been demonstrated to be a moderate risk factor with some studies suggesting a roughly doubled relative risk in these patients. Interestingly obesity has more recently been identified as an independent risk factor for development of RCC, relative risk being increased by as much as 2.3 by the sixth decade of life for patients in the highest quartile of BMI (Chiu et al. 2006). This may partly explain the high incidence noted in North America compared to other parts of the globe.

There are many hereditary forms of RCC; however, these syndromes only represent 2–3 % of all RCC diagnosed today. Von Hippel-Lindau warrants mention given its nature as an autosomal dominant disorder which results in an RCC incidence of 50 % in patients affected. RCC in these patients is often multifocal and bilateral and these patients are at higher risk for recurrence. As such, renal sparing intervention is particularly important. Of note, these patients are at risk for nonrenal cancers as well such as cerebellar hemangioblastomas, retinal angiomas, and pheochromocytomas, among others. These patients when identified should be referred for genetic counseling.

Physical Exam

A physical exam can provide additional information about the signs and symptoms associated with RCC. A physical exam in a patient with suspected malignancy or a known mass demonstrated on imaging should always include a blood pressure measurement as well as a thorough lymph node examination. An abdominal examination should be performed to determine if the kidney mass is palpable. Rarely large masses will be palpable on abdominal or flank examination. Additionally in males the presence of a nonreducing varicocele, particularly right sided, may indicate the presence of a retroperitoneal mass. Unilateral lower extremity edema may be a result of venous compression, but like most physical findings caused by renal masses, denotes advanced disease. The presence or absence of spinal tenderness should be documented as the spine is most frequently involved by bony metastases. Hypertension may be secondary to increased renin secretion and can improve with surgical excision of tumors.

Diagnostic Tests

Laboratory Evaluation

The purpose of laboratory testing is to rule out paraneoplastic syndromes, identify other potential sites of metastases, and determine the overall health of the patient. Laboratory analysis in patients with a renal mass should include renal function as measured by BUN and Cr, a serum calcium level, CBC, liver function panel, alkaline phosphatase, and urinalysis.

Imaging Studies

The minimum standard imaging in all cases of renal masses suspicious for malignancy should include abdominal and pelvic imaging in the form of either CT or MRI with intravenous contrast and a chest x-ray.

Ultrasonography (US) Ultrasound is a useful imaging modality which utilizes a transducer that both creates and receives high frequency sound waves to create grayscale images. It has the advantage of being a radiation-free modality and is adequate for diagnosis of benign simple cysts. Additional benefits include patient tolerance, wide clinical availability, and low cost. Clinically it is often used to follow mildly complex cysts, such as Bosniak IIF lesions, to assess for interval growth or changes in complexity. It is important to remember however that complex or echogenic cysts detected by ultrasound must be further investigated with either CT or MRI imaging modalities.

Computed Tomography (CT) A thin-slice CT scan collects data based on how much various tissues attenuate radiation and generates an axial image based on this data. For evaluation of a renal mass, CT is obtained with and without IV contrast to evaluate for enhancement. Enhancement is defined as an increase in Hounsfield units (a measure of attenuation) of 10 or more after administration of contrast. Enhancing renal masses are considered RCC until proven otherwise.

Magnetic Resonance (MRI) MRI generates cross-sectional imaging based on both hydrogen ion density in various tissues as well as the response of these ions to the presence of a strong magnetic field. It has the distinct advantage of higher sensitivity for tumor thrombus and venous involvement, making it the study of choice when either of these entities is suggested by CT. Along the same lines it provides greater clarity of soft tissue planes helping delineate potentially locally invasive disease. MRI is additionally radiation-free. The studies do however take longer to perform, during which time patients must remain still to ensure image quality. Not all patients can undergo MRI imaging as they may have magnetic material in their body in the form of pacemakers or neurostimulators, among other medical devices.

Positron Emission Tomography (PET) This imaging modality involves injection of a radiotracer intravenously and subsequent imaging to determine areas of increased molecular uptake and activity. Currently with regard to RCC, it is best used as an adjunct when traditional imaging is equivocal for the presence of metastatic disease, in patients for whom the diagnosis of metastatic disease would influence further management.

Bone Scan Additionally, laboratory abnormalities such as elevated calcium or alkaline phosphatase should raise suspicion for metastatic disease and may prompt a bone scan.

Chest X-Ray A chest x-ray is a mandatory study in the initial evaluation of these patients. If the chest x-ray is abnormal or if pulmonary symptoms such as new onset cough or hemoptysis are present, this should prompt a CT of the chest, however CT chest is not required in all patients

Intravenous Pyelogram (IVP) It is worth noting that axial imaging in the form of CT or MRI has essentially entirely replaced IVP as an imaging modality for renal masses. Nonetheless it is of historical significance. A scout plain x-ray film is obtained followed by administration of intravenous iodinated contrast and serial radiographs at timed intervals provide an image of the renal unit as the kidney takes up and ultimately excretes the contrast.

Percutaneous Biopsy

Historically renal mass biopsy has been avoided in most cases of enhancing renal masses due to previously reported high false negative rates as well as concern for cancerous seeding of the biopsy tract and other complications such as bleeding

(Abel et al. 2012). More recently however percutaneous biopsy has been enjoying a renaissance of sorts. Roughly 20 % of T1a masses (<4 cm) are actually benign, and an accurate biopsy can spare these patients the morbidity of surgical intervention. It has been reported that greater than 90 % of needle core biopsies are sufficient to render a diagnosis (Wang et al. 2009; Millet et al. 2012). More importantly, in biopsies which have sufficient tissue for diagnosis several studies have reported near or up to 100 % accuracy (Wang et al. 2009; Menogue et al. 2013), which has alleviated the historical concern of false negative and potentially not intervening in the case of a missed cancerous tumor. Complication rates are satisfactorily low and as more biopsies are performed, tract seeding has been shown to be exceedingly rare. It is now generally recommended by the American Urological Association that renal biopsy be offered to patients who are surgical candidates for whom a diagnosis has the potential to change management, with the understanding that some patients when faced with a renal mass will consider even low levels of diagnostic uncertainty unacceptable.

Management

Management of suspected malignant renal masses is directed by numerous variables such as tumor size, stage, patient comorbidities, life expectancy, and biopsy results, among others. A discussion of management requires a basic understanding of tumor, node, and metastasis (TNM) staging which is presented for review in Table 18.3.

Surveillance of Renal Masses

With the frequency of body imaging an increasing number of small, incidental renal masses have been discovered in elderly patients who are poor surgical candidates and this has granted insight into the natural history of such masses in the absence of intervention. It has been demonstrated that these tumors have relatively slow growth rates and low risks for metastases, with only 1.1 % progression to metastatic disease for lesions <4 cm in size at 28 months follow-up and a growth rate of roughly 0.1 cm per year (Jewett et al. 2011). As such, the American Urological Association (AUA) 2009 guidelines state active surveillance is "a reasonable option for patients with limited life expectancy or for those who are unfit for or do not desire intervention."

Surgical Intervention

There have been novel treatments introduced, some of which will be discussed, however surgical excision remains a mainstay in the management of localized renal tumors.

Table 18.3 TNM staging of kidney cancer as published by American Joint Committee on Cancer (AJCC)

Primary tumor (T)	
Tx	Primary tumor cannot be assessed
T0	No evidence of primary tumor
T1	Tumor ≤7 cm confined to kidney
T1a	Tumor ≤4 cm confined to kidney
T1b	Tumor 4–7 cm confined to kidney
T2	Tumor >7 cm confined to kidney
T2a	Tumor 7–10 cm confined to kidney
T2b	Tumor >7 cm confined to kidney
T3	Tumor extends into major veins or perinephric tissue but not ipsilateral adrenal gland and not beyond Gerota's fascia
T3a	Tumor grossly extends into renal vein or its segmental branches or invades perirenal fat (not beyond Gerota's)
T3b	Tumor extends into vena cava below diaphragm
T3c	Tumor extends into vena cava above diaphragm or invades wall of vena cava
T4	Tumor invades beyond Gerota's fascia or into ipsilateral adrenal
Regional lymph nodes (N)	
NX	Regional nodes cannot be assessed
N0	No regional lymph node metastasis
N1	Metastasis present in regional lymph nodes
Distant metastasis (M)	
M0	No distant metastasis
M1	Distant metastasis

Radical Nephrectomy

Radical nephrectomy (RN) has been a long-standing gold standard surgical procedure for localized RCC. This involves removing the entire kidney and all of the contents within Gerota's fascia. Traditionally this included removal of the adrenal but it has been demonstrated more recently for the majority of kidney tumors the ipsilateral adrenal can be spared during radical nephrectomy. RN is often performed laparoscopically at many institutions and offers excellent oncologic outcomes with shortened hospital stays while avoiding the morbidity of open surgery.

Partial Nephrectomy

Recently more attention has been paid to the health consequences of CKD, specifically increased cardiovascular morbidity, and subsequent mortality (Go et al. 2004). Not surprisingly, radical nephrectomy leads to CKD in a higher number of patients than partial nephrectomy. PN entails clamping of the renal vessels and excision of the tumor with removal of a rim of normal renal parenchyma. When performed via an open surgical approach, cold ischemia in the form of ice on the kidney is used, but laparoscopically this is not as feasible and is usually done without cold ischemia. Given our understanding of the potential for CKD and its sequelae, for patients with T1 tumors and a normal contralateral kidney, there has been a push in recent years to perform partial nephrectomy given that the mass is amenable to this approach. This decision is based largely on feasibility as determined by the individual surgeon. Partial nephrectomy (PN) can be performed via open, laparoscopic, or robotic-assisted approaches and management will vary based on surgeon expertise. It has been demonstrated that PN does carry with it an increased morbidity in terms of potential for bleeding and urinary leak which are complications not seen as often after RN; however, with the benefit of better preserved renal function.

Important preoperative considerations for both radical and partial nephrectomy are those common to most surgical interventions. All patients should receive preoperative medical clearance from either an internist or cardiologist, and further preoperative risk stratification and testing will be obtained at their discretion. Coordination of care across specialties is an important principle of preoperative surgical care.

Thermal Ablation

Thermal ablation for renal masses encompasses a variety of minimally invasive procedures done either percutaneously with CT guidance or laparoscopically including cryotherapy, radiofrequency ablation, among others. The literature regarding these is limited by short-term follow-up and the absence of standardized methodology; however it suggests roughly equivalent cancer-specific survival when compared to traditional surgical management, albeit with short follow-up. Recurrence-free survival, while high, does not match the rates noted with surgical management. It is important to note that these studies have been performed mostly on elderly patients who are considered high surgical risk and on small renal masses generally <3 cm in size. In summary, they are recognized as a reasonable minimally invasive alternative in patients who are poor surgical candidates who are willing to accept the higher recurrence rate and need for additional procedures in exchange for potentially less morbidity. Decision making regarding these alternative options is complex and the urologist should play an integral role in patient counseling.

Follow-Up

After surgical excision of RCC, continued follow-up is essential given the estimation that 20–30 % of patients will experience relapse. Patients are at various risks of relapse depending on stage, grade, and size of tumor at resection, and thus there is no standard follow-up protocol which can be applied to all patients. NCCN Guidelines recommend a history and physical exam every 6 months for the first 2 years for every patient, along with annual visits thereafter. At all visits a comprehensive metabolic panel should be obtained which includes liver enzymes. Additionally patients with solitary kidneys or those with risk factors for renal insufficiency should be screened annually with 24 h urine protein measurements, as proteinuria is often the first sign of progressing renal disease. When detected a nephrology referral is appropriate.

With regard to imaging the lung is the most common site of distant recurrence, and as such, a chest x-ray is reasonable to obtain at these 6-month visits. The frequency of abdominal CT scans will vary based on T-stage and grade of the primary tumor. AUA guidelines recommend for T1 tumors a baseline CT scan be obtained within the first year. For higher risk tumors and higher stages, (T2-T4), the AUA recommendation is that abdominal imaging and chest imaging of some sort be obtained every 6 months for 3 years, initially with CT and moving forward with either CT or ultrasound and CXR at the discretion of the physician. Greater detail on follow-up recommendations can be found both at the NCCN and AUA links provided in the resources section.

Clinical Pearls
- Many renal tumors are found incidentally during evaluation for other issues; the classic triad (flank mass, hematuria, pain) is now rare.
- Angiomyolipoma is the only solid renal mass which can reliably be diagnosed as benign on imaging alone; this is determined by the presence of macroscopic fat.
- Renal US is adequate to diagnose simple renal cysts for which reassurance is appropriate, but more complex renal cysts require CT or MRI to further evaluate.
- Biopsy is not necessary before excision of primary solid renal mass.
- 20–30 % of patients may demonstrate paraneoplastic syndrome (elevated ERS, cachexia, fever, anemia, hypertension, elevated serum calcium and alkaline phosphatase, polycythemia)

Resources for the Nurse Practitioner

Practical and readily accessible resources exist for nurse practitioners working in the field of Urology. AUA guidelines present best practice statements regarding the workup and management of renal masses, as well as concise summaries of current evidence in the literature. Additionally algorithms are presented which are of great clinical utility. These can be accessed at auanet.org under the guidelines tab and are an excellent resource for further education, with guidelines for clinical management as well as follow-up imaging.

http://www.auanet.org/education/clinical-practice-guidelines.cfm
http://www.nccn.org/professionals/physician_gls/f_guidelines.asp#site

Resources for the Patient

http://www.urologyhealth.org/urologic-conditions/kidney-cancer
http://www.nccn.org/patients/default.aspx
http://www.urologyhealth.org/urologic-conditions/kidney-cancer
http://www.nccn.org/patients/default.aspx

References

Abel EJ et al (2012) Limitations of preoperative biopsy in patients with metastatic renal cell carcinoma: comparison to surgical pathology in 405 cases. BJU Int 110(11):1742–1746

Chiu BC et al (2006) Body mass index, physical activity, and risk of renal cell carcinoma. Int J Obes (Lond) 30(6):940–947

Go AS et al (2004) Chronic kidney disease and the risks of death, cardiovascular events, and hospitalization. N Engl J Med 351:1296

Gudbjartsson T, Thoroddsen A, Petursdottir V et al (2005) Effect of incidental detection for survival of patients with renal cell carcinoma: results of population-based study of 701 patients. Urology 66:1186

Hanash KA (1982) The nonmetastatic hepatic dysfunction syndrome associated with renal cell carcinoma (hypernephroma): Stauffer's syndrome. Prog Clin Biol Res 100:301

Hock LM et al (2002) Increasing incidence of all stages of kidney cancer in the last 2 decades in the United States: an analysis of surveillance, epidemiology and end results program data. J Urol 16:57

Israel GM, Bosniak MA (2005) An update of the Bosniak Renal Cyst Classification system. Urology 66:484

Jamel A et al (2010) Cancer statistics, 2010. CA Cancer J Clin 60:277

Jewett MA et al (2011) Active surveillance of small renal masses: progression patterns of early stage kidney cancer. Eur Urol 60(1):39–44

Menogue SR et al (2013) Percutaneous core biopsy of small renal mass lesions: a diagnostic tool to better stratify patients for surgical intervention. BJU Int 111(4 Pt B):E146–E151

Millet I et al (2012) Can renal biopsy accurately predict histological subtype and Fuhrman grade of renal cell carcinoma? J Urol 188(5):1690–1694

Nguyen MM, Gill IS (2009) Effect of renal cancer size on the prevalence of metastasis at diagnosis and mortality. J Urol 181(3):1020–1027

Pantuck AJ et al (2000) Incidental renal tumors. Urology 56(2):190–196

Romis L et al (2004) Frequency, clinical presentation and evolution of renal oncocytomas: multicentric experience from a European database. Eur Urol 45:53

SEER Stat Fact Sheet: Kidney and Renal pelvis. http://seer.cancer.gov/statfacts/html/kidrp.html

Siegel R, Ward E, Brawley O, Jemal A (2011) Cancer statistics, 2011: the impact of eliminating socioeconomic and racial disparities on premature cancer deaths. CA Cancer J Clin 61:212

Wang R et al (2009) Accuracy of percutaneous core biopsy in management of small renal masses. Urology 73(3):586–590

Neoplasms of the Penile and Testis

19

Susanne A. Quallich

Contents

Objectives
1. Describe penile and testicular neoplasms.
2. Identify populations that benefit from screening for penile and testicular neoplasms.
3. Appropriately order imaging studies and relevant labs to make the diagnosis of penile or testicle testicular neoplasm.
4. Discuss surveillance issues unique to these malignancies.

S.A. Quallich, ANP-BC, NP-C, CUNP, FAANP
Division of Andrology and Urologic Health, Department of Urology, University of Michigan Health System, Ann Arbor, MI, USA
e-mail: quallich@umich.edu

© Springer International Publishing Switzerland 2016
M. Lajiness, S. Quallich (eds.), *The Nurse Practitioner in Urology*,
DOI 10.1007/978-3-319-28743-0_19

Penile Neoplasms

Neoplasms of the penis arise from the squamous epithelium of the glans and penile shaft. These cancers are rare in the United States, with an expected 1820 cases for 2015. Although other cell types may occur, the most prominent subtype is squamous cell carcinoma, and these lesions develop from the mucosal surface of the penis in the prepuce making the primary risk for this condition in the presence of the foreskin. This tends to be a particularly aggressive type of neoplasm with lesions that arise typically to the glans, prepuce, and penile shaft and infiltrate through lymphatic dissemination. Treatment for penile cancer commonly involves surgery, radiation, and chemotherapy.

Epidemiology and Risk Factors

The greatest risk for penile cancer is seen in men between the ages of 50 and 70. Industrialized nations have a much lower rate of penile cancer; among nonindustrialized countries, prevalence rates are up to five to ten times higher than that seen in the United States. It is an uncommon disease in children and young men, with exceptions seen among men who have human immunodeficiency virus and human papilloma virus (HPV).

Several distinct risk factors have been associated with penile cancer including phimosis, lack of circumcision, HPV infection, lower socioeconomic status, chronic inflammatory conditions such as balanitis, smoking, and overall poor genital hygiene. Uncircumcised men continue to have the highest risk, as a group, for penile cancer. Circumcision as an infant can prevent almost all penile cancer from developing. A lack of circumcision can contribute to chronic inflammatory states such as phimosis and balanitis, with these conditions present in 45–85 % of men with penile cancers. This is compounded by poor hygiene, tobacco use, and other chronic inflammatory states. HPV infection has also gained recognition as a causative factor for penile cancer, with serotypes 16 and 18 remaining the most common influences on the malignant conversion of cells.

Clinical Diagnosis and Staging

Most penile cancers are superficial and low grade. Previous nomenclature for penile cancers have included terms such as carcinoma in situ (CIS), Bowen's disease, and erythroplasia of Queyrat, but have been more recently termed penile intraepithelial neoplasia (PeIN). Further subdivision is based upon morphologic and microscopic characteristics. When the penile cancer is diagnosed, it can be termed superficial spreading, described by vertical growth, and can be described as verruciform, multicenter, and mixed. Squamous cell carcinoma remains the most common type of penile cancer and is seen up to two-thirds of cases. The most important predictors for metastatic spread and survival remain as diagnosed tumor grade, depth of

Table 19.1 TMN staging of penile cancer

TX	Primary tumor cannot be assessed
T0	No evidence of primary tumor
Tis	Carcinoma in situ
Ta	Noninvasive verrucous carcinoma
T1a	Invasion into subepithelial connective tissue, no lymph vascular invasion; *not* poorly differentiated
T1b	Invasion into subepithelial connective tissue, with lymph vascular invasion, or *is* poorly differentiated
T2	Invasion into corpus spongiosum or cavernosum
T3	Invasion into the urethra
T4	Invasion to other adjacent structures
Regional lymph nodes (N) *clinical stage definition*	
cNX	Regional lymph nodes cannot be assessed
cN0	No palpable or visibly enlarged inguinal lymph nodes
cN1	Palpable mobile unilateral inguinal lymph node
cN2	Palpable mobile multiple or bilateral inguinal lymph nodes
cN3	Palpable fixed inguinal nodal mass or pelvic lymphadenopathy unilateral or bilateral
Regional lymph nodes (N) *pathologic stage definition*	
X	Regional lymph nodes cannot be assessed
pN0	No regional lymph node metastasis
pN1	Metastasis in a single inguinal lymph node
pN2	Metastases in multiple or bilateral inguinal lymph nodes
pN3	Extranodal extension of lymph node metastasis or pelvic lymph node(s) unilateral or bilateral
Distant metastasis (M)	
0	No distant metastasis
M1	Distant metastasis

Adapted from AJCC (2010)

invasion, and presence or absence of perineural invasion. Clinical staging is assigned using the 2010 AJCC TMN staging for penile cancer (Table 19.1).

Metastasis occurs in a predictable stepwise fashion; it spreads from the penis to the sentinel node, the superficial inguinal nodes, to deep inguinal nodes, to pelvic nodes, and then to distant metastasis sites. This stepwise progression is because the lymphatics of the penis do not drain directly to the pelvic lymph nodes.

History and Physical Examination

The focused history includes age at circumcision (if relevant), history of balanitis or other chronic inflammatory conditions, history of prior penile trauma, and history of sexually transmitted infections (especially HPV), along with questions about tobacco use and personal hygiene habits. An individual's history should also be reviewed for previous treatment for dermatologic conditions such as lichen sclerosis or balanitis xerotica obliterans (BXO). A delay in seeking treatment is common, and men may present with paraneoplastic syndromes such as hypercalcemia.

Physical examination involves careful inspection of the penis, penile shaft, and bilateral inguinal regions. The foreskin should be retracted when possible. Each lesion must be assessed by including the diameter, whether it is fixed or mobile, location relative to the phallus and other anatomical structures, and obvious morphological features (keratinization, ulceration, nodular). Inguinal lymph nodes should be characterized as well, e.g., mobile versus fixed; the most common site of metastasis is the inguinal lymph nodes. Note should be made of potential underlying infection. Excisional biopsy or punch biopsy may be performed in clinic to confirm diagnosis.

Other conditions can present with lesions to the male genitals. A Buschke-Lowenstein tumor (giant condyloma) is a large exophytic mass that can occur in the genital, inguinal or anorectal region. It is benign but can be locally invasive, and surgical excision may be quite extensive. Bowenoid papulosis presents as red-brown papules to the glans or shaft and is similar in appearance to carcinoma in situ. It is commonly treated with topical medications or laser ablation. Zoon's balanitis is a well-circumscribed, red, flat lesion, and it contains darker red spots. It looks similar to carcinoma in situ and is diagnosed by biopsy. It is also treated with topical preparations or laser ablation.

Lichen sclerosis (LS) results from a chronic infection, trauma, or inflammation to the male genitals. Two to nine percent of men diagnosed with lichen sclerosis progress to penile cancer. LS presents as flat white patches on the glans and prepuce. It may feel fibrotic and is usually asymptomatic, although men may complain of burning and itching, and painful erections.

Diagnostic Tests

Initial evaluation will include a biopsy of the primary lesion. If the patient is appropriate for organ-sparing (penis-sparing) therapy, a penile ultrasound or MRI with contrast may help determine the extent of any tissue invasion. A biopsy of the sentinel lymph node may also be helpful. Patients at risk for cancer in the regional lymph nodes should also undergo a chest x-ray, CT scan of the abdomen and pelvis, and routine blood tests including serum chemistries including calcium and liver function tests. If the patient has bone pain, elevated calcium or alkaline phosphatase, a bone scan is indicated.

Management

The suitability of an individual patient for various therapies is determined by the clinical stage of his lesion(s). The American Urological Association offers guidelines for managing primary penile tumors (see Appendix). Tis and Ta primary tumors can be managed with topical treatments (5 % imiquimod, 5-fluorouracil) with or without local resection. Men with higher-stage penile tumors should be offered wide local excision, penile-preserving surgery with skin grafts, and/or possibly laser ablation surgery. Penile-sparing surgery is heavily dependent on the grade, stage, and location of the primary tumor, but has a higher local recurrence rate. Surgery may take the form of penectomy or glansectomy; penectomy is considered when a penile stump of >2 cm cannot be preserved. A regional lymph node dissection may also be indicated, and emphasis on negative margins is paramount.

Chemotherapy is indicated when the primary tumor or inguinal node metastasis are unresectable. Regimens usually include 5-FU and cisplatin.

Perioperative Management

All team members caring for patients with penile cancer must be sensitive to the fact that this treatment can have significant psychosocial and sexual implications for men, independent of the stage of their tumor. Men may benefit from psychosocial counseling and possibly counseling with a specialized sex therapist as well.

Ongoing management involves intensive follow-up over the first 2 years, although there is a paucity of scientific literature supporting rigid follow-up guidelines. Men should be taught self-examination of the penis and inguinal lymph nodes. Men should be examined by clinician every 3–6 months over the first 2 years. If they undergo a lymph node dissection, men will need serial chest imaging (every 6 months) and abdominal/pelvic CT or MRI (every 3 months for the first year, every 6 months for the second year). Prognosis depends on surgical staging; men with invasion of the corpus spongiosis appear to have a better prognosis. Relative survival rate for cancers combined to the penis is 85 % at 5 years.

Metastatic disease at time of diagnosis is treated with a multimodal approach than can include chemotherapy with consolidative surgery (preferably), radiotherapy, or chemoradiation, but prognosis is poor.

Long-Term Follow-Up

Men who have undergone penile-sparing surgery will be seen closely for the first 2 years (every 3 months), while those who have undergone partial/total penectomy will be seen every 6 months for the first 2 years (Clark et al. 2013). If there were bulky lymph nodes, men will need a physical examination and abdominal/pelvic imaging (CT or MRI) every 3 months for the first year and then every 6 months during year 2; chest x-ray is added according to this same imaging schedule. If there were negative lymph nodes, men will need a physical examination every 3–6 months for 2 years and then every 6–12 months for another 3 years. Imaging will target men whose examination is challenging (e.g., obesity). Management of local recurrences is poorly explored, but can include surgical resection, external beam radiotherapy, and/or systemic chemotherapy.

Testis Neoplasms

Neoplasms of the testes are relatively uncommon and are rare in the United States with an expected 8430 cases for 2015. Over 95 % are germ cell tumors, with the remaining types split among germ cell tumors. These germ cell tumors are also classified as seminoma or non-seminoma germ cell tumors (NSGCT) and are the most common malignancy seen in men between the ages of 20–40. Only 10–30 % of men present with metastatic disease; most men present with a localized testicular seminoma.

Epidemiology and Risk Factors

The well-recognized risk factors for testicular cancer include cryptorchidism, family or personal history of testicular cancer, or intratubular germ cell neoplasia (ITGCN). For men with a history of cryptorchidism, a higher risk for testicular cancer is associated with a higher location of the testes, meaning highest risk occurs in men with a history of intra-abdominal testis. Relative risk in men with cryptorchidism remains at 4–6 when compared with a matched cohort (Albers, et al. 2011). Other conditions also increase risk for testis cancer including HIV infection, gonadal dysgenesis, male infertility, Klinefelter's syndrome, and testicular feminization after 30 years of age. The incidence of testicular cancer is highest among non-Hispanic whites and lowest among African Americans. Men ages 50 or greater are more likely to have a spermatocytic seminoma.

Anatomy

Testicular neoplasms are more common on the right, because cryptorchidism is more common on the right. Retroperitoneal lymph nodes are the most common site of metastasis; lymphatic spread occurs in a stepwise pattern. Within normal lymphatics, right testis tumors spread to interaortocaval retroperitoneal nodes, while left testis tumors are to be para-aortic retroperitoneal nodes. Distant metastasis, in the order of most common to least common, includes lung, and liver, brain, bone, kidney, adrenal, gastrointestinal, and spleen.

Clinical Diagnosis and Staging

The most common presentation is painless mass or swelling in the testis, usually found incidentally by the patient or his partner. Physical examination will reveal a firm, tender, or nontender testis mass. Five to ten percent of men may present with a hydrocele which can obscure examination of any potential tumor. Other presenting symptoms can include clues to metastatic disease such as abdominal mass, supraclavicular mass, shortness of breath, or hemoptysis. Back pain can occur with bulky retroperitoneal metastasis and is more commonly seen with non-seminomas. Clinical staging is assigned using the 2010 AJCC TMN staging for testis cancer (Table 19.2).

Table 19.2 TMN staging of testicular tumors

Primary tumor (T)	
pTx	Primary tumor cannot be assessed
pT0	No evidence of primary tumor
pTis	Intratubular germ cell neoplasia
pT1	Tumor limited to the testis and epididymis without lymphovascular invasion; may invade the tunica albuginea but not the tunica vaginalis
pT2	Tumor limited to the testis and epididymis with lymphovascular invasion or tumor involving the tunica vaginalis
pT3	Invasion into spermatic cord with or without lymphovascular invasion
pT4	Invasion of scrotum with or without lymphovascular invasion
Regional lymph nodes (clinical) (N)	
Nx	Regional lymph nodes cannot be assessed
N0	No regional lymph node metastasis
N1	Metastasis within one or more lymph nodes <2 cm in size
N2	Metastasis within one or more lymph nodes >2 cm but <5 cm in size
N3	Metastasis within one or more lymph nodes >5 cm in size
Regional lymph nodes (pathologic) (N)	
Nx	Regional lymph nodes cannot be assessed
N0	No regional lymph node metastasis
N1	Metastasis within 1–5 lymph nodes; all node masses <2 cm in size
N2	Metastasis within a lymph node >2 cm but not >5 cm in size, or >5 lymph nodes involved, none >5 cm; none demonstrating extranodal extension
N3	Metastasis within one or more lymph nodes >5 cm in size
Distant metastasis (M)	
Mx	Distant metastasis cannot be assessed
M0	No distant metastasis
M1	Distant metastasis
M1a	Nonregional nodal or pulmonary metastasis
M1b	Distant metastasis at site other than nonregional lymph nodes or the lung
Serum tumor markers (S)	
Sx	Tumor markers not available or performed
S0	Tumor markers within normal limits
S1	LDH <1.5 × normal, hCG <5000 IU/L, AFP <1000 ng/ml
S2	LDH 1.5–10 × normal, hCG 5000–50,000 IU/L, AFP 1000–10,000 ng/ml
S3	LDH >10 × normal, hCG >50,000 IU/L, AFP >10,000 ng/ml

Adapted from AJCC Cancer Staging Manual (2010)

History and Physical Examination

A key point in the history of men presenting with a testis mass is their personal history of cryptorchidism: where the testicle was located and at what age they underwent orchiopexy. There can be a typical delay in seeking treatment from 3 to 6 months after a nodule is noticed by the individual; length of delay correlates with the risk for metastasis. A history of acute testicular pain may be an indication of intratesticular hemorrhage or infarction.

Physical examination includes careful examination of the genitals, lymph nodes, abdomen, and breast tissue. A mass may be readily noted on examination of the testis; if the mass is sizable enough, there may also be erythema and pain associated with the examination due to distention of the scrotal skin. Transillumination of the scrotum will yield no evidence of light passing through scrotum. The patient abdomen may reveal bulky retroperitoneal disease, if the patient is thin enough. Gynecomastia may also be present.

Diagnostic Tests

A scrotal ultrasound is mandatory when physical exam reveals any testicular mass. If the scrotal ultrasound confirms a mass, tumor markers (Table 19.3) should be ordered along with liver function tests, creatinine, and CBC. Testosterone, FSH, and LH may be added if the patient is particularly interested in his fertility status pre- and posttreatment. Chest x-ray should also be ordered; if the clinician's suspicion is high for a testicular neoplasm, a CT scan of the abdomen and pelvis with contrast can be ordered, anticipating the need for staging studies. It is important to note that abdominal CT scan has a 30 % false negative rate – some men will have tumor in the retroperitoneal nodes. Additional workup is performed after a radical inguinal orchiectomy and confirmation of tumor pathology.

Table 19.3 Discussion of testicular cancer tumor markers

Marker	Non-seminoma germ cell tumors (NSGCT)	Yolk sac tumor	Seminoma	Embryonal carcinoma	Choriocarcinoma
Alpha-fetoprotein (AFP)	Elevated in 50–80 %	Produced	Not produced	Not produced	Not produced
β-Human chorionic gonadotropin (bHCG)	Elevated in 20–60 %	Never produced	Elevated in 15%	Produced	High levels
Lactate dehydrogenase (LDH)	Elevated but nonspecific	Nonspecific but produced	Nonspecific but produced	Nonspecific but produced	Nonspecific but produced

Management

Radical inguinal orchiectomy is the standard of treatment when a primary testis cancer is suspected. This involves complete removal of the testicle and spermatic cord to the level of the internal inguinal ring, through inguinal incision. Management and surveillance are based on type of and stage of the tumor and can involve surveillance (Table 19.4), radiation therapy, or chemotherapy. Platinum is the most effective chemotherapeutic agents against germ cell tumors, but can result in long-term arrest of spermatogenesis.

Some men may need retroperitoneal lymph node dissection (RPLND) for bulky disease; this eliminates possible relapse and a simpler regimen for follow-up. Some centers may offer this option laparoscopically. In many men RPLND leads to ejaculatory dysfunction.

Perioperative Management

All men preparing to be treated for a testicular mass should be offered the opportunity for sperm cryopreservation. Many men with a diagnosis of testicular neoplasm suffer from pretreatment subfertility, meaning that their sperm production has been in some way adversely affected by the presence of the testicular neoplasm. In the majority of patients, their sperm production will rebound; however, if they are treated with radiation or chemotherapy, this rebound can be unpredictable and may occur over 5 years.

All team members caring for patients with testicular cancer must be sensitive to the fact that this treatment can have significant psychosocial and sexual implications for men, independent of their age and independent of the stage of their tumor. Men may benefit from psychosocial counseling and possibly counseling with a specialized sex therapist as well. Emphasis should be placed on a curability of testicular neoplasms, regardless of stage. Men may be offered information about a testicular prosthesis, although there may be issues relative to insurance coverage of these devices.

Long-Term Management

Specific long-term follow-up is dependent on the biology of the tumor, in conjunction with the tumor markers and their changes after removal of the testicle. The

Table 19.4 Recommendations for a stage I seminoma surveillance

Year	1	2	3	4	5
History and physical exam	Every 3–6 months	Every 6–12 months	Every 6–12 months	Every 12 months	Every 12 months
Beta-HCG, AFP, and LDH	Optional	Optional	Optional	Optional	
Abdominal/pelvic CT	At 3, 6, 12 months	Every 6–12 months	Every 6–12 months	Every 12–24 months	Every 12–24 months
Chest x-ray	As clinically indicated				

highest risk for recurrence is generally in the first 2 years after initial treatment. For germ cell tumors, follow-up involves regular tumor markers, imaging, and physical examinations. Men should be taught self-examination of the remaining testis. Any evidence of recurrence on imaging studies will require surgical resection.

Because of the success of treatment for testicular neoplasms, there can be issues of survivorship for these men, especially relative to the late effect of treatments. This can include monitoring for risk of cardiovascular disease, secondary malignancies such as leukemia, ongoing sub- or infertility, kidney dysfunction, lung toxicity, anxiety, or depression.

Cultural Considerations with Penile and Testicular Neoplasms

Because of the private nature and reproductive and sexual functions inherent to the genitals, all team members caring for these men should be sensitive to the potential for cultural, religious, and social implications involved with treatment. Penile cancer is very rare in Jewish men where circumcision is an accepted ritual and higher in Muslim populations where circumcision at puberty is a ritual. These factors may influence their comfort level with providers of the opposite gender and influence an individual's choice to seek treatment. Survivorship for men with testicular cancer is vital, as the disease is curable at almost every stage of presentation.

Clinical Pearls
All testicular masses should be considered tumors until proven otherwise.
A scrotal ultrasound is mandatory for any suspected testicular mass.
Penile cancer is strongly linked to HPV strains, especially HPV-16.
Clinical staging for testicular cancers is very important.
Men undergoing surgery for penile or testicular cancer may benefit from psychosocial support, due to the disfiguring nature of the surgery.

Resources for the Nurse Practitioner
American Cancer Society: www.cancer.org
NCCN Clinical Practice Guidelines in Oncology (NCCN Guidelines®) www.nccn.org
Testicular prosthesis: http://www.coloplast.us/torosa-en-us.aspx
RESOLVE: The National Infertility Association: www.resolve.org
American Society for Reproductive Medicine: http://www.reproductivefacts.org

Resources for the Patient
American Cancer Society: www.cancer.org
The Urology Care Foundation: www.urologyhealth.org/urologic-conditions/penile-cancer

Testicular Cancer Foundation: www.testicularcancer.org
RESOLVE: The National Infertility Association: www.resolve.org
American Society for Reproductive Medicine: http://www.reproductivefacts.org

References

American Joint Committee on Cancer: Penis (2010) In: Edge SB, Byrd DR, Compton CC, et al (eds) AJCC cancer staging manual, 7th edn. Springer, New York, pp 447–455

Albers P, Albrecht W, Algaba F, European Association of Urology et al (2011) EAU guidelines on testicular cancer: 2011 update. Eur Urol 60:304–319

Bleeker MC, Heideman DA, Snijders PJ, Horenblas S, Dillner J, Meijer CJ (2009) Penile cancer: epidemiology, pathogenesis and prevention. World J Urol 27(2):141–150

Castellasgue X, Bosch FX, Munoz N, Meijer CJ, Shah KV, de Sanjose S et al (2002) Male circumcision, penile human papillomavirus infection, and cervical cancer in female partners. N Engl J Med 346(15):1105–1112

Clark PE, Spiess PE, Agarwal N, Biogioli MC, Eisenberger M, Greenberg RE, Herr HW, Inman BA, Kuban DA, Kuzel TM, Lele SM, Michalski J, Pagliaro L, Pal SK, Patterson A, Plimack ER, Pohar KS, Porter MP, Richie JP, Sexton WJ, Shipley WU, Small EJ, Trump DL, Wile G, Wilson TG, Dwyer M, Ho M (2013) Penile cancer: clinical practice guidelines in oncology. J Natl Compr Canc Netw 11(5):594–615

Edge SE, Byrd DR, Compton CC (2010) AJCC cancer staging manual, 7th edn. Springer, New York, pp 469–473

Groll RJ, Warde P, Jewett MA (2007) A comprehensive systematic review of testicular germ cell tumor surveillance. Crit Rev Oncol Hematol 64:182

International Germ Cell Cancer Collaborative Group (1997) International Germ Cell Consensus Classification: a prognostic factor-based staging system for metastatic germ cell cancers. J Clin Oncol 15:594–603

Procedures for the Nurse Practitioner in Urology

20

Heather Schultz and Sarah R. Stanley

Contents

H. Schultz, FNP-C (✉)
Department of Urology, University of North Carolina at Chapel Hill, Chapel Hill, NC, USA
e-mail: hschultz@med.unc.edu

S.R. Stanley, MS, MHS, PA-C
Department of Urology, University of North Carolina, Chapel Hill, NC, USA

© Springer International Publishing Switzerland 2016
M. Lajiness, S. Quallich (eds.), *The Nurse Practitioner in Urology*,
DOI 10.1007/978-3-319-28743-0_20

Objectives
1. Describe indications for specific office-based procedure appropriate to the urology patient.
2. Review both provider and patient preparation.
3. Discuss necessary post-procedure monitoring and follow-up.

Introduction

Physician shortages have opened the doors for advanced practice nurses to enter into the field of urology. As a surgical subspecialty, urology provides opportunities for providers to perform procedures in both the OR and office. This chapter on clinic based urologic procedures is not meant to be instructive on how to perform the procedures themselves. Rather this chapter is meant to be a discussion of indications, follow-up, potential insurance issues, and resources for the advanced practice nurse (APN). This chapter will act as a guide for the APN to begin their journey in learning procedures.

The procedures that are reviewed in this chapter are certainly not exhaustive and there are many other procedures that APNs are performing that are not included. According to the 2010 AUA survey sent to the APRN/PA/allied health membership database with 205 respondents (included APNs, PAs, RNs, and other allied health members) and a 30 % response rate, the APRN/PA was found to be performing urodynamics, stent removal, urethral dilation, vasectomy, injection treatment for priaprism, bladder biopsy (prostate biopsy and cystoscopy were not reported). Quallich reported in a survey from 2011 (53 surveys and 46.7 % response rate) that showed that ANPs were performing a wide variety of procedures some at very advanced levels. The primary cultural and religious considerations relative to these procedures relate to providers of the opposite sex performing procedures and need to be addressed as the situation requires.

For the purposes of this chapter, the following procedures will be the focus: cystoscopy (diagnostic and stent removal), prostate biopsy, Testopel®, Vantas®, urethral dilation, penile block, reduction of paraphimosis, and penile injection for Peyronie's disease.

This chapter should not act as the only consideration of reference for a procedure. Rather this chapter should act as a guide that will supplement the hands on training that you may get from national organization meetings and most importantly the training that you will get from your supervising/collaborating physician. Every practice will have their own intricacies/protocols for performance. Every state and institution will have their own laws/rules of the APN performing procedures. This would need to be researched through your local board, credentialing committee, hospital committee, supervising/collaborating physician, and/or practice manager.

The AUA consensus statement on utilization of APNs in urologic practice (http://www.auanet.org/advocacy/advanced-practice-providers.cfm) may also be referenced when thinking of how the APN role can be utilized.

Questions to Keep in Mind When Considering Learning Procedures
1. Is this part of my practice agreement with my supervising/collaborating physician?
2. Does the state and practice I work in allow me to perform procedures?
3. If I am allowed, is there any training/tracking of progress that is required by either my state or practice?
4. Do I work in a supportive environment that will be willing to teach the skill?
5. How would I incorporate this skill into my practice and is there a need?

Two other important articles/statements that should be kept in mind that support the role of APNs in practice:

1. Institute of Medicine (2010)
2. Fairman et al. (2010)

Objectives
1. The learner will be able to identify three resources for beginning their didactic training.
2. The learner will be able to identify three pre-procedure considerations.
3. The learner will be able to name three post-procedure instructions.

Urethral Dilation

Define Procedure

Dilation of urethral strictures on awake patient with the goal of draining bladder and temporally treat stricture until a more formal surgical repair can be performed. These techniques may include the use of filiforms/followers, flexible cystoscopy, and glide wires.

Indications

The most common reason for the need for catheter placement is the need for bladder emptying. The most common reasons for difficult urinary catheter placement are enlarged prostate, urethral stricture(s), bladder neck contracture, or false passage.

Prep Required

1. Ensure that patient does not have an active UTI, and if suspicious, treat.
2. Antibiotic prophylaxis according to institution policy.

Pre-procedure Considerations

1. Urethral dilation in setting of infection can lead to sepsis.
2. Urethral dilation in setting of anticoagulation can lead to bleeding.
3. Urethral dilation is a painful procedure for awake patients.
4. Urethral dilation can cause rectal perforation in post prostatectomy and pelvic radiation patients, for example.
5. If uncircumcised male, replace foreskin in the reduced position to prevent paraphimosis.
6. Trauma to the urethra can occur with use of Heyman or filiforms and followers.
7. Consider not performing dilation in unstable patient.
8. Consider not performing dilation in patient with pelvic fracture.
9. Vagal response can occur and can present with orbital numbness, hypotension, tachycardia, diaphoresis, syncope, and weakness.

Post-procedure Instructions to Call Clinic

1. Fevers >101
2. Foley blockage
3. Severe abdominal pain or rectal pain/drainage

Follow-Up

1. Urethral stricture may be assessed with Uroflow, international prostatic symptom score.

Discussion

The trend is that urethral dilation on the awake patient is a temporary option until formal surgery can be achieved. With that said, the provider placing the catheter or perhaps in performance of diagnostic cystoscopy may run into the stricture etiology, such as a urethral stricture. Then the provider would have to decide how to proceed.

Referral Suggestions

1. Formal surgical repair can be considered after urethral dilation of either urethroplasty or bladder neck contracture repair) and should be with a urethral surgeon.
2. Urethral dilation may make formal surgical repair more difficult.
3. Urethral surgeon may want imaging in the form of:
   (a) Retrograde urethrogram
   (b) Voiding cystogram

Insurance Issues

Reimbursement for urethral dilation has been low. So low that urologist will at times look for alternatives for a difficult urinary catheter placement. There are Foley catheter teams that have been put in place at some institutions to help meet this need by trained nurses or APN/PAs. There has been a report that with the use of APN/PAs quality of life of urologist can be better Urethral dilation can be seen as emergent at times, preauthorization typically not required

1. Reimbursement has been reported low.
2. Can be an emergent procedure: prior authorization not indicated.

Guidelines

1. No current guidelines exist for urethral dilation.

Option for Difficult Urinary Catheterization
1. http://www.percuvision.com/index.html for Direct vision ® that is meant for nurses to have a visual guide for difficult urethral catheterization (DUC) in patients that have a history of DUC to help prevent the need for use of guide wires in the case of false passages.

Resources for Learning

AUA Core Curriculum Available at Auanet.org with Membership
1. Anatomy and physiology of the lower urinary tract

CME Review Article

1. AUA update series paid subscription. 2011 Urethral Dilation: Tricks of the trade Carlos Villanueva, M.D. and George P. Hemstreet III, M.D., Ph.D. vol 30 lesson 5.
   (a) Blitz technique is reviewed here for placement of glide wire through Foley

National and Local Meeting Courses

2. UAPA and SUNA National Meetings: Cystoscopy Course
   (a) Check specific details of course for urethral dilation or if just for performing cystoscopy depending on learning needs.

Book Chapters

3. Mendez-Probst et al.
4. Duffey and Monga
5. Chung et al.
6. Fulgham and Bishoff
7. Gerald and McCammon

General Urethral Stricture Management

1. Blitz (1995)
2. Mendez-Probst et al. (2012)
3. Villanueva and Hemstreet (2008).
4. Athanassopoulos et al. (2005)
5. Beaghler et al. (1994)
6. Chelladurai et al. (2008)
7. Krikler (1989)
8. Villanueva and Hemstreet (2010)
9. Freid and Smith (1996)

Journal Articles on Local Anesthetic Use

1. Tzortzis et al. (2009)
2. Ho et al. (2003)
3. Patel et al. (2008)

Cystoscopy

Define the Procedure

Identifying lower urinary tract pathology by directly visualizing the anterior urethra, posterior urethra, and the bladder

Indications

- Gross and microscopic hematuria
- Recurrent UTIs

- Trauma
- Obstructive voiding symptoms
- Irritative voiding symptoms
- Dysuria
- Atypical cytologies
- Bladder abnormalities on imaging studies
- Obstruction after TURP
- Interstitial cystitis (or chronic pelvic pain syndrome)
- Known history of bladder cancer
- Incontinence
- Urethral stricture disease
- Hematospermia
- Pelvic mass
- Bladder stones
- Removal of foreign bodies
- Facilitate catheter insertion
- Suprapubic tube, Foley, or clean intermittent catheterization >5–10 years

Prep Required

1. Rule out active UTI.
2. Counsel patient regarding indications for procedure/informed consent.
3. Sterilely prep and drape.
4. Supine position for flexible cystourethroscopy (with a slight frog-leg position for females).
5. 5–10 mL of lubricant-anesthetic jelly should be instilled into the urethra before the procedure.

Pre-procedure Considerations

1. Stability of patient.
2. Active bleeding (may require irrigation).
3. Will urine for cytology be collected (if for diagnostic cystoscopy)?
4. Will antibiotics be given based on patient risk or facility policy?
   (a) High risk: Anatomic anomalies of the urinary tract, poor nutritional status, smoking, chronic corticosteroid use, immunodeficiency, externalized catheters, colonized endogenous/exogenous material, distant coexistent infection, and prolonged hospitalization (Wolf et al. 2008) otherwise can be avoided. If patient is not high risk but there is need for fulguration, biopsy, or catheterization, antibiotic should be used (Wolf et al. 2008).

Discussion/Pearls of Cystoscopy

1. Preventing procedural discomfort: Most studies will state that lubrication does not make a difference (Patel et al. 2008). Male patients may report more of a benefit, while female may not (Patel et al. 2008; Taghizadeh et al. 2006). Viewing the monitor and talking may benefit the patient, relieving anxiety and helping him/her feel more in control of the situation. This is most helpful for men when reaching the membranous urethra and prostate and encouraging relaxation (Taghizadeh et al. 2006).
   (a) Water-soluble lubricant-anesthetic
   (b) Male: urethral clamp – 30 ml of lubricant
   (c) Position video tower in patient view.
   (d) Explain procedure in real time.
   (e) During entrance into membranous urethra, have patient relax pelvic floor muscles and wiggle toes.
2. Technique: Finding the female urethral meatus is the challenging aspect for the female patient. Obesity, estrogen-deficient tissue, and anatomic anomalies can make this a challenge. For the male patient, ensure penile stretch throughout the procedure for maximum visibility of the fossa navicularis, penile urethra, and bulbar urethra (Duffey and Monga).
   (a) Obese female may need assistance with positioning and visualization of the meatus.
   (b) Penile stretch: of 90° angle to the abdominal wall.
   (c) Penile stretch: The glans is held by the third and fourth digits, and the thumb and forefinger will remain free for guiding scope into the meatus.
   (d) Turn irrigation on once the tip is in the meatus.
   (e) With flexible scope: more anterior angulation aid in passage over the bladder neck in men.
   (f) You can drain the bladder for comfort once inspection is complete.
3. Special considerations:
   (a) Suprapubic tubes:
      (i) You may be able to navigate through the urethra but when not able may be through the mature suprapubic tract.
      (ii) Guide wire through the suprapubic tract to aid the endoscope in difficult cases (Duffey and Monga).
   (b) Continent urinary diversions:
      (i) Understanding of construction.
         • Type and location of ureteroenteric anastomosis
         • Presence or absence of an afferent limb
         • Continence mechanism employed (Duffey and Monga)
      (ii) Mucus, debris, bowel peristalsis, and mucosal folding may inhibit visualization.
4. Stent removal:
   (a) The process is similar to diagnostic cystoscopy.

Post-procedure Instructions/Red Flags

1. Fever over 101
2. Profuse urethral bleeding
3. Inability to void
4. Significant dysuria or abdominal pain

Referral Suggestions

1. For any findings that would require general anesthesia
2. For any finding that the APN is not trained in performing, e.g., urethral dilation and removal of small stone in the bladder

Resources for Learning and Suggested Reading

Joint AUA/SUNA White Paper on the reprocessing of flexible cystoscopes 2013: https://www.auanet.org/education/other-aua-clinical-guidance-documents.cfm   or https://www.suna.org/resource/clinical-practice?page=1

National and Local Meeting Courses
1. UAPA and SUNA national meetings: cystoscopy course.
   (a). Check specific details of course for stent removal or if just for performing cystoscopy depending on your learning needs.

Guidelines
2. No current US guidelines exist for cystoscopy.
3. UK guidelines: http://www.baus.org.uk/Updates/publications-new/flexi-cystoscopy.

AUA Core Curriculum Available at Auanet.org with Membership
1. Anatomy and physiology of the lower urinary tract

Book Chapters
1. Mendez-Probst et al.
2. Duffey and Monga
3. Chung et al.
4. Gerald and McCammon

Local Anesthetic Use and Discomfort
1. Tzortzis et al. (2009)
2. Ho et al. (2003)
3. Patel et al. (2008)

4. Patel et al. (2008)
5. Taghizadeh et al. (2006)

Antibiotic Prophylaxis
1. Herr (2014)
2. Jiménez-Pacheco et al. (2012)
3. Wilson et al. (2005)
4. Latthe et al. (2008)
5. Wolf et al. (2008)

Role of ANP in Cystoscopy
1. Kleier (2009)
2. Quallich (2011)
3. Schultz (2011)
4. Chatterton (2010)
5. Fagerberg and Nostell (2005)
6. Gidlow et al. (2000)
7. Radhakrishnan et al. (2006)

Artificial Urinary Drainage and Surveillance
8. Subramonian et al. (2004)
9. Hess et al. (2003)

Complications
10. Sung et al. (2005)

Testopel® (Testosterone Pellets)

Define the Procedure

In-office procedure on awake patients, using local anesthetic for insertion of testosterone (each pellet 75 mg) into subcutaneous tissue of dissolvable testosterone into the gluteal area

Indications

Testosterone replacement therapy in adult males for conditions associated with low or absent testosterone from either primary hypogonadism (congenital or acquired) or hypogonadotrophic hypogonadism (congenital or acquired)

Contraindications

1. Men with known breast cancer and/or known or suspected prostate cancer
2. Pregnant women (not approved for use in women)

Warnings/May Cause

- Gynecomastia
- DVT/PE
- Edema
- BPH
- Prostate cancer
- With high doses for long periods of time, may cause peliosis hepatitis or hepato-cellular carcinoma
- Hirsutism
- Male pattern baldness
- Abnormal liver function studies
- Polycythemia
- Prolonged erection
- Acne
- Increase or decrease in libido
- Depression and or anxiety
- Generalized paresthesia
- Breast discomfort
- Decreased sperm count
- Rarely anaphylaxis
- Decreased size in testicles
- Decrease insulin dosage need

Site Reactions

1. Pain to insertion site
2. Scar development (site rotation decreases risk)
3. Infection
4. Bleeding
5. Expulsion of pellets

Patient Prep

1. Pre labs as indicated: hematocrit/hemoglobin, PSA, total and free testosterone, liver function studies, and cholesterol.
2. Physical male GU exam as indicated.
3. Assess the skin for scar.
4. Informed consent.
5. Sterile prep of the skin.
6. Each pellet is supplied in a glass ampule. Careful inspection should be made of each ampule. When opening, care should be taken to open away from the sterile field to prevent small shards of glass from dropping on pellet tray.

Post-procedure Instructions/Red Flags

1. No soaking in water for 72 h.
2. No vigorous exercise for 72 h.
3. Bruising is typical.
4. Discomfort for the first couple of days may occur.
5. Leave bandage on for 24–48 h.
6. Steri-Strips will fall off in about 4–5 days.
7. No showering for 24 h.
8. Ice for about 15 min to help decrease swelling/pain.
9. Patient should report bleeding that is continuous, hematoma, expulsion of pellets from the site, fluid discharge from the site, exquisite tenderness to the site or discomfort that persists for more than 5 days, and erythema to the site that lasts longer than 5 day.

Discussion

The use of subcutaneous testosterone can be a great way to reduce risk of exposure to others and eliminate the need for biweekly injection or daily application. Typical training is onsite at the facility, with instruction from seasoned provider performing the task.

Dose adjustment is less flexible with Testopel® than with other products; if treatment needs to be discontinued, surgical removal of the pellets may be necessary. If patient is testosterone replacement naïve, consideration should be made for shorter-acting modalities, such as topical gels, that can be discontinued without the need for an invasive procedure. Starting with another product will also help establish a beginning dose for Testopel®. Dose adjustment can vary from patient to patient, based on sensitivity to medication and absorption rates. Starting doses can vary, but between 10 and 12 pellets is common (McCullough 2014; Mechlin et al. 2014; Pastuszak et al. 2012) with the higher end of dosing at 6 pellets. The maximum treatment number of pellets can be debated, and when considering dose adjustment, there should be continued communication with the provider-mentor in Testopel® management. There are no formalized guidelines on starting dose or dose adjustment; it is up to the patient/provider and joint decision making. There is certainly an "art" to finding the therapeutic dose for each individual patient. Counseling the patient that there may be a "trial and error" period of dose adjustment is helpful to set expectations when initially starting Testopel®.

Expulsion of pellets is rare and can be avoided with proper technique in depth of pellet placement and use of proper aseptic technique (Kelleher et al. 1999). Stitches are not required and typically Steri-Strips are applied but one suture can be used. If at any point there are side effects, they may be reported at www.fda.gov/medwatch.

Referral

1. Polycythemia: hematology
2. Surgical removal of pellets if discontinuation is needed
3. Maximum pellet allowance with suboptimal objective or subjective outcome

Insurance

1. Prior authorization recommended https://www.testopel.com/reimbursement for prior authorization forms and letter of medical necessity/appeals
2. Testopel® reimbursement hotline: 1–800–897–9006
3. Claim form: http://www.auanet.org/advnews/hpbrief/view.cfm?i=364&a=873

Billing Codes

CPT1 (procedure) code	11,980	Subcutaneous hormone pellet implantation (implantation of testosterone pellets beneath the skin)
HCPCS code (private insurance)	S0189	Testosterone pellet, 75 mg
HCPCS code (Medicare)	J3490	Unclassified drugs
NDC (for Medicare claims except CA and NV)	66,887–004–20	100-count box. Use in Box 19 of CMS 1500 form
NDC (for Medicare claims, CA and NV)	66,887–004–10	10-count box. Use in Box 19 of CMS 1500 form

(Retrieved from https://www.testopel.com/reimbursement)

1. Coding hotline: AUA's coding hotline at 866-746-4282, option 2, or e-mail at codinghotline@AUAnet.org

Resources

Training Videos
1. Cartoon video: https://www.youtube.com/watch?v=KeS395ePpX4
2. Patient video: https://www.youtube.com/watch?v=O3kOY46ZakE
3. Other multiple videos available with search of Testopel® video

Guidelines: Currently no guidelines exist for management or placement of Testopel®

Seminars
1. SUNA, UAPA, and AUA (regional and national) meetings with search of "Hands on Course"

Patient Satisfaction
Kovac et al. (2014)
Smith et al. (2013)

Dosing
1. McCullough et al. (2012)
2. McCullough (2014)
3. Mechlin et al. (2014)
4. Pastuszak et al. (2012)
5. Kelleher et al. (2004)

Complications
1. Kelleher et al. (1999)

Book Chapters
1. Morales
2. Paul

Vantas® (Histrelin Acetate)

Define the Procedure

In-office procedure using a local anesthetic for subcutaneous placement of long-term LHRH agonist (histrelin acetate) into the upper inner aspect of the nondominant arm. It requires removal and replacement yearly.

Indications

Metastatic prostate cancer with treatment of Vantas®, intended to help alleviate symptoms, but not cure

Contraindications

1. Hypersensitivity to gonadotropin-releasing hormone
2. Pregnant women

Warnings/May Cause

- Hot flashes/night sweats
- Osteoporosis
- Decreased size of testicles
- If disease to the bone/spine, may cause increase in pain
- Gynecomastia
- Erectile dysfunction/decreased libido
- Fatigue
- Voiding complaints
- Constipation
- Increase in blood sugar
- Implant site reactions
- Convulsions
- Pituitary apoplexy
- Drug-induced liver injury
- Decrease in cognitive function
- Anemia
- Change in body habitus

Patient Prep

1. Pre labs as indicated
2. Physical male GU exam as indicated
3. Assess the skin for scar
4. Informed consent
5. Sterile prep of the skin

Post-procedure Instructions/Red Flags

1. No soaking in water for 72 h.
2. No vigorous exercise for 72 h.
3. Bruising can occur.
4. Discomfort for the first couple of days may occur.
5. Leave bandage on for 24–48 h.
6. Steri-Strips will come off in about 4–5 days/suture; follow up based on type used.
7. No showering for 24 h.
8. Ice for about 15 min to help decrease swelling/pain.
9. Patient should report bleeding that is continuous, hematoma, expulsion of pellets from the site, fluid discharge from the site, exquisite tenderness to the site or discomfort that persists for more than 5 days, and erythema to the site that lasts longer than 5 days.

Insurance/Coding

Endo Pharmaceuticals Reimbursement Services: 1-800-462-ENDO
NDC #: 67,979-500-01, J code: J9225
Administration (CPT Codes):
- 11981 insertion, nonbiodegradable drug delivery implant
- 11982 removal, nonbiodegradable drug delivery implant
- 11983 removal, with reinsertion, nonbiodegradable drug delivery implant
ICD-9-CM Code: 185 Prostate Cancer

Discussion

The use of yearlong impact can help in those who do not want surgical castration, compliance, decreased visits, and decreased injections (Shore et al. 2012). It has been found that histrelin can be efficacious for several years for PSA suppression (Chertin et al. 2000), but one would need to consider cost-effectiveness. In one study that included 97 men who were on LHRH agonist for or greater than 10 year period, there was a greater than 10.7–3.2 times the cost compared to that of bilateral orchiectomy (Mariani et al. 2001). It has been found that orchiectomy and the use of LHRH agonist are both just as efficacious in the treatment for prostate cancer (Mariani et al. 2001). In the setting of the prostate cancer patient that only has a few months to live, the use of LHRH agonist compared to bilateral orchiectomy is more cost-effective (Mariani et al. 2001). There are many reasons for patient decision for chemical versus surgical castration with the most common psychological implications of orchiectomy perhaps with the permanence of and body image issues (Nelson 2013).

Other considerations should be made with initiation of luteinizing hormone-releasing hormone (LHRH) agonist in setting of metastatic disease to the spine and bones (in symptomatic patients) and the LH flare (Weckermann and Harzmann 2004). With this there may need to be consideration of complete androgen blockage with the use of antiandrogens prior to the use of LHRH agonist to decrease risks associated with flare in particular pain (Labrie et al. 1987; Kuhn et al. 1989).

In regard to technique, anecdotally, if there is difficulty with removal of previous implant, transverse incision versus traditional horizontal incision may aid in the removal. With the obese patient, it may be difficult to palpate for the previous implant, and some facilities have the ability to ultrasound the arm in the room to help in the identification for removal. Stitches may be used for closure or use of surgical tape.

Cultural/Religious Considerations

1. Views of foreign body implantation for medical use

Referrals

1. Other urologic provider if unable to extract implant
2. Medical oncology in setting of castrate resistance

Resources and References

Websites
1. Vantas® official website: http://www.vantasimplant.com
2. Vantas® website for video of placement: http://www.vantasimplant.com/hcp/administration/
3. Vantas® website for patient brochures: http://www.vantasimplant.com/hcp/resource-center/

Dose Efficacy
1. Djavan et al. (2010)
2. Altarac (2011)
3. Schlegel (2009)
4. Chertin et al. (2000)
5. Schlegel and Histrelin Study Group (2006)
6. Mariani et al. (2001)
7. Weckermann and Harzmann (2004)

Tolerability
1. Shore et al. (2012)

Patient Safety
1. Ricker et al. (2010)
2. Labrie et al. (1987)
3. Kuhn et al. (1989)

Book Chapter
1. Nelson (2013)

Other Suggested Readings
1. Messing et al. (1999)
2. Prostate Cancer Trialists' Collaborative Group (2000)

Seminars

1. Local national meetings for SUNA, UAPA, and AUA with search of "Hands on Course"

Penile Nerve Block

Define the Procedure

Many in-office urologic procedures require regional anesthesia. A penile nerve block involves local infiltration of an injectable anesthetic into the base of the penis prior to proceeding with other penile procedures (Yachia 2007a, b).

Indications

- Circumcision
- Paraphimosis
- Dorsal slit
- Priapism
- Penile laceration
- Meatotomy
- Optical urethrotomy

Pre-procedure Preparation

- Informed consent should be obtained from the patient or patient's guardian prior to proceeding.
- Aseptic precautions should be used when prepping the patient.
- Avoid the use of epinephrine due to risk of ischemia.

Post Doral Penile Block Complications

- Pain at the injection site.
- Hematoma.
- Edema.
- Compression or vasospasm is rare but can occur with large volumes of anesthetic.

Follow-Up

- As directed, based on the indication for the nerve block

Insurance Coverage

- Issues of coverage may come into play for the procedure being conducted, i.e., circumcision.

Resources

Online Videos
- Several videos are available through www.youtube.com.

Guidelines
- No current guidelines exist for dorsal penile block.

Book Chapters
- Lewis and Stephan (1997)
- Yachia (2007a, b)

Journal Articles on Penile Nerve Block
- Choe (2000)
- Serour et al. (1995)
- Kirya and Werthmann (1978)
- Stav et al. (1995)
- Snellman and Stang (1995)

Online Resources
- Up to date: Management of Zipper Injuries

References
1. Choe (2000)
2. Serour et al. (1995)
3. Kirya and Werthmann (1978)
4. Stav et al. (1995)
5. Snellman and Stang (1995)
6. Lewis and Stephan (1997)
7. Yachia (2007a)
8. Bothner (2014)

Reduction of Paraphimosis

Define the Procedure

Paraphimosis is a condition where the foreskin of the penis is retracted for a prolonged period of time, preventing normal advancement of the foreskin. This urologic emergency causes engorgement of the glans that can eventually result in infection, ischemia, and gangrene of the glans (Wein 2012b; Vunda et al. 2013).

Indications

Reduction should be performed immediately once paraphimosis has been identified (Vunda et al. 2013).

Procedure

Paraphimosis reduction requires reducing the edema in the glans, ultimately allowing placement of the foreskin to its normal anatomical position (Turner et al. 1999; Dubin and Davis 2011; Pohlman 2012). Paraphimosis and reduction techniques can be very painful and should be conducted with analgesics (Turner et al. 1999; Pohlman 2012). Noninvasive manual compression and reduction should be attempted first; this procedure requires steady compression of the distal penis with a gloved hand for several minutes followed by manual traction applied to the foreskin by the provider's fingers. Traction with Babcock or Adson forceps can also be used to aid in reduction (Turner et al. 1999; Chambers 2008). If no ischemia is present, adjunctive methods can aid in reducing swelling and include ice, compression bandages, and osmotic agents (Houghton 1973; Dubin and Davis 2011; Cahill and Rane 1999, Pohlman 2012, Kerwat et al. 1998; Anand and Kapoor 2013). Invasive techniques include puncture techniques, glans aspiration, and dorsal slit (Little and white 2005; Reynard and Barua 1999; Barone and Fleisher 1993; Hamdy and Hastie 1990; Raveenthiran 1996; Choe 2000).

Pre-procedure Preparation
- Careful examination of the penis should be done to rule out other causes of edema.
- Informed consent should be obtained from the patient or patient's guardian prior to proceeding.
- A topical or a local anesthetic is used to anesthetize the area (Vunda et al. 2013). Some patients may also need oral opioids or anxiolytics to help with pain and anxiety.

Post-procedure Instruction
- The foreskin should not be retracted for 1 week after procedure (Vunda et al. 2013).
- If minor tears occur during the procedure, topical antibiotics can be applied to prevent infection.

Follow-Up

- Patients should have a follow-up appointment 1 week after reduction to reevaluate the penis. Patient education should be provided concerning proper hygiene of the penis and gentle retraction of the foreskin to avoid recurrence (Vunda et al. 2013).
- Patients are at risk of scarring and recurrence of paraphimosis. Circumcision may be needed.

Insurance Coverage

Since this is a medical emergency, prior authorization is not warranted.

Resources

Online Videos
- Vunda et al. (2013)

Guidelines
No current guidelines exist for paraphimosis reduction.

Book Chapters
- Chapter 36: Surgery of the Penis and Urethra
- Chambers (2008)
- Yachia (2007a, b)

Journal Articles on Paraphimosis Reduction
- Reynard and Barua (1999)
- Dubin and Davis (2011)
- Vunda et al. (2013)
- Cahill and Rane (1999)
- Choe (2000)
- Turner et al. (1999)
- Little and White (2005)
- Houghton (1973)
- Pohlman et al. (2013)
- Ganti et al. (1985)
- Kerwat et al. (1998)
- Anand and Kapoor (2013)
- Coutts (1991)
- Barone and Fleisher (1993)
- Hamdy and Hastie (1990)
- Kumar and Javle (2001)
- Raveenthiran (1996)

Online Resources
- Up to date: Paraphimosis Reduction

Paraphimosis References

1. Reynard and Barua (1999)
2. Dubin and Davis (2011)
3. Vunda et al. (2013)
4. Cahill and Rane (1999)
5. Choe (2000)

6. Turner et al. (1999)
7. Little and White (2005)
8. Houghton (1973)
9. Pohlman et al. (2013)
10. Ganti et al. (1985)
11. Kerwat et al. (1998)
12. Anand and Kapoor (2013)
13. Coutts (1991)
14. Barone and Fleisher (1993)
15. Hamdy and Hastie (1990)
16. Kumar and Javle (2001)
17. Raveenthiran (1996)
18. Vunda et al. (2013)
19. Wein (2012b)
20. Chambers (2008)
21. Yachia (2007b)
22. Tews (2013)

Penile Duplex Doppler Ultrasound

Description of Procedure

Penile duplex Doppler ultrasound uses high-resolution real-time ultrasound with color-pulsed Doppler to analyze the blood flow of the deep penile arteries. It can assess for arterial obstruction and venous leak (Wein 2012c).

Indications

- Evaluation of erectile dysfunction
- Evaluation of priapism
- Evaluation of penile trauma
- Evaluation of Peyronie's disease

Pre-procedure Preparation

- None unless indication requires injection or anesthetic prior to proceeding with study.
- Erectile dysfunction evaluation generally requires intracavernous injection with vasodilator(s). Informed consent should be obtained and risks of priapism should be discussed (Wein 2012d).

Post-procedure Instruction

- Dependent on indication.
- If patients are given intracavernous injection, the patient should not leave until the penis is flaccid (Wein 2012e).

Follow-Up

- As directed based on the indication for the penile duplex Doppler ultrasound

Insurance Coverage

- Prior authorization may be required for evaluation of ED and Peyronie's disease.
- Documentation of both the images and interpretation is vital for reimbursement. Images of all areas should be recorded and variations from normal should be measured and documented. The images should have the patient's name, date, anatomical location, and right vs. left (Martino et al. 2014).
  - More information can be found on the AUA website at: http://www.auanet.org/resources/billing-for-ultrasound.cfm

Resources

National and Local Meeting Courses
- 2014 Doppler and Advances Techniques in Urologic Ultrasound Video (must purchase course)

Online Videos

- AUA Videos and CME Videos:
  - 2014 Doppler and Advanced Techniques in Urologic Ultrasound Video (must purchase)
- Several videos are available for penile duplex Doppler ultrasound and intracavernous injections through www.youtube.com.

Book Chapters
- Chapter 24: Evaluation and Management of Erectile Dysfunction
- Chapter 25: Priapism

Journal Articles on Penile Duplex Doppler Ultrasound
- Martino et al. (2014)
- Wilkins et al. (2003)
- Chiou et al. (1998)
- Mihmanil and Faith (2007)

- Fitzgerald et al. (1992)
- Bhatt et al. (2005)
- Sadeghi-Nejad et al. (2004)

Online Resources
Up To Date Topics
- Evaluation of male sexual dysfunction
- Surgical management of Peyronie's disease
- Priapism

  AUA Core Curriculum: Available at auanet.org with membership

- Uroradiology: Ultrasound
- Sexual Medicine: Peyronie's Disease Epidemiology, Pathophysiology, Evaluation
- Sexual Medicine: ED Patient Evaluation, Investigations

Guidelines
No current guidelines exist for penile duplex Doppler ultrasound but, there are AUA guidelines discussing the use of this procedure with priapism.

Penile Duplex Doppler Ultrasound References
1. Wein (2012c)
2. Wein (2012d)
3. Martino et al. (2014)
4. Wilkins et al. (2003)
5. Chiou et al. (1998)
6. Mihmanli and Kantarci (2007)
7. Fitzgerald et al. (1992)
8. Bhatt et al. (2005)
9. Sadeghi-Nejad et al. (2004)
10. Cunningham (2015)
11. O'Brant (2014)
12. Deveci (2014)
13. Figler
14. Muhlhall
15. Shindell

Xiaflex® (Collagenase Clostridium Histolyticum) Injections

Description of Procedure

Several injectable therapies have been used to manage Peyronie's disease but collagenase clostridium histolyticum (Xiaflex) became the first FDA-approved agent in 2013. Penile plaques are infused with the medication followed by wrapping the penis with an elastic bandage for a few hours.

Indications

- Peyronie's disease

Pre-procedure Preparation

- Patient should be repeatedly reminded, and this should be documented that sexual activity is strongly advised against both intercourse and masturbation from after the first injection to at least 14 days after the second injection of the series, depending on the degree of ecchymosis and swelling.
- Patients should be advised that the bruising that can occur is very deep purple, described as "eggplant."
- The medication must be stored according to manufacturer's instructions.
- Documentation prior to the procedure must include degree of curvature, to ensure the patient meets the criteria for the medication.
- If the is no previous documentation, induce a penile erection with an intracavernous injection of a 10–20 ug of alprostadil. Anesthetic can be injected prior to intracavernous injection.
- Lyophilized Xiaflex powder must be reconstituted with the sterile diluent provided with the medication.

Post-procedure Instruction/Red Flags

- Sexual activity for 2 weeks after the second in the series of two injections is prohibited.
- Daily at-home penile modeling activities shown in the office for 6 weeks after the injection.
- Immediate follow-up is needed if penile facture or anaphylaxis occurs.
- Most common reactions include bruising/hematoma at the injection site.

Follow-Up

- 1–3 days after the first injection, the provider performs in-office penile modeling and performs the second Xiaflex injection to complete one cycle. Up to four cycles can be completed for each patient.

Insurance Coverage

Treating with Xiaflex can be very costly. Prior authorization should be completed so patients are informed about their out-of-pocket expenses. Some insurance companies consider the procedure experimental and submission of the above journal articles and a letter of necessity may be required. Some insurance companies require documented failure of two non-FDA-approved treatments prior to accepting preauthorization paperwork. Auxilium Pharmaceuticals has information concerning CPT codes and financial assistance for patients at https://peyronies-disease.xiaflex.com/hcp/copay-program.php.

Resources

Online Videos
- Xiaflex website: https://peyronies-disease.xiaflex.com/hcp/

Book Chapters
- Campbell-Walsh Chapter 28: Peyronie's Disease

Journal Articles on Penile Duplex Doppler Ultrasound
- Jordan (2008)
- Gelbard et al. (1993)
- Gelbard et al. (2013)

Online Resources
- Up To Date Topics: Peyronie's Disease (diagnosis and medical management)

  AUA Core Curriculum: Available at auanet.org with membership

- Sexual Medicine: Peyronie's Disease Medical Treatment

Guidelines

- No current guidelines exist for Xiaflex.

Collagenase Clostridium Histolyticum (Xiaflex) Injections References
1. Treatment of Peyronie's Disease: Curved or Bent Penis
2. Wein (2012e)
3. Jordan (2008)
4. Gelbard et al. (1993)
5. Gelbard et al. (2013)
6. O'Brant (2013)

Transrectal Ultrasound (TRUS)-Guided Prostate Needle Biopsy

Description of Procedure

TRUS prostate biopsy remains the gold standard for diagnosing prostate cancer and uses ultrasound to aid in removing core samples of tissue from the prostate to be analyzed for cancer. An ultrasound probe is inserted into the rectum to visualize the prostate while a spring-driven biopsy gun is passed through the needle guide of the ultrasound probe into the prostate to obtain tissue core samples (Wein 2012a).

Indications

- Elevated or rising PSA
- Abnormal prostate exam
- Inadequate initial sampling on prior prostate biopsy

Pre-procedure Preparation

- Prophylactic antibiotics: To help lower the risk of post-biopsy infection, prophylactic antibiotics are recommended. Typically, a fluoroquinolone or first-, second-, or third-generation cephalosporin antibiotic has been the standard practice (Kapoor et al. 1998; Aron et al. 2000; Sabbagh et al. 2004; Shigemura et al. 2005). Studies have also show that a single dose of antibiotics is as effective as 1- or 3-day regimens (Sabbagh et al. 2004; Shigemura et al. 2005). The AUA Best Practice Policy on antimicrobial prophylaxis was updated on 1/1/2014 to include trimethoprim-sulfamethoxazole as an alternative therapy, and when using an IM/IV aminoglycoside or aztreonam, clindamycin or metronidazole is no longer required. Bacterial resistance to fluoroquinolones contributes to infectious complications following prostate biopsy. One study showed that 22 % of patients undergoing a rectal swab prior to a prostate biopsy harbored fluoroquinolone-resistant bacteria (Liss et al. 2011). However, at this time the AUA guidelines do not recommend rectal swabs prior to prostate biopsy.
- Bowel prep: A standard bowel preparation has not been established due to limited research. One study found a decreased number of infectious complications with the use of a bisacodyl rectal suppository done the night prior to the biopsy (Jeon et al. 2003). However, two studies found no benefit with the use of sodium bisphosphonate enema or pre-procedural povidone-iodine (Otrock et al. 2004; Carey and Korman 2001). Mechanical enema in conjuncture with antimicrobial prophylaxis decreases the risk of bacteremia according to the literature. However, it does not reduce the risk of fever (Zani et al. 2011).
- Anticoagulation medications: Per AUA best practice statement, 1–4 % of patients experience signification post prostate biopsy bleeding. However, a significant number of patients experience some post-procedure bleeding whether it be hematuria, hematospermia, or rectal bleeding (Kariotis et al. 2010; Halliwell et al. 2006; Ihezue et al. 2005; Carmignani et al. 2011). Literature reviews are mixed on the use of anticoagulant/antiplatelet medication during biopsy, but given the high number of patients experiencing some bleeding, discontinuation of anticoagulation medication may be warranted.

Post-procedure Complications

- Infection: All patients should be instructed to call if they develop a fever.
- Bleeding: Patients should be counseled on the bleeding risk.
- Urinary retention: Although rare, occurring in 0.2–1.1 % of men, patients should be instructed to call their urologist or proceed to the ER if they are in retention (Berger et al. 2004; Raaijmakers et al. 2002; Zaytoun et al. 2011; Kakehi et al. 2008).
- Hematospermia.

Follow-Up

- Pending biopsy results or if post-procedure complications occur.

Insurance Coverage

- Prior authorization may be required for coverage.
- The AUA has information about CPT coding for TRUS prostate biopsy at:
  - www.auanet.org/resources/biopsy-procedures.cfm

Resources

Online Videos
- AUA Videos and CME Videos:
  - 2008 Transrectal Ultrasound of the Prostate (must purchase)
  - Basic Urologic Ultrasound (must purchase)

National and Local Meeting Courses
- AUA National Meeting: Hands on Urologic Ultrasound
  - Check for course offerings on AUA website.
- SUNA National Meeting: Prostate Ultrasound Workshop
  - Check for course offerings on SUNA website.
- UAPA National Meeting: Ultrasound Breakout Session
  - Check for course offerings on UAPA website.

Book Chapters
- Chapter 97: Ultrasound and Biopsy of the Prostate
- Wieder

Journal Articles on TRUS and Prostate Biopsy
- Matlaga et al. (2003)
- El-Hakim and Moussa (2010)

Journal Articles on Ultrasound of the Prostate
- Martino et al. (2014)
- Boczko et al. (2006)

Online Resources
- Up To Date Topics: Prostate Biopsy

  AUA Core Curriculum: Available at auanet.org with membership

- Uroradiology: Ultrasound

Guidelines

AUA/SUNA White Papers
- Optimal Techniques of Prostate Biopsy and Specimen Handling
- AUA Quality Improvement Summit 2014: Conference Proceedings on Infectious Complications of Transrectal Prostate Needle Biopsy
- The Incidence, Prevention, and Treatment of Complications Related to Prostate Needle Biopsy

TRUS Prostate Biopsy Resources
1. Kapoor et al. (1998)
2. Aron et al. (2000)
3. Sabbagh et al. (2004)
4. Shigemura et al. (2005)
5. American Urological Association. Prostate-Specific Antigen Best Practice Statement. Revised (2014)
6. Roberts et al. (2014)
7. Liss et al. (2011)
8. Jeon et al. (2003)
9. Otrock et al. (2004)
10. Carey and Korman (2001)
11. Zani et al. (2011)
12. Halliwell et al. (2008)
13. Kariotis et al. (2010)
14. Halliwell et al. (2006)
15. Ihezue et al. (2005)
16. Carmignani et al. (2011)
17. Raheem et al. (2011)
18. Berger et al. (2004)
19. Raaijmakers et al. (2002)
20. Zaytoun et al. (2011)
21. Kakehi et al. (2008)
22. Biopsy Procedures: American Urological Association

23. https://www.auanet.org/university/product-detail-cme.cfm?typeID=1&produc tID=474
24. https://www.auanet.org/university/product-detail-cme.cfm?typeID=1&produc tID=476
25. Wein (2012a)
26. Weider (2010)
27. Matlaga et al. (2003)
28. El-Hakim and Moussa (2010)
29. Martino et al. (2014)
30. Boczko et al. (2006)
31. Benway (2014)
32. Gonzolez et al. (2012)
33. Averch et al. (2014)
34. Samir et al. (2015)

References

Altarac S (2011) [Histrelin acetate--the first once yearly LHRH agonist]. Lijec Vjesn 133((9–10)):320–322. Croatian

American Urological Association. Prostate-Specific Antigen Best Practice Statement. Revised (2014). Available at: http://www.auanet.org/common/pdf/education/clinical-guidance/Antimicrobial-Prophylaxis.pdf. Accessed 2 Jan 2015

Anand A, Kapoor S (2013) Mannitol for paraphimosis reduction. Urol Int 90.106

Aron M, Rajeev TP, Gupta NP (2000) Antimicrobial prophylaxis for transrectal needle biopsy of the prostate: a randomized controlled study. BJU Int 85:682

Athanassopoulos A, Liatsikos EN, Barbalias GA (2005) The difficult urethral catheterization: use of a hydrophilic guidewire. BJU Int 95:192

Averch T et al (2014) AUA quality improvement summit 2014: conference proceedings on infectious complications of transrectal prostate needle biopsy. AUA White Paper. American Urological Association Education and Research, Inc

Barone JG, Fleisher MH (1993) Treatment of paraphimosis using the "puncture" technique. Pediatr Emerg Care 9:298

Beaghler M, Grasso M 3rd, Loisides P (1994) Inability to pass a urethral catheter: the bedside role of the flexible cystoscope. Urology 44:268

Benway B (2014) Prostate biopsy. Retrieved 8 Feb 2015, from http://www.uptodate.com/contents/prostate-biopsy?source=search_result&search=prostate biopsy&selectedTitle=1~42

Berger AP, Gozzi C, Steiner H et al (2004) Complication rate of transrectal ultrasound guided prostate biopsy: a comparison among 3 protocols with 6, 10 and 15 cores. J Urol 171:1478

Bhatt S, Kocakoc E, Rubens DJ, Seftel AD, Dogra VS (2005) Sonographic evaluation of penile trauma. J Ultrasound Med 24:993–1000

Biopsy Procedures: American Urological Association (n.d.) Retrieved 8 Feb2015, from http://www.auanet.org/resources/biopsy-procedures.cfm

Blitz BF (1995) A simple method using hydrophilic guide wires for the difficult urethral catheterization. Urology 46:99

Boczko J, Messing E, Dogra V (2006) Transrectal sonography in prostate evaluation. Radiol Clin North Am 44:679

Bothner J (2014) Management of zipper injuries. Retrieved 31 Jan 2015, from http://www.uptodate.com/contents/management-of-zipper-injuries?source=search_result&search=management of zipper injuries&selectedTitle=1~4

Cahill D, Rane A (1999) Reduction of paraphimosis with granulated sugar. BJU Int 83:362

Carey JM, Korman HJ (2001) Transrectal ultrasound guided biopsy of the prostate. Do enemas decrease clinically significant complications? J Urol 166:82

Carmignani L, Picozzi S, Bozzini G et al (2011) Transrectal ultrasound-guided prostate biopsies in patients taking aspirin for cardiovascular disease: a meta-analysis. Transfus Apher Sci Off J World Apheresis Asso Off J Eur Soc Haemapheresis 45:275–280

Chambers P (2008) Paraphimosis reduction. In: King C, Henretig FM (eds) Textbook of pediatric emergency procedures, 2nd edn. Lippincott, Williams & Wilkins, Philadelphia, p 904

Chatterton K (2010) A bladder cancer nurse-led flexible cystoscopy service. Europ Urol Today 22(3). Retrieved from http://www.uro.web.org/news/?act=showfull&aid=104

Chelladurai AJ, Srirangam SJ, Blades RA (2008) A novel technique to aid urethral catheterization in patients presenting with acute urinary retention due to urethral stricture disease. Ann R Coll Surg Engl 90:77

Chertin B, Spitz IM, Lindenberg T, Algur N, Zer T, Kuzma P, Young AJ, Catane R, Farkas A (2000) An implant releasing the gonadotropin hormone-releasing hormone agonist histrelin maintains medical castration for up to 30 months in metastatic prostate cancer. J Urol 163(3):838–844

Chiou RK, Pomeroy BD, Chen WS, Anderson JC, Wobig RK, Taylor RJ (1998) Hemodynamic patterns of pharmacologically induced erection: evaluation by Color Doppler sonography. The Journal of Urology 159(1):109–112

Choe JM (2000) Paraphimosis: current treatment options. Am Fam Physician 62:2623

Chung B, Sommer G, Brooks JD Chapter 2: Anatomy of the lower urinary tract and male Genitalia. In: Wein AL, Kavoussi LR, Partin AW & Peters CA (EDs.) Campbell-Walsh Urology, 11th ed. Philadelphia, PA: Elsevier. pp 33–70.e2

Coutts AG (1991) Treatment of paraphimosis. Br J Surg 78:252

Cunningham G (2015) Evaluation of male sexual dysfunction. Retrieved 31 Jan 2015, from http://www.uptodate.com/contents/evaluation-of-male-sexual-dysfunction?source=search_result&search=evaluation of male sexual dysfunction&selectedTitle=1~150

Deveci S (2014) Priapism. Retrieved 31 Jan 2015, from http://www.uptodate.com/contents/priapism?source=search_result&search=Priapism&selectedTitle=1~14

Djavan B, Schlegel P, Salomon G, Eckersberger E, Sadri H, Graefen M (2010) Analysis of testosterone suppression in men receiving histrelin, a novel GnRH agonist for the treatment of prostate cancer. Can J Urol 17(4):5265–5271

Dubin J, Davis JE (2011) Penile emergencies. Emerg Med Clin North Am 29:485

Duffey B, Monga M. Chapter 8: Principles of endoscopy. In: Wein AL, Kavoussi LR, Partin AW & Peters CA (EDs.) Campbell-Walsh Urology, 11th ed. Philadelphia, PA: Elsevier. pp 192–203.e3

El-Hakim A, Moussa S (2010) CUA guidelines on prostate biopsy methodology. Can Urol Assoc J 4(2):89–94

Fagerberg M, Nostell PO (2005) Follow up of urinary bladder cancer – a task for the urology nurse? Lakartidningen 102:2149–2150

Fairman JA, Rowe JW, Hassmiller S, Shalala DE (2010) Broadening the scope of nursing practice. N Engl J Med 364(3):193–196

Figler B (n.d.) Uroradiology: ultrasound. Retrieved 31 Jan 2015, from https://www.auanet.org/university/core_topic.cfm?coreid=67

Fitzgerald SW, Erickson SJ, Foley WD, Lipchik EO, Lawson TL (1992) Color Doppler sonography in the evaluation of erectile dysfunction. Radiographics 12:3–17

Freid RM, Smith AD (1996) The Glidewire technique for overcoming urethral obstruction. J Urol 156:164

Fulgham PF, Bishoff JT Chapter 4: Urinary tract imaging: ultrasonography of penis and urethral tact. In: Wein AL, Kavoussi LR, Partin AW & Peters CA (EDs.) Campbell-Walsh Urology, 11th ed. Philadelphia, PA: Elsevier. pp 99–139.e3

Ganti SU, Sayegh N, Addonizio JC (1985) Simple method for reduction of paraphimosis. Urology 25:77

Gelbard MK, James K, Riach P et al (1993) Collagenase versus placebo in the treatment of Peyronie's disease: a double-blind study. J Urol 149:56

Gelbard M, Goldstein I, Hellstrom WJ et al (2013) Clinical efficacy, safety and tolerability of collagenase clostridium histolyticum for the treatment of peyronie disease in 2 large double-blind, randomized, placebo controlled phase 3 studies. J Urol 190:199

Gerald J, McCammon KA Chapter 36: Surgery of the penis and urethra: anatomy of the penis and male perineum. In: Wein AL, Kavoussi LR, Partin AW & Peters CA (EDs.) Campbell-Walsh Urology, 11th ed. Philadelphia, PA: Elsevier. pp 956–1000.e5

Gidlow AB, Laniado ME, Ellis BW (2000) The nurse cystoscopist: a feasible option? Br J Urol Int 85:651–654

Gonzolez CM et al (2012) AUA/SUNA white paper on the incidence, prevention and treatment of complications related to prostate needle biopsy. AUA White Paper. American Urological Association Education and Research, Inc

Halliwell OT, Lane C, Dewbury KC (2006) Transrectal ultrasound-guided biopsy of the prostate: should warfarin be stopped before the procedure? Incidence of bleeding in a further 50 patients. Clin Radiol 61:1068–1069

Halliwell OT, Yadegafar G, Lane C, Dewbury KC (2008) Transrectal ultrasound-guided biopsy of the prostate: aspirin increases the incidence of minor bleeding complications. Clin Radiol 63:557–561

Hamdy FC, Hastie KJ (1990) Treatment for paraphimosis: the 'puncture' technique. Br J Surg 77:1186

Herr HW (2014) Should antibiotics be given prior to outpatient cystoscopy? A plea to urologists to practice antibiotic stewardship. Eur Urol 65(4):839–842

Hess MJ, Zhan EH, Foo DK, Yalla SV (2003) Bladder cancer in patients with spinal cord injury. J Spinal Cord Med 26:335–338

Ho KJ, Thompson TJ, O'Brien A et al (2003) Lignocaine gel: does it cause urethral pain rather than prevent it? Eur Urol 43:194–196

Houghton GR (1973) The "iced-glove" method of treatment of paraphimosis. Br J Surg 60:876

Ihezue CU, Smart J, Dewbury KC, Mehta R, Burgess L (2005) Biopsy of the prostate guided by transrectal ultrasound: relation between warfarin use and incidence of bleeding complications. Clin Radiol 60:459–463; discussion 7–8

Institute of Medicine (2010) The future of nursing: leading change, advancing health. National Academies Press, Washington, DC. Retrieved from http://www.iom.edu.libproxy.lib.unc.edu/Reports/2010/The-Future-of-Nursing-Leading- Change-Advancing-Health.aspx

Jeon SS, Woo SH, Hyun JH, Choi HY, Chai SE (2003) Bisacodyl rectal preparation can decrease infectious complications of transrectal ultrasound-guided prostate biopsy. Urology 62(3):461–466

Jiménez-Pacheco A, Lardelli Claret P, López Luque A, Lahoz-García C, Arrabal Polo MA, Nogueras Ocaña M (2012) Arch randomized clinic trial on antimicrobial prophylaxis for flexible urethrocystoscopy. Esp Urol 65(5):542–549

Jordan GH (2008) The use of intralesional clostridial collagenase injection therapy for Peyronie's disease: a prospective, single-center, non-placebo-controlled study. J Sex Med 5:180

Kakehi Y, Naito S, Japanese Urological Association (2008) Complication rates of ultrasound-guided prostate biopsy: a nation-wide survey in Japan. Int J Urol 15:319

Kapoor DA, Klimberg IW, Malek GH, Wegenke JD, Cox CE, Patterson AL et al (1998) Single-dose ciprofloxacin versus placebo for prophylaxis during transrectal prostate biopsy. Urology 52:552

Kariotis I, Philippou P, Volanis D, Serafetinides E, Delakas D (2010) Safety of ultrasound-guided transrectal extended prostate biopsy in patients receiving low-dose aspirin. Int Braz J Urol Off J Braz Soc Urol 36:308–316

Kelleher S, Turner L, Howe C, Conway AJ, Handelsman DJ (1999) Extrusion of testosterone pellets: a randomized controlled clinical study. Clin Endocrinol (Oxf) 51(4):469–471

Kelleher S, Howe C, Conway AJ, Handelsman DJ (2004) Testosterone release rate and duration of action of testosterone pellet implants. Clin Endocrinol (Oxf) 60(4):420–428

Kerwat R, Shandall A, Stephenson B (1998) Reduction of paraphimosis with granulated sugar. Br J Urol 82:755

Kirya C, Werthmann M (1978) Neonatal circumcision and penile dorsal nerve block: a painless procedure. J Pediatr 92:998–1000

Kleier JA (2009) Procedure competencies and job functions of the urologic advanced practice nurse. Urologic Nursing 29(2):112–7. Retrieved from http://search.proquest.com/docview/220 160997?accountid=14244

Kovac JR, Rajanahally S, Smith RP, Coward RM, Lamb DJ, Lipshultz LI (2014) Patient satisfaction with testosterone replacement therapies: the reasons behind the choices. J Sex Med 11(2):553–562. doi:10.1111/jsm.12369. Epub 2013 Nov 6

Krikler SJ (1989) Flexible urethroscopy: use in difficult male catheterization. Ann R Coll Surg Engl 71:3

Kuhn JM, Billebaud T, Navratil H, Moulonguet A, Fiet J, Grise P, Louis JF, Costa P, Husson JM, Dahan R et al (1989) Prevention of the transient adverse effects of a gonadotropin-releasing hormone analogue (buserelin) in metastatic prostatic carcinoma by administration of an antiandrogen (nilutamide). Engl J Med 321(7):413–418

Kumar V, Javle P (2001) Modified puncture technique for reduction of paraphimosis. Ann R Coll Surg Engl 83:126

Labrie F, Dupont A, Belanger A, Lachance R (1987) Flutamide eliminates the risk of disease flare in prostatic cancer patients treated with a luteinizing hormone-releasing hormone agonist. J Urol 138(4):804–806

Latthe PM, Foon R, Toozs-Hobson P (2008) Review – infections antibiotic prophylaxis in urologic procedures: a systematic review. Eur Urol 54:1270–1286

Lewis LS, Stephan M (1997) Local and regional anesthesia. In: Henretig FM, King C (eds) Textbook of pediatric emergency procedures. Williams & Wilkins, Baltimore

Liss MA, Chang A, Santos R et al (2011) Prevalence and significance of fluoroquinolone resistant Escherichia coli in patients undergoing transrectal ultrasound guided prostate needle biopsy. J Urol 185:1283

Little B, White M (2005) Treatment options for paraphimosis. Int J Clin Pract 59:591

Mariani AJ, Glover M, Arita S (2001) Medical versus surgical androgen suppression therapy for prostate cancer: a 10-year longitudinal cost study. J Urol 165(1):104–107

Martino P, Galosi AB, Bitelli M, Imaging Working Group-Societa Italiana Urologia (SIU); Società Italiana Ecografia Urologica Andrologica Nefrologica (SIEUN) et al (2014) Practical recommendations for performing ultrasound scanning in the urological and andrological fields. Arch Ital Urol Androl 86(1):56–78

Matlaga BR, Eskew AL, McCullough DL (2003) Prostate biopsy: indications and technique. J Urol 169(1):12–19

McCullough A (2014) A review of testosterone pellets in the treatment of hypogonadism. Curr Sex Health Rep 6(4):265

McCullough AR, Khera M, Goldstein I, Hellstrom WJ, Morgentaler A, Levine LA (2012) A multi-institutional observational study of testosterone levels after testosterone pellet (Testopel ®) insertion. J Sex Med 9(2):594–601. doi:10.1111/j.1743-6109.2011.02570.x. Epub 2012 Jan 12

Mechlin CW, Frankel J, McCullough A (2014) Coadministration of anastrozole sustains therapeutic testosterone levels in hypogonadal men undergoing testosterone pellet insertion. J Sex Med 11(1):254–261

Mendez-Probst C, Razvi H, Denstedt JD Chapter 7: Fundamental of instrumentation and urinary tract drainage. In: Wein AL, Kavoussi LR, Partin AW & Peters CA (EDs.) Campbell-Walsh Urology, 11th ed. Philadelphia, PA: Elsevier. pp 177–191.e4

Mendez-Probst CE, Razvi H, Denstedt JD (2012) Management of the difficult-to-catheterize patient. In: Wein AL, Kavoussi LR, Partin AW & Peters CA (EDs.) Campbell-Walsh Urology, 11th ed. Philadelphia, PA: Elsevier. pp 177–191.e4

Messing EM, Manola J, Sarosdy M et al (1999) Immediate hormonal therapy compared with observation after radical prostatectomy and pelvic lymphadenectomy in men with node-positive prostate cancer. N Engl J Med 341:1781–1788

Mihmanil I, Faith K (2007) Erectile dysfunction. Seminars in ultrasound, CT and MRI. Semin Ultrasound CT MR 28(4):274–286

Morales A Chapter 29: Androgen deficiency in aging male. In: Wein AL, Kavoussi LR, Partin AW & Peters CA (EDs.) Campbell-Walsh Urology, 11th ed. Philadelphia, PA: Elsevier. pp 810–822.e3

Muhlhall J (n.d.) Sexual medicine: peyronie's disease epidemiology, pathophysiology, evaluation. Retrieved 31 Jan 2015, from https://www.auanet.org/university/core_topic.cfm?coreid=103

Nelson JB (2013) Chapter 109: Hormone therapy for prostate cancer. In: Wein AL, Kavoussi LR, Partin AW & Peters CA (EDs.) Campbell-Walsh Urology, 11th ed. Philadelphia, PA: Elsevier. pp 2934–2953

O'Brant W (2013) Peyronie's disease: diagnosis and medical management. Retrieved 6 Feb 2015, from http://www.uptodate.com/contents/peyronies-disease-diagnosis-and-medical--management?source=search_result&search=peyronies disease diagnosis and medical management&selectedTitle=1~150

O'Brant W (2014) Surgical management of peyronie's disease. Retrieved 31 Jan 2015, from http://www.uptodate.com/contents/surgical-management-of-peyronies-disease?source=search_result&search=surgical management of peyronie's&selectedTitle=1~150

Otrock ZK, Oghlakian GO, Salamoun MM, Haddad M, Bizri AR (2004) Incidence of urinary tract infection following transrectal ultrasound guided prostate biopsy at a tertiary-care medical center in Lebanon. Infect Control Hosp Epidemiol 25:873

Pastuszak AW, Mittakanti H, Liu JS, Gomez L, Lipshultz LI, Khera M (2012) Pharmacokinetic evaluation and dosing of subcutaneous testosterone pellets. J Androl 33(5):927–937. Epub 2012 Mar 8

Patel AR, Jones JS, Babineau D (2008) Lidocaine 2% gel versus plain lubricating gel for pain reduction during flexible cystoscopy: a meta-analysis of prospective, randomized, controlled trials. J Urol 179:86

Patel AR, Jones JS, Babineau D (2008c) Impact of real-time visualization of cystoscopy findings on procedural pain in female patients. J Endourol 22:2695–2698

Paul JT. Chapter 20. Male reproductive physiology. In: Wein AL, Kavoussi LR, Partin AW & Peters CA (EDs.) Campbell-Walsh Urology, 11th ed. Philadelphia, PA: Elsevier. pp 591–615.e5

Pohlman GD, Phillips JM, Wilcox DT (2013) Simple method of paraphimosis reduction revisited: point of technique and review of the literature. J Pediatr Urol 9:104

Prostate Cancer Trialists' Collaborative Group (2000) Maximum androgen blockade in advanced prostate cancer: an overview of randomized trials. Lancet 255:1491–1498

Quallich SA (2011) A survey evaluating the current role of the nurse practitioner in urology. Urologic Nursing 31(6):328–6. Retrieved from http://search.proquest.com/docview/911434605?accountid=14244

Raaijmakers R, Kirkels WJ, Roobol MJ, Wildhagen MF, Schrder FH (2002) Complication rates and risk factors of 5802 transrectal ultrasound-guided sextant biopsies of the prostate within a population-based screening program. Urology 60:826

Radhakrishnan S, Dorkin TJ, Johnson P, Menezes P, Greene D (2006) Nurse-led flexible cystoscopy: experience from one UK center. Br J Urol Int 98(2):256–258

Raheem O, Casey RG, Lynch TH (2011) Does anticoagulant or antiplatelet therapy need to be discontinued for transrectal ultrasound-guided prostate biopsies? A systematic literature review. Curr Urol 5:121–124

Raveenthiran V (1996) Reduction of paraphimosis: a technique based on pathophysiology. Br J Surg 83:1247

Reynard JM, Barua JM (1999) Reduction of paraphimosis the simple way – the Dundee technique. BJU Int 83:859

Ricker JM, Foody WF, Shumway NM, Shaw JC (2010) Drug-induced liver injury caused by the histrelin (Vantas) subcutaneous implant. South Med J 103(1):84–86

Roberts MJ, Williamson DA, Hadway P, Doi SA, Gardiner RA, Paterson DL (2014) Baseline prevalence of antimicrobial resistance and subsequent infection following prostate biopsy using empiric or altered prophylaxis: a bias-adjusted meta-analysis. Int J Antimicrob Agents 43(4):301–309

Sabbagh R, McCormack M, Péloquin F, Faucher R, Perreault JP, Perrotte P et al (2004) A prospective randomized trial of 1-day versus 3-day antimicrobial prophylaxis for transrectal ultrasound guided prostate biopsy. Can J Urol 11:2216

Sadeghi-Nejad H, Dogra V, Seftel AD, Mohamed MA (2004) Priapism. Radiol Clin N Am 42:427–443

Samir ST et al (2015) Optimal Techniques of Prostate Biopsy and Specimen Handling. AUA White paper. Retrieved from www.AUAnet.org.

Schlegel P (2009) A review of the pharmacokinetic and pharmacological properties of a once-yearly administered histrelin acetate implant in the treatment of prostate cancer. BJU Int 103(Suppl 2):7–13

Schlegel PN, Histrelin Study Group (2006) Efficacy and safety of histrelin subdermal implant in patients with advanced prostate cancer. J Urol 175(4):1353–1358

Schultz II (2011) Practical and legal implications of nurse practitioners and physician assistants in cystoscopy. Urologic Nursing 31(6);355–8. Retrieved from http://search.proquest.com/docvie w/911434610?accountid=14244

Serour F, Reuben S, Ezra S (1995) Circumcision in children with penile block alone. J Urol 153(2):474–476

Shigemura K, Tanaka K, Yasuda M, Ishihar S, Muratani T, Deguchi T et al (2005) Efficacy of 1-day prophylaxis medication with fluoroquinolone for prostate biopsy. World J Urol 23:356

Shindell A (n.d.) Sexual medicine: ED patient evaluation, investigations. Retrieved 31 Jan 2015, from https://www.auanet.org/university/core_topic.cfm?coreid=98

Shore N, Cookson MS, Gittelman MC (2012) Long-term efficacy and tolerability of once-yearly histrelin acetate subcutaneous implant in patients with advanced prostate cancer. BJU Int 109(2):226–232. doi:10.1111/j.1464-410X.2011.10370.x, Epub 2011 Aug 18

Smith RP, Khanna A, Coward RM, Rajanahally S, Kovac JR, Gonzales MA, Lipshultz LI (2013) Factors influencing patient decisions to initiate and discontinue subcutaneous testosterone pellets (Testopel) for treatment of hypogonadism. J Sex Med 10(9):2326–2333

Snellman L, Stang H (1995) Prospective evaluation of complications of dorsal penile nerve block for neonatal circumcision. Pediatrics 95:705–708

Stav A, Gur L, Gorelik U, Ovadia L, Isaakovich B, Sternberg A (1995) Modification of the penile block. World J Urol 13:251–253

Subramonian K, Cartwright RA, Harnden P, Harrison SC (2004) Bladder cancer in patients with spinal cord injuries. BJU Int 93:739–743

Sung JC, Springhart WP, Marguet CG et al (2005) Location and etiology of flexible and semirigid ureteroscope damage. Urology 66:958–963

Taghizadeh AK, El Madani A, Gard PR et al (2006) When does it hurt? Pain during flexible cystoscopy in men. Urol Int 76:301–303

Tews M (2013) Paraphimosis reduction. Retrieved 3 Jan 2015, from http://www.uptodate.com/contents/paraphimosis-reduction?source=search_result&search=paraphimosis reduction&sele ctedTitle=1~3

Treatment of peyronie's disease: curved or bent penis (n.d.) Retrieved 6 feb 2015, from https://peyronies-disease.xiaflex.com/hcp/

Turner CD, Kim HL, Cromie WJ (1999) Dorsal band traction for reduction of paraphimosis. Urology 54:917

Tzortzis V, Gravas S, Melekos MM, de la Rosette JJ (2009) Intraurethral lubricants: a critical literature review and recommendations. J Endourol 23:821–826

Villanueva C, Hemstreet GP 3rd (2008) Difficult male urethral catheterization: a review of different approaches. Int Braz J Urol 34:401

Villanueva C, Hemstreet G (2010) Experience with a difficult urethral catheterization algorithm at a university hospital. Curr Urol 4:152

Vunda A, Lacroix LE, Schneider F et al (2013) Videos in clinical medicine. Reduction of paraphimosis in boys. N Engl J Med 368:e16

Weckermann D, Harzmann R (2004) Hormone therapy in prostate cancer: LHRH antagonists versus LHRH analogues. Eur Urol 46(3):279–283

Weider A (2010) Prostate cancer. 4th edn. Caldwell, ID: Griffith Publishing, p 113–117

Wein A (2012a) Ultrasound and biopsy of the prostate, vol 3, e-book, 10th edn. Saunders, an imprint of Elsevier, Philadelphia

Wein A (2012b) Surgery of the penis and urethra. In: Campbell-Walsh urology, vol 3, e-book, 10th edn. Saunders, an imprint of Elsevier, Philadelphia

Wein A (2012c) Evaluation and management of erectile dysfunction. In: Campbell-Walsh urology, vol 3, e-book, 10th edn. Saunders, an imprint of Elsevier, Philadelphia

Wein A (2012d) Priapism. In: Campbell-Walsh urology, vol 3, 10th edn. Saunders, an imprint of Elsevier, Philadelphia

Wein A (2012e) Peyronie's disease. In: Campbell-walsh urology, vol 3, e-book, 10th edn. Saunders, an imprint of Elsevier, Philadelphia

Wilkins CJ, Sriprasad S, Sihus PS (2003) Colour doppler ultrasound of the penis. Clin Radiol 58(7):14–23

Wilson LR, Thelning C, Masters J, Tuckey J (2005) Is antibiotic prophylaxis required for flexible cystoscopy? A truncated randomized double-blind controlled trial. J Endourol 19(8):1006–1008

Wolf JS, Bennett CJ, Dmochowski RR et al (2008) Best practice policy statement on urologic surgery antimicrobial prophylaxis. J Urol 179:1379–1390

Yachia D (2007a) Chapter 2: Anesthesia for Penile Surgery. Text Atlas of Penile Surgery. Boca Raton, FL: CRC Press. pp. 9–11

Yachia D (2007b) Chapter 4: Paraphimosis. In: Text atlas of penile surgery. Informa Healthcare, pp 17–19

Yachia D Chapter 2: Anesthesia for penile surgery. In: Text atlas of penile surgery

Yachia D. Chapter 4: Paraphimosis. In: Text atlas of penile surgery

Zani EL, Clark OA, Rodrigues NN Jr (2011) Antibiotic prophylaxis for transrectal prostate biopsy. Cochrane Database Syst Rev (5):CD006576

Zaytoun OM, Anil T, Moussa AS, Jianbo L, Fareed K, Jones JS (2011) Morbidity of prostate biopsy after simplified versus complex preparation protocols: assessment of risk factors. Urology 77(4):910–914

Further Reading

Wieder JA (Ed.) (2014) Pocket guide to urology. 5th edn. Oakland: J. Wieder Medical

Susanne A. Quallich, Sherry M. Bumpus,
and Shelly Lajiness

Contents

Reprinted by permission Quallich SA, Bumpus SM, Lajiness S (2015) Competencies for the nurse practitioner working with adult urology patients. Urologic Nursing 35(5):221–230. doi: 10.7257/1053-816X.2015.35.5.221

S.A. Quallich, ANP-BC, NP-C, CUNP, FAANP (✉)
Division of Andrology and Urologic Health, Department of Urology,
University of Michigan Health System, 3875 Taubman Center,
1500 E. Medical Center Drive, Ann Arbor, MI 48109-5330, USA
e-mail: quallich@umich.edu

S.M. Bumpus, PhD, RN, FNP-BC
School of Nursing, Eastern Michigan University, Ypsilanti, MI, USA

S. Lajiness, MSN, FNP-BC
Department of Urology and Department of Infectious Disease,
Beaumont Health System, Royal Oak, MI, USA

Table 21.1 Comparison of NP competencies and the AUA milestone concepts

Nurse practitioner competency	Urology milestone concepts
Scientific foundation	Foundation in urologic/medical and scientific knowledge
Leadership	Leadership
Quality, scientific foundation	Evidence-based practice
Practice inquiry	Quality improvement and research
Technology and information literacy	Use of technology in patient care
Policy	Healthcare policy, regulation
Health delivery system, quality, ethics, health, delivery system	Organizational practice/resource allocation
Independent practice, healthcare delivery system	Role as part of healthcare delivery team
Ethics, quality	Patient care/professional ethics
Independent practice	Scope of practice
Independent practice, scientific foundation	Procedural competencies

Adapted from AUA Consensus Statement on Advanced Practice Providers (2014), p. 7–8

Introduction

It is widely recognized that with the aging population in the USA, there is a growing need for urologic care that exceeds the capacity of presently available urologists (American Urological Society [AUA] 2014). Nurse practitioners (NPs) are ideally situated to fill this mounting need that has been created, in part, by changes in resident training programs and funding for graduate medical education. In response to this need, the AUA (2014) has published a consensus statement on the role of advanced practice providers (APPs) (NPs and physician assistants) within the specialty. However, the only urology competencies that exist are from the AUA (2014) *Milestones* project for assessing and evaluating resident physicians and are not constructed for NP practice (see Table 21.1) (Accreditation Council for Graduate Medical Education [ACGME] & the American Board of Urology 2012).

This increasing demand for urology services in the USA and the decline in available urologists, combined with restrictions on resident work hours and changes to primary care training requirements at a time of decreasing reimbursement for graduate medical education, has created an opportunity for NPs. The Institute of Medicine ([IOM] 2010) supports NP expansion to specialty services. However, this movement is happening without formal didactic education within NP programs, which has been cited as a barrier to practice (Albaugh 2012), as well as to assessing and evaluating the urology NP.

A growing body of literature supports the high-quality, cost-effective, patient-centered care that NPs provide (Newhouse et al. 2011). According to the American Association of Nurse Practitioners (AANP) (2015), NPs are becoming the healthcare provider of choice for millions of Americans and including specialty populations. NPs are now practicing in a number of subspecialty areas from allergy and immunology to urology; in 2012, there were 3,338 NPs functioning in urology (AUA 2014). The present document proposes a set of 24 urology NP competencies that define the continuum between novice and expert and that are consistent with both the AUA Advanced Practice Provider consensus statement and primary care NP competencies.

Education and Certification for Advance Practice Urology Nurses

As highly educated and qualified providers, NPs provide comprehensive health care. They are clinical experts in managing disease and promoting heath of the whole person (AANP 2015). They are registered nurses who complete advanced education and clinical training (minimum of 500 h) at the master's or doctoral level. Nurse practitioners must pass a National Certification Exam upon completion of their program of study and must be licensed in the state where they practice as both a registered nurse and a nurse practitioner (or state equivalent).

Specialty designation as a urology NP requires additional postgraduate education and training both independently and as part of a urology team. The new graduate NP has significant knowledge deficits when entering this specialty field since genitourinary (GU) issues are minimally covered in the NP curricula. Albaugh (2012) highlighted this lack of standardized curricula for advanced nursing roles in urology. His discussion of the various educational backgrounds encountered across the globe that represented "urology APNs" included 33 distinct titles across the world, with NP the most common. Crowe (2014) brought this lack of education for nurse practitioners and others in advanced nursing practice in urology to the forefront in her opinion piece, noting that this expansion of nursing into urology has occurred without any formal role definitions or curricula changes to formally incorporate didactic content. Therefore, NPs working in urology environments (or other specialty environments) or seeking to move into urology environments must pursue information from a variety of sources in order to deliver high-quality care to these special populations. In response, the AUA has developed educational modules on topics such as overactive bladder, sexual dysfunction, surgical assistance, and stone management to augment the knowledge base of APPs.

For experienced urology NPs, the Certification Board for Urologic Nurses and Associates (CBUNA) offers a specialty certification for NP recognition as a *Certified Urology Nurse Practitioner (CUNP)*. To be eligible to sit for this exam, the NP must have completed their educational program, hold a national certification and be state licensed as an NP, have worked for 2 years as an NP, and have a minimum of 800 clinical practice hours in providing urology care (www.CBUNA.org). Certification is valid for three years, and there are currently 160 CUNPs in the USA (M. Borch, May 21, 2015, personal communication).

Role and Scope of Practice for the Urology Nurse Practitioner

Access to subspecialty services is improved by NPs working within specialty environments. A nursing specialty is characterized by a unique body of knowledge and skill set, with nurses providing care focused on phenomena unique to the practice (Stewart-Amidei et al. 2010). Urology nursing is recognized as "a unique nursing specialty that addresses the needs of individuals with urologic healthcare concerns due to injury, aging, cancer, neurologic, genetic, reproductive and medical illnesses"

(Society of Urologic Nurses and Associates [SUNA] 2013, p. 6). However, a similar concise definition for the role of the *urology nurse practitioner* does not yet exist. In the rapidly evolving environment of the Patient Protection and Affordable Care Act (2010) and other healthcare demands, formal acknowledgment of the specialty practice of NPs in urology becomes imperative.

The 24 competencies presented here help establish standards for practice, which are currently absent for urology NPs except as represented by extrapolation from generalist NP certification. The AUA (2014) recognizes APPs as integral members of a physician-led team to provide high-quality urological care. Their specific role, however, is highly variable and will be dependent on the type of practice, setting, location, and the experience of both the urologist and the NP (AUA 2014). A wide range of expected activities in the urology environment can be completed by NPs, such as comprehensive history and physical exams, ordering and interpreting diagnostic studies, diagnosing and treating illness, promoting wellness, and providing patient and family education and counseling. In addition, NPs also engage in GU research, advocacy, and administration, all while functioning as part of an interdisciplinary collaborative team. Further, urology NPs may perform procedures such as prostate ultrasounds, urodynamics, cystoscopy, vasectomy, and stent removal as part of their role (AUA 2014). Such activities will require additional education, training, and supervision as designated uniquely by each state's scope of practice. Despite training and licensing differences, NPs are held to the same level of care as physicians.

Theoretical Framework

These urology NP competencies represent expectations along a continuum from the graduate NP to those of an experienced NP. As such, this framework is deeply rooted in the work of Benner (1982). Her influence can be seen in the progression from a novice to an expert urology clinician. This distinction in progress is so vital to the urology nursing specialty that her theory provides the foundation for the Certification Board for Urologic Nurses and Associates (CBUNA) certification examinations (Quallich 2011), an important step in defining urology nursing and urology NP practice. Although these proposed competencies do not fully depict the gradual progression detailed by Benner (1982), they are consistent with advanced beginner, proficient, and expert levels described in her work.

Benner's theory (1982) provides an impetus for describing and detailing the nuances of expert urology NP practice. The categorization of expertise described herein acknowledges the difference between "practical and theoretical knowledge" (Cash 1995, p. 527) in clinical applications. We acknowledge that within the context of these proposed guidelines, progression between the three tiers is not guaranteed. Yet practice-based experience is vital to the ongoing growth and development of the expert urology practitioner. Benner's (1982) model supports lifelong learning as a clinician; this is a reflection of the position which is not only of nurse practitioner practice but of nursing practice as well.

Process of Competency Development

Providing care to urology patients requires a thorough understanding of GU pathophysiology, knowledge of medical and surgical treatment options, as well as the ability to preserve the nursing role in effective patient management, especially education. It involves knowledge of acute and chronic urologic disease and the capacity to manage specialty and primary care needs simultaneously. These proposed urology NP competencies represent a synthesis of multiple resources, including the National Organization of Nurse Practitioner Faculties (NONPF) 2014 NP core competencies, the 2010 Adult-Gerontology NP competencies, the 2013 Family NP competencies, the AANP (2013) "Standards of Practice for Nurse Practitioners," and the Society of Urologic Nurses and Associates (SUNA 2013) "Urologic Nursing: Scope and Standards of Practice" (2nd edition). The Adult-Gerontology and Family NP competencies were included as these two NP groups comprise the majority of NPs who self-identify as a "urology NP" (Quallich 2011).

These urology-specific competencies are modeled after the American Medical Directors Association (2011) paper and the AUA consensus statement on Advanced Practice Providers (2014) and informed by *The Urology Milestone Project* (Accreditation Council for Graduate Medical Education [ACGME]/AUA 2012). These new urology NP-specific competencies maintain fidelity with the SUNA competencies and serve to move specialty urology practice forward for NPs by creating a framework for assessing and acquiring skills essential to the discipline. The SUNA competencies are not NP focused and do not accommodate the more advanced patient interaction skills of the NP or the NP post-graduation GU knowledge deficit. These 24 urology NP-specific competencies fill a gap in knowledge and practice and are also consistent with NONPF and the Advanced Practice Registered Nurses (APRN) Consensus Work Group and the National Council of State Boards of Nursing APRN Advisory Committee (2008) consensus guidelines. These competencies offer congruency with existing APRN regulatory model and are consistent with the nurse practitioners' focus on providing "nursing and medical services to individuals, families and groups accordant with their practice specialties…diagnosing and managing acute episodic and chronic illnesses, NPs emphasize health promotion and disease prevention" (AANP 2013).

Overview of the Proposed Advanced Practice Urology Nursing Competencies

These 24 urology NP competencies compliment the AUA (2014) White Paper as well as the NONPF documents and APRN consensus model. The competencies cover three general content areas (patient care, professional issues, and health system role) and three levels of progression for the urology NP from advanced beginner to proficient and finally to expert. This detailed description of responsibilities offers a more in-depth manner in which to establish "mentorship, a baseline assessment of clinical skill and knowledge in general urology or a specific dimension within an area of urology" (AUA 2014, p. 8). This provides guidance to relate the population-based skills and knowledge of an NP's generalist certification toward urology care while building upon the core competencies for all NPs (NONPF 2014). These competencies address the specific care needs of a urology population, reflecting the knowledge base, scope of practice, and interdisciplinary nature of the emerging model for care delivery, and emphasize the NP's ability to provide both chronic and acute GU care. The competencies acknowledge the independent role of the NP while accommodating the role of professional collaboration and a urology team in the efficient and cost-effective care of urology patients.

These 24 competencies represent specific aspects of NP practice unique to the care of patients with GU issues and promote the NP role in the care of GU patients. Many of the issues and concerns are related to parts of the body or their functions that may be considered taboo in many cultures and religious contexts. Therefore these competencies reflect the vital role of cultural sensitivity in the care of urology patients, highlighting the approach of the NP in recognizing the unique needs of GU patients.

These urology NP competencies offer a framework for progression rather than offering distinct criteria for measurement. Each level includes and builds upon the tenants of the previous level (see Table 21.2). No specific time frame is proposed for transition between levels. In fact, progression along this continuum will be unique to each practice environment. Progression through these competencies may not be linear; that is, some NPs may attain "level 2" in a short time for some of the competencies but not others.

These competencies represent another step toward describing and detailing the nuances of expert urology NP practice and work toward defining specialty NP practice; few specialty NP groups have competency documents (e.g., oncology). These competencies offer evidence that urology NPs can offer increasingly complex care in a variety of primary, acute, and tertiary settings.

Limitations

While these competencies offer guidance, they *must* be viewed in the context of individual state laws and individual state practice acts, which must be considered when utilizing these competencies. Because there is no national NP license, individual State Boards of Nursing regulate entry into NP practice and determine the legal scope of practice for NPs in each state. These competencies do not describe a scope of practice, as that is a legal description of NP practice determined by individual states and national certifying bodies. Further, these competencies are not permission to expand one's NP practice beyond the bounds of the original generalist certification; that is, they are not a mechanism for a women's health nurse practitioner to care for adult male patients with urology concerns. These

Table 21.2 Proposed urology NP competencies for adult populations (age > 18)

Competency (NONPF competency)	Level 3 (newly graduated and/or new to urology)	Level 2 (experienced NP new to urology)	Level 1 (expert urology NP)
Patient care activities			
1. Obtains relevant health history, focused to genitourinary complaints, as comprehensive as needed to evaluate present issue (*scientific foundation, independent practice*)	Incorporates knowledge of pediatric urologic issues and their impact on the care of adult urology patients Evaluates signs and symptoms within context of a GU complaint to formulate plan of care Developing skill with male and female GU examination	Sensitive to complex patient and family needs when transitioning from pediatric urology to adult urology environment Prioritizes history and physical findings within context of GU complaint Recognizes relevant history to prioritize evaluation of complaint Developing skill in recognizing specifics of male and female GU examination, appropriately targeted to a patient's genitourinary complaints and medical condition Developing skill with recognition of subtle GU physical exam findings	Distinguishes GU complaints that are a symptom of other health concerns from GU complaints that represent a specific GU health issue Able to routinely identify subtle or unusual physical findings within context of GU complaints Highly efficient at gathering pertinent information necessary to formulate specific GU plan of care
2. Integrates diagnostic tests and procedures into culturally sensitive genitourinary care (*scientific foundation, independent practice*)	Selects appropriate diagnostic tests and/or imaging procedures pertinent to current GU complaints, in the context of relevant comorbidities Revises plan of care in consultation with a urologist or more experienced colleague as appropriate	Demonstrates understanding of appropriate application of advanced GU imaging and procedures Continues to revise plan of care and clinical decisions in consultation with a urologist or more experienced colleague as needed	Integrates routine and advanced diagnostic tests and imaging procedures based on GU complaints and comorbidities Revises plan of care in consultation with a urologist as needed Assesses concerns relative to sexual function and fertility issues with GU diagnoses

(continued)

Table 21.2 (continued)

Competency (NONPF competency)	Level 3 (newly graduated and/or new to urology)	Level 2 (experienced NP new to urology)	Level 1 (expert urology NP)
3. Analyzes data and formulates and initiates plan of care for urology-based complaint (scientific foundation, independent practice)	Recognizes deviance from normal Formulates and validates differential diagnosis and plan of care based on common GU presentations Prepares plans that acknowledge an individual's risk factors with specific urologic health conditions Implements specific GU screening as appropriate for the individual	Formulates differential diagnosis and plan of care based on common and uncommon GU presentations Develops increasingly comprehensive GU differentials when evaluating patients Prioritizes list of differentials based on suspected GU etiology	Synthesizes data to arrive at management, consultation, and/or education plan Formulates differential diagnosis and plan of care based on complex knowledge of common and uncommon GU presentations Able to generate complex differentials and an appropriate strategy to finalize plan of care Incorporates the potential role of polypharmacy on GU complaints and management
4. Develops a plan of care that includes medical, surgical, and/or radiological interventions as appropriate (scientific foundation, independent practice)	Develops plan for routine GU clinical problem with typical treatment recommendations in individuals who are otherwise healthy Addresses GU disease prevention, GU health promotion, GU health maintenance issues Provides informed consent for routine, low-risk interventions Prescribes medication with consideration for GU specifics (e.g., renal excretion, bladder effects)	Promotes GU self-care as appropriate (e.g., post coital antibiotics, low purine diet) Manages complex GU problems in the patient with multiple comorbid conditions Identifies impact of GU treatment on normal physiology Provides informed consent for routine and intermediate risk urologic interventions	Extensive knowledge of age and age-related changes and their potential impact on GU conditions and management Develops plan for individuals experiencing multiple or complex GU clinical problem(s) while incorporating patient comorbid conditions Provides informed consent and counsels patients for urologic interventions that are considered high risk Emphasizes quality-of-life impact throughout discussions

5. Integrates knowledge of urologic issues with nursing principles to provide perioperative management from the nurse practitioner perspective (*scientific foundation, independent practice*)	Identifies common postoperative issues Manages common perioperative complaints, with input of urologist or more experienced colleague as needed Promotes return to maximum functional status	Identifies and manages common postoperative issues Independently identifies and manages most outpatient postoperative complaints and surgical complications with input of urologist or more experienced colleague as needed	Identifies and manages common post-discharge and postoperative complaints and surgical complications Identifies and manages later complications of urologic interventions and procedures Collaboration with urologist as needed
6. Acknowledges role of cognition, culture, spirituality, and ethnicity when communicating in the healthcare setting (*health delivery system*)	Displays effective communication skills in establishing therapeutic relationships with patients and families Effectively communicates in non-stressful situations	Consistently exhibits effective communication skills in a variety of clinical and team contexts Adjust communication style to each individual patient interaction Adapts teaching to environment and resources	Adjust communication style to be respectful of cultural, ethnic or cognitive status Provides model of effective communication for other team members
7. Manages established plan of GU care, assuming leadership as appropriate (*independent practice, leadership*)	Recognizes need for consistent and concise communication in prevention of patient harm Cognizant of medicolegal perspectives regarding accurate GU documentation	Functions largely independently, seeking input from more senior team members, urologists, or other disciplines for management of complex GU patients as necessary Works to ensure continuity in GU care whenever possible Develops mastery in responding to the changing demands of GU patient care needs	Mainly collaborative relationship with urologist(s) due to high skill level and experience Partners with other healthcare professionals in specific aspects of patient management Able to anticipate the needs of a particular clinical or patient situation

(continued)

Table 21.2 (continued)

Competency (NONPF competency)	Level 3 (newly graduated and/or new to urology)	Level 2 (experienced NP new to urology)	Level 1 (expert urology NP)
8. Incorporates compassion, integrity, and respect for spiritual and cultural beliefs into genitourinary care (ethics, independent practice)	Assists diverse panel of patients to obtain GU care Honors requests for same gender provider when possible Sensitive to psychological factors in GU conditions Identifies need for background information (e.g., SES, sexual orientation) as issues emerge in GU patient care	Demonstrates sensitivity to cultural, ethnic, and spiritual context when faced with patient or family emotions, within context of providing GU care	Willingness to express concerns regarding team behaviors that are inconsistent with culturally and spiritually sensitive care
9. Strives for patient-centered care based on respect and collaboration among team members (health delivery system, leadership)	Responsive to patient needs and consistent follow-up based on results of evaluation Communicates and coordinates plan of care with appropriate team members	Consistently prompt and responsive to patient care issues Completes tasks and charting on time Communicates with patient and family and other team members, as needed	Consistent in maintaining obligations to patient care Always accepts feedback willingly Plan of care issues completed in a careful and thorough manner, and communicated to patient and family
10. Demonstrates respect for the autonomy of the patient in negotiating his/her own genitourinary care (ethics, independent practice)	Almost always mindful of patient respects patient autonomy and right to refuse plan of care Honors requests for same gender provider when possible	Recognizes and honors patient privacy concerns, especially in GU care context Seeks to balance patient autonomy and patient safety issues	Education of other team members in prevention of behaviors that threaten patient privacy or autonomy
Professional activities			
11. Seeks training and privileging for office-based procedures as permitted by practice environment (independent practice, policy)	Performs routine GU and generalist NP procedures (e.g., suture removal, wound culture, catheter change postoperatively)	Performs routine outpatient procedures under supervision, or as specified by state practice act or state collaborative practice requirements (e.g., wound incision and drainage)	Performs GU outpatient procedures, independently or under supervision, or as specified by state practice act or state collaborative practice requirements (e.g., cystoscopy with stent removal)

12. Provides genitourinary care in cost-aware fashion while accommodating risk-benefit issues (*independent practice, health delivery system*)	Understands coding issues that are specific to GU care Acknowledges socioeconomic barriers that influence patient-centered GU care Minimizes unnecessary care by adhering to established guidelines	Understands and follows established guidelines for GU management Focuses on patient-centered care by assessing economic impact of commonly performed GU procedures Able to envision long-term goals of GU care, and plan for patients and their support systems	Well-versed in coding issues specific to NP role within urology Leads and explores mechanism for cost containment, such as utilization of urologic supplies Practices within GU environment in a cost-effective fashion, including minimizing inappropriate medical resource use
13. Evaluates one's practice against established standards for NP care, locally/regionally/nationally (*quality, ethics*)	Responds productively to feedback from all members of the healthcare team and patients Performs continuous self-assessment	Responds to the needs of the team and clinical environment Demonstrates improvement via self-assessment	Incorporates feedback from all members of the healthcare team into self-improvement Reflects on feedback to ensure highest quality of care Participates in development of guidelines and professional standards for GU care
14. Evaluates evidence for value and appropriateness to decision-making for individual patients, to generate knowledge and improve clinic practice and patient outcomes (*practice inquiry, quality, scientific foundation*)	Understands basic research designs used in clinical research Uses research evidence to guide clinical decision-making in individual patients, asking for clarification as needed	Formulates evidence-based plan of care, based on knowledge from previous clinical scenarios Incorporates evidence into patient-centered GU care Relates clinical evidence to an individual GU patient Seeks to integrate a body of evidence for a specific clinical question in reaching a clinical decision Demonstrates knowledge of relevant GU epidemiology	Appraises a specific clinical context, patient's values and preferences, and the quality of evidence to develop a plan of care Distinguishes roles of various stakeholders (e.g., family, insurance payors) in patient management Identifies process issues on the system level and proposes interventions to facilitate patient care

(continued)

Table 21.2 (continued)

Competency (NONPF competency)	Level 3 (newly graduated and/or new to urology)	Level 2 (experienced NP new to urology)	Level 1 (expert urology NP)
15. Continuously strives for evidence-based practice (practice inquiry, quality, scientific foundation)	Able to identify and utilize resources that promote evidenced based practice Identifies and refers patients as appropriate	Demonstrates ability to perform searches of the literature for evidence-based information Collaborates for GU research Aware of appropriate clinical trials or research studies, recruiting patients as appropriate	Synthesizes information by effectively and efficiently performing relevant reviews of literature Incorporates evidence base into helping patients to make informed decisions about GU care Promotes translational research to benefit GU patients
16. Advocates for quality care for GU patients (ethics, policy, health delivery system)	Develops knowledge of regulatory issues unique to urology Interfaces with insurance companies on behalf of GU patients as necessary and appropriate Identifies safety issues, both real and potential Committed to high-quality GU care	Works with team to develop evidence-based, team-based quality improvement interventions Formulates teaching plans specific to the NP role in the care of GU patients	Collaborates with providers within the system and informal caregivers to promote a plan of care Seeks to improve the processes and outcomes of care Contributes to knowledge development relative to the overall care of GU patients
17. Acts as clinical preceptor and promotes the education of all team members (practice inquiry, leadership)	Seeks educational opportunities to advance own working knowledge of urology	Precepts NP and nursing students and other health profession students Acts as a mentor for other team members Provides education and support to caregivers of GU patients	Involved in developing education for all team members, including APRNs, residents, and PAs Contributes to knowledge and development of the urology NP role Disseminates knowledge specific to the urology NP via publication and presentation

18. Practices with highest ethical standards *(ethics, policy, independent practice)*	Demonstrates critical thinking Acknowledges legal limits of NP scope Asks for input and help from colleagues as needed Uses both internal (e.g., risk management) and external resources (e.g., professional organizations) to resolve issues	Works with more experienced colleagues to improve skills and knowledge base Seeks opportunities for learning and improving own skills Seeks specialty certification as a urologic NP (CUNP)	Monitors quality of own practice as an NP within urology Expresses concerns regarding team behaviors that are below accepted standard and represents inappropriate task selection or scope of practice issues Seeks and/or maintains specialty certification as a urologic NP (CUNP)
19. Applies tenets of nursing science to diverse populations (e.g., gender, age, culture, race, religion, disabilities, sexual orientation) demonstrating cultural sensitivity and responsiveness to their unique needs *(independent practice, scientific knowledge)*	Strives for sensitivity to diversity issues Recognizes own comfort level with issues of diversity Identifies potential GU health issues in families and individuals	Sensitive to potential ethical dilemmas related to cultural differences Comfortable managing needs of diverse patient groups within GU context	Always provides culturally sensitive care Mentors team members and students regarding observed behaviors that threaten acknowledgment of diversity or culturally sensitivity care

Health system activities

20. Demonstrates leadership in the clinical environment *(leadership, practice inquiry)*	Participates in development of own orientation to urologic clinical environment Takes responsibility for actions and admits mistakes Recognizes conflicts of interest Seeks mentorship from GU providers with a complementary skill set	Seeks feedback on clinical role and emerging expertise Consistent in timely completion of medical records and patient communications	Willingness to function in an oversight capacity of the care team in the clinical environment Provides leadership for quality improvement initiatives

(continued)

Table 21.2 (continued)

Competency (NONPF competency)	Level 3 (newly graduated and/or new to urology)	Level 2 (experienced NP new to urology)	Level 1 (expert urology NP)
21. Uses knowledge of healthcare environment to provide care within and across a health delivery system in order to deliver both patient-centered and population-centered GU care (policy, health delivery system)	Provides guidance regarding access to care based on identified GU needs Develops knowledge of community-based resources (e.g., support groups for GU cancers)	Manages and coordinates care across delivery systems, as appropriate to specific clinical role Advocates for patient-centered GU care Bases care plan on analysis of multiple factors (age, SES, comorbidities)	Promotes non-pharmacologic and non-procedural patient management options (e.g., physical therapy, alternative medicine providers) with patients and families as culturally appropriate Participates fully in interdisciplinary teams
22. Demonstrates collaborative approach to communication with other health professionals and health-related agencies (health delivery system, leadership, policy)	Delivers necessary information as required by established system protocols and standards Uses appropriate GU terminology	Maintains patient privacy and autonomy managing conflicts Consistent and effective communication in a wide variety of clinical scenarios Works with community organizations in the care of GU patients	Relays appropriate information to necessary stakeholders to promote GU patient care issues
23. Uses technology, such as electronic medical records (EMR), to accomplish safe healthcare delivery within specific work environment (practice inquiry, technology)	Efficient and competent in the use of EMR while considering risks and limitations common with EMR	Demonstrates increased efficiency and competency in the use of EMR, compensating for the risks and limitations common with EMR	Demonstrates consistently high-quality care with efficient use of EMR and other technology Skilled at using data management systems to improve clinical practice
24. Effective member or leader of a healthcare team and/or other professional group(s) (health delivery system, leadership)	Demonstrates communication and interpersonal behaviors that foster effective teamwork Promotes current and evolving urology NP role to other providers in the public	Works toward creation and maintenance of shared values and mutual respect among urologic care team Expresses him/herself in an objective, straightforward manner Demonstrates respect for team members during disagreements or conflicts	Demonstrates reliable leadership skills, including managing conflict Leads by example, focusing on collaborative relationships Promotes collaboration among all members of care team, by fostering the culture of shared values and promotion of highest-quality GU care Exemplifies urology NP role

Note. *GU* genitourinary, *SES* socioeconomic status, *PA* physician assistant, *APRN* advanced practice registered nurse, *EMR* electronic medical records, *NP* nurse practitioner, *NONPF* national organization of nurse practitioner faculties competencies are designed to support nurse practitioners seeking a role, or clarifying a current role, within urology practice environments. These 24 competencies can be placed in the additional setting of community and institutional practice environments, employer needs, and employer requirements. While these competencies could be adapted for other APRN groups with roles in urology environments, there may be potential reimbursement issues related to the individual's primary certification and licensure. There may also be considerations related to the degree of detail that may be required, by other APRN groups, within the competencies themselves.

These competencies do not suggest specific didactic or practice content that may be beneficial to an NP working in urology. Such content would be inspired by a particular work environment and job description or agreed upon in consultation with colleagues and team members. This reflects the need for an NP to both recognize the need for specific didactic content and be responsible to the needs of a particular clinic population.

Summary

These 24 urology NP competencies will standardize and improve urology education for NPs, as they blend the nursing and medical aspects of the NP role. Keough et al. (2011) highlighted the "importance of assessing NP proficiency with core-based competencies and developing a plan to provide additional education and mentoring" (p. 199) because NPs are moving into nontraditional clinical settings (not specific to their population-based certification). Primary care nurse practitioner programs prepare NPs with sufficient clinical and didactic components to be effective primary care providers. These urology-specific competencies take that groundwork and focus the primary care skills toward GU care and management. Many GU conditions benefit from episodic but long-term medical management, which is a role well suited to the nurse practitioner. As the role of the urology NP continues to evolve, we can anticipate increasing responsibility and interdisciplinary collaboration in clinical decision-making and patient management.

Proficiency in patient management comes with time and exposure: "clinical judgments and human responses to patients are developed through habits of thought and practice rather than through the mastery of information or technical skills alone" (Benner 2011, p. 8). These 24 competencies are intended to describe and promote urology NP practice across the entire spectrum of adult (>18)-older adult care, with the goal of providing cost-effective, patient-centered quality genitourinary care while creating a hallmark for advancing urology NP practice.

Acknowledgment The authors wish to thank MiChelle McGarry, MSN, CPNP, CUNP, for her support and input.

References

Accreditation Council for Graduate Medical Education and the American Board of Urology (2012) The urology milestone project. Retrieved from http://acgme.org/acgmeweb/Portals/0/PDFs/Milestones/UrologyMilestones.pdf

Advanced Practice Registered Nurses (APRN) Consensus Work Group & the National Council of State Boards of Nursing APRN Advisory Committee (2008) Consensus model for APRN regulation: licensure, accreditation, certification, and education. Retrieved from http://www.aacn.nche.edu/education/pdf/APRNReport.pdf

Albaugh JA (2012) Urology nursing practice educational preparation, titles, training, and job responsibilities around the globe. Urol Nurs 32(2):79–85

American Association of Nurse Practitioners (2013) Standards of practice for nurse practitioners. Retrieved from http://www.aanp.org/images/documents/publications/standardsofpractice.pdf

American Association of Nurse Practitioners (2015) Nurse practitioners in primary care. Retrieved from http://www.aanp.org/images/documents/publications/primarycare.pdf

American Medical Directors Association (2011) Collaborative and supervisory relationships between attending physicians and advanced practice nurses in long-term care facilities. Geriatr Nurs 32(1):7–17

American Urological Association (2014) AUA consensus statement on advanced practice providers. Retrieved from http://www.auanet.org/common/pdf/advocacy/advocacy-by-topic/AUA-Consensus-Statement-Advanced-Practice-Providers-Full.pdf

Benner P (1982) From novice to expert. Am J Nurs 82(3):402–407

Benner P (2011) Formation in professional education: an examination of the relationship between theories of meaning and theories of the self. J Med Philos 36(4):342–53. doi:10.1093/jmp/jhr030

Cash K (1995) Benner and expertise in nursing: a critique. Int J Nurs Stud 32:527–535

Crowe H (2014) Advanced urology nursing practice. Nat Rev Urol 11(3):178–182

Institute of Medicine (2010) The future of nursing: leading change, advancing health. National Academies Press, Washington, DC

Keough VA, Stevenson A, Martinovich Z, Young R, Tanabe P (2011) Nurse practitioner certification and practice settings: implications for education and practice. J Nurs Scholarsh 43(2):195–202

National Organization of Nurse Practitioner Faculties (2010) Adult-gerontology primary care nurse practitioner competencies. Washington, DC. Retrieved from http://c.ymcdn.com/sites/www.nonpf.org/resource/resmgr/competencies/adult-geroaccompsfinal2012.pdf

National Organization of Nurse Practitioner Faculties (2013) Population-focused nurse practitioner competencies. Washington, DC. Retrieved from http://c.ymcdn.com/sites/www.nonpf.org/resource/resmgr/Competencies/CompilationPopFocusComps2013.pdf

National Organization of Nurse Practitioner Faculties (2014) Nurse practitioner core competencies content. Washington, DC. Retrieved from http://c.ymcdn.com/sites/nonpf.site-ym.com/resource/resmgr/Competencies/NPCoreCompsContentFinalNov20.pdf

Newhouse RP, Stanik-Hutt J, White KM, Johantgen M, Bass EB, Zangaro G, Wilson RF, Fountain L, Steinwachs DM, Heindel L, Weiner JP (2011) Advanced practice nurse outcomes 1990–2008: a systematic review. Nurs Econ 29(5):1–21

Patient Protection and Affordable Care Act of 2010, & Pub. L. No. 111–148, 124 Stat. 119. (2010)

Quallich SA (2011) A survey evaluating the current role of the nurse practitioner in urology. Urol Nurs 31(6):328–336

Society of Urologic Nurses and Associates (2013) Urologic nursing: scope and standards of practice, 2nd edn. Anthony J. Jannetti, Inc. Pitman; NJ

Stewart-Amidei C, Villanueva N, Schwartz RR, Delemos C, West T, Tocco S, Cartwright C, Jones R, Blank-Reid C, Haymore J (2010) American Association of Neuroscience Nurses Scope and Standards of Practice for Neuroscience Advanced Practice Nurses. J Neurosci Nurs 42(3):E1–E8

Additional Reading

National Organization of Nurse Practitioner Faculties (NONPF) (2010) Adult-gerontology primary care nurse practitioner competencies. Retrieved from http://c.ymcdn.com/sites/www.nonpf.org/resource/resmgr/competencies/adult-gero accompsfinal2012.pdf

National Organization of Nurse Practitioner Faculties (NONPF) (2013) Population-focused nurse practitioner competencies. Retrieved from http://c.ymcdn.com/sites/www.nonpf.org/resource/resmgr/Competencies/CompilationPopFocusComps2013.pdf

Appendix: Resources, PSA Screening, Urologic Emergencies

Summary of PSA screening guidelines by organization

Organization	Baseline testing (age)	Invitation to screening[a] (age)	High-risk groups[b] (age)	Screening interval	PSA threshold for biopsy (ng/mL)
American Cancer Society (2010)	None	Beginning at 50 years while life expectancy ≥10 years	Beginning at 40 years while life expectancy ≥10 years	Annually if PSA ≥2.5 ng/mL	2.5 ng/mL in select patients
				Every 2 years if PSA <2.5 ng/mL	4.0 ng/mL in most patients
U.S. Preventive Services Task Force (2012)	None	None	None	None	None
American Urological Association (2013)	None	55–69 years	40–69 years	Every 2 years	None specified
European Association of Urology (2013)	40–45 years	Any age while life expectancy ≥10 years	Any age while life expectancy ≥10 years	Every 2–4 years if baseline PSA >1 ng/mL	None specified
				Every 8 years if baseline PSA ≤1 ng/mL	
American College of Physicians (2013)	None	50–69 years	40–69 years	Annually if PSA ≥2.5 ng/mL	None specified
National Comprehensive Cancer Network (2014)	45–49 years	50–70 years	Consider change in biopsy threshold	*For 40–49 years*: every 1–2 years if PSA >1 ng/mL	3.0 ng/mL *or*
		70–75 years if life expectancy ≥10 years		Repeat at age 50 if PSA ≤1 ng/mL	<3.0 ng/mL with excess risk based on multiple factors (family history, race, PSA kinetics)
				For 50–70 years:- every 1–2 years	

[a]For men who are well informed on the risks and benefits of PSA screening
[b]African American race and first-degree relatives diagnosed with PCa

© Springer International Publishing Switzerland 2016
M. Lajiness, S. Quallich (eds.), *The Nurse Practitioner in Urology*,
DOI 10.1007/978-3-319-28743-0

Key points from PSA screening studies

The Göteborg screening study	European randomized study of screening for prostate cancer (ERSPC) results	Prostate, lung, colorectal, and ovarian (PLCO) cancer screening trial
Trial invited 10,000 randomly selected men for prostate-specific antigen (PSA) testing every 2 years since 1995	Prostate cancer screening can be cost-effective when limited to two or three screens between ages 55 and 59 years	76,693 men randomly assigned to receive annual screening or usual care
Showed organized screening reduces PCa mortality but is associated with overdiagnosis	Screening above age 63 years is less cost-effective because of loss of quality-adjusted life years (QALY) due to overdiagnosis	Updates for 13-year follow-up show no difference in PCa-specific mortality but a persistent excess of cases, suggesting overdiagnosis
If, after careful counseling, a man chooses to participate in PSA screening, it should be in an organized program at sufficient intervals and with adequate follow-up	Most favorable results for screening cessation below age 60 years	Shows that a systematic program of annual screening is no better than a less intense or opportunistic screening program
	Incremental cost-effectiveness ratios of these strategies were $31467 to $72971 per QALY gained	Mass annual screening of population of men aged 55–74 unlikely to decrease death from PCa

Urologic emergencies overview

Red flags	Sudden onset of acute testicular pain → think torsion
	Cellulitic or necrotic changes to the skin of the scrotum, penis, perineal region → think Fournier's gangrene
	Complaints of an erection lasting >60 min after cessation of sexual activity → think priapism
	Complaints of issues with the foreskin → think paraphimosis
	Complaints of inability to urinate → think acute retention
	Complaints of new, painful, or newly painful mass in scrotum → think testicular tumor
	Complaints of sudden pain, bruising, possible "pop" during intercourse → think penile fracture

Testicular torsion: see Chap. 3

Testicular tumor: see Chaps. 3 and 19

Priapism	History	Signs/symptoms	Evaluation	Therapeutic interventions
	38–42 % of adult patients with sickle cell disease reported at least one episode of priapism	Persistent, painful erection (low-flow or veno-occlusive priapism)	Penile Doppler	Provide analgesia and sedation as needed
	Overall incidence is 1.5 cases per 100,000 person-years	Present for hours or days	Penile blood gases	Manage any underlying conditions
	Erection that has lasted >4 h beyond cessation of sexual activity	Erect but nontender penis (high-flow or nonischemic priapism)	Arteriography	Epinephrine, phenylephrine, pseudoephedrine, or terbutaline can be injected into the penis to help reverse engorgement
	Common for men to delay seeking evaluation and treatment for several hours		CBC if malignancy suspected	The corpora may also be irrigated with normal saline
	Direct penile trauma may result in priapism (cycling)			Urgent urologic consultation
	Recent illicit drug use (cocaine, ecstasy, marijuana)			The patient may need a needle aspiration to remove trapped blood
				If this does not improve the condition, a shunt may be attempted
				If this is unsuccessful, the patient may be taken to the operative room for a more aggressive shunt procedure

	History	Signs/symptoms	Evaluation	Therapeutic interventions
Acute retention	Recent GU instrumentation Use of over-the-counter cold medicines (men on α-blockers) Recent back injury that may have compromised lumbosacral spine In men, symptoms consistent with acute prostatitis In the elderly, recent general anesthesia	Lower abdominal discomfort/increasing size Bladder distention (palpable just above symphysis pubis)	Bladder ultrasound Catheterization Eventual spine imaging as indicated	Insert an indwelling urinary catheter for immediate relief Rapid drainage avoids stretch injury to the bladder Investigate the cause and treat as indicated Consider consultation with urologist to further investigate functional status of the bladder Establish why this occurred
Fournier's gangrene	Progressive necrotizing infection of the external genitalia or perineum 1.6/100,000 males Peaks in males 50–79 years old (3.3/100,000) Highest rate in the south (1.9/100,000) Overall case fatality rate 7.5% Also happens in women, incidence is much less Obesity Possible history of some break in the skin within the preceding 48 h Recent poor blood sugar control, with recent rising levels/difficulty managing levels	**Signs/symptoms:** Painful swelling, erythema, and induration of the genitalia Cellulitis, odor, tissue necrosis Fever/chills and other systemic complaints, such as anxiety Pain that seems in excess of the visible skin changes Essential to appreciate that the degree of *internal* necrosis is much greater than suggested by the external signs; adequate (repeated) surgical debridement is necessary to save patient's life	**Evaluation:** Typically a type 1 necrotizing fasciitis that is polymicrobial in origin, including *Staphylococcus aureus*, *Streptococcus* sp., *Klebsiella* sp., *Escherichia coli*, and anaerobic bacteria Plain films or computed tomography may demonstrate gas in the subcutaneous tissue Elevated WBC Serum blood sugar or finger stick	**Therapeutic interventions** Broad spectrum antibiotics – antibiotic treatment should be given that covers all causative organisms and can penetrate inflammatory tissue Provide analgesia and sedation Admission to hospital Plan for extensive debridement Surgical consultations: urology, general surgery, plastics

	History	Signs/symptoms		Therapeutic interventions
Penile fracture	Erect penis became disengaged from the vagina and hits some impervious part of the female anatomy causing an acute bend in the penis Rupture or tear to tunica albuginea Male patient (and partner) may report feeling and/or hearing a "pop," followed by pain to penile shaft and immediate loss of erection and subsequent penile ecchymosis May also report bright red blood from urethra	Ecchymosis to site of injury, may extend to much of penile shaft May result in deviation of the shaft Edema Pain Urinary function typically unaffected Ecchymosis fo lows genital fascial barriers along the lines of those involved with trauma to the urethra This is a clinical diagnosis	*True urologic emergency* Evaluation Penile Doppler	Therapeutic interventions Immediate surgical repair of the tunica albuginea defect is necessary – ideally within 24–36 h after injury Many men do not present within this time frame, due to embarrassment or belief that injury is less severe If injury was minor (no loss of erection) and hematoma is confined to penile skin, supportive measures such as ice and (NSAIDs) Reassurance this will improve with time
Paraphimosis	Phimosis, with increasing difficulty advancing the foreskin History of recent increased phimosis History of frequent catheterizations, poor hygiene, and/or chronic balanoposthitis leading to phimosis	Swollen, painful edematous glans Tight ring of skin apparent behind glans on examination Discolored, necrotic areas may be noted to the glans	*True urologic emergency* Necrosis of glans may occur secondary to arterial occlusion	Therapeutic interventions Provide nonsteroidal anti-inflammatory drugs for pain management Initiate antibiotic therapy as indicated *Manual reduction can be attempted, by applying pressure with the thumbs to reduce the edema and advance the foreskin* If this is unsuccessful, local anesthetic may be given so that a small incision can be made in order to correct the restriction Advise patient to consider a circumcision or dorsal slit to prevent further episodes

		History	Signs/symptoms	Evaluation	Therapeutic interventions
GU trauma	Urethral	History Rare in females Commonly occurs in setting of pelvic fracture (posterior) Anterior urethral injury occurs in setting of blunt or penetrating trauma, also with saddle injury	Signs/symptoms Blood at meatus Penile, perineal, or scrotal hematoma Anterior urethral injury can present with "butterfly hematoma" to perineum, ± a scrotal hematoma	Evaluation All patients need a retrograde pyelogram (RUG)	Therapeutic interventions Do not place catheter in the context of suspected urethral injury Posterior injury: urology consult for immediate repair, except in setting or need for rectal/bladder neck injury Anterior urethral injury is managed by bladder drainage, such as suprapubic tube, catheter, and deferred repair
	Renal	History Most common GU organ injured Usually due to blunt trauma Increased risk with existing renal cysts	Signs/symptoms If diagnosis delayed, can see hematoma, urinoma, infection, pain, renovascular hypotension	Evaluation Diagnosed by CT scan with both IV and oral contrast	Therapeutic interventions: Depends on the grade of the injury More severe injuries require surgical exploration Less severe injuries can be managed by embolization
	Bladder	History Commonly occurs in setting of pelvic fracture: ~5 % of patients Usually in setting of motor vehicle accident (especially if wearing lap belt)	Signs/symptoms Gross hematuria Pelvic fracture Suprapubic discomfort Motor vehicle accident If diagnosis delayed, can see ileus, urinary ascites, rising BUN/creatinine	Evaluation Diagnosed by cystogram – will demonstrate extravasation	Therapeutic interventions Open surgical repair
	Ureteral	History Usually involves pelvic ureter Can occur during abdominal or pelvic surgery Due to penetrating wound Sudden deceleration injury Classified by site of injury, e.g., ureteral pelvic junction	Signs/symptoms Identification can be difficult Hematuria Flank mass Prolonged ileus postoperatively Hydronephrosis Elevated BUN/creatinine Prolonged output from drains postoperatively If diagnosis delayed, can see persistent flank pain, urinoma, infection, fistula, renal loss, death	Evaluation Diagnosed by IVU, retrograde pyelogram, CT scan of abdomen/pelvis with both IV and oral contrast, CT urogram	Therapeutic interventions Surgical exploration and repair If prolonged time to diagnosis, stricture may form

Suggested Reference Books

American Urological Association (2010) Guidelines-at-a-glance; a quick reference for Urologists-2010. Also available on line: http://www.auanet.org/content/guidelines-and-qualitycare/clinicalguidelines

Goldstein M, Schlegel MN (2013) Surgical and medical management of male infertility. Cambridge University Press, New York

Gomella L (ed) (2014) The 5-minute urology consult, 3rd edn. Lippincott Williams & Wilkins., Philadelphia

Goolsby MJ, Grubbs L (eds) (2014) Advanced assessment: interpreting findings and formulating differential diagnoses, 3rd edn. F.A. Davis, Philadelphia

Gray M, Moore K (2008) Urologic disorders: adult and pediatric care. Elsevier Mosby, St. Louis

Hanno P, Guzzo TJ, Malkowicz SB, Wein A (eds) (2014) Penn clinical manual of urology, 2nd edn. McGraw-Hill, New York

Heidelbaugh JJ (ed) (2008) Clinical men's health: evidence in practice. Saunders Elsevier, Philadelphia

Kirby RS, Carson CC, White A, Kirby MG (2010) Men's health, 3rd edn. Informa Healthcare USA, Inc., New York

Newman DK, Wein AJ (2009) Managing and treating urinary incontinence, 2nd edn. Health Professions Press, Baltimore

Porst H, Reisman Y (eds) (2012) The ESSM syllabus of sexual medicine, 2nd edn. Medix Publishers, Amsterdam

Tanagho EA, McAninch JW (eds) (2012) Smith's general urology, 18th edn. Lange Medical Books/McGraw-Hill Medical Publishing Division: New York

Wein AJ, Kavoussi LR, Partin AW, Peters CA (2015) Campbell-walsh urology, 11th edn. Elsevier, St. Louis

Wieder JA (ed) (2014) Pocket guide to urology, 5th edn. J. Wieder Medical, Oakland

Web-Based Resources

Agency for Health Care Research and Quality National Guideline Clearing House. http://www.guideline.gov/

American Association of Sexuality Educators, Counselors and Therapists (AASECT). www.aasect.org

American Herbal Pharmacopoeia. www.herbal-ahp.org

American Urological Association (AUA) Consensus Statement on Advanced Practice Providers (2014)   www.auanet.org/common/pdf/advocacy/advocacy-by-topic/AUA-Consensus-Statement-Advanced-Practice-Providers-Full.pdf

American Urological Association Advanced Practice Provider education series. www.auanet.org/education/education-for-allied-health.cfm

American Urological Association. Urodynamics: documentation and coding. www.auanet.org/advnews/hpbrief/view.cfm?i=2678&a=5368

American Urological Association/Society of Urodynamics, Female Pelvic Medicine & Urogenital Reconstruction Urodynamics guidelines. www.auanet.org/education/guidelines/adult-urodynamics.cfm

American Urological Association Prostate Cancer Screening Decision Tool. http://urologyhealth.org//Documents/Product%20Store/Prostate-Cancer-Screening-Decision-tool-english.pdf

American Urological Association Guidelines. http://www.auanet.org/education/aua-guidelines.cfm

Australian Men's Health Forum. http://www.amhf.org.au/

Blackmores Institute for Complementary and Alternative Medicine. www.blackmoresinstitute.org

Bladder diary. www.ics.org/public/bladderdiaryday/download

Centers for Disease Control and Prevention- Men's Health. http://www.cdc.gov/men/

Certification Board for Urologic Nurses and Associates (CBUNA)
Certified Urologic Nurse Practitioner (CUNP) examination information: www.cbuna.org/certification/exam-criteria-description-and-objectives
Hartford Institute for Geriatric Nursing. www.hartfordign.org
Herb Research Foundation. www.herbs.org
International Continence Society terminology. www.ics.org/Terminology
Jeff Bauer, PhD- Health Futurist & Medical Economist. www.jeffbauerphd.com
National Institute of Diabetes and Digestive and Kidney Diseases (NIDDK) Multidisciplinary Approach to the Study of Chronic Pelvic Pain (MAPP) Research Network. www.mappnetwork.org
National Institutes of Health- Men's Health. http://health.nih.gov/search_results.aspx?terms=Men%27s+Health, https://www.nlm.nih.gov/medlineplus/menshealth.html
Society of Urologic Nurses and Associates. www.SUNA.org
Urologic nursing: scope and standards of practice, guide to urologic medications. www.suna.org/resources/suna-store

Coding Tips Specifically for Urology

https://www.auanet.org/resources/coding-tips.cfm
https://www.auanet.org/resources/aua-coding-resources.cfm
https://www.auanet.org/resources/other-coding-assistance.cfm

Printed by Printforce, the Netherlands